W9-AQD-505

ETHICAL ISSUES IN HEALTH CARE

MARGOT JOAN FROMER, R.N., M.A., M.Ed.

Assistant Professor, University of Delaware,
College of Nursing, Newark, Delaware

The C. V. Mosby Company

ST. LOUIS • TORONTO • LONDON   1981

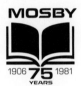

MOSBY

1906 **75** 1981
YEARS

A TRADITION OF PUBLISHING EXCELLENCE

Copyright © 1981 by The C. V. Mosby Company

All rights reserved. No part of this book may be reproduced
in any manner without written permission of the publisher.

Printed in the United States of America

The C. V. Mosby Company
11830 Westline Industrial Drive, St. Louis, Missouri 63141

Library of Congress Cataloging in Publication Data

Fromer, Margot Joan
    Ethical issues in health care.

    Bibliography: p.
    Includes index.
    1. Nursing ethics.   2. Medical ethics.
I. Title.   [DNLM: 1. Ethics, Nursing.   WY 85
F931e]
RT85.F76   174′.2   80-25058
ISBN 0-8016-1728-6

C/M/M 9 8 7 6 5 4 3 2 1   01/A/031

ETHICAL ISSUES
IN HEALTH CARE

KANSAS SCHOOL OF RELIGION
UNIVERSITY OF KANSAS
1300 OREAD AVENUE
LAWRENCE, KANSAS 66044

To

those who will not be caged

As I listened to all this, I recalled the hare which Makar once caught in a trap. He was a fine large animal. One could sense in him a drive for freedom, for powerful leaps, playful tumbles, and swift escapes. Locked in a cage he raged, stamped his feet, beat against the walls. After a few days Makar, furious over his restlessness, threw a heavy tarpaulin over him. The hare struggled and fought under it, but finally gave up. Eventually he became tame and ate from my hand. One day Makar got drunk and left the door of the cage open. The hare jumped out and started toward the meadow. I thought he would plunge into the tall grass with one huge leap and never be seen again. But he seemed to savor his freedom and just sat down, with ears pricked up. From the distant fields and woods came sounds that only he could hear and understand, smells and fragrances that only he could appreciate. It was all his own; he had left the cage behind.

Suddenly there was a change in him. The alert ears flopped, he sagged somehow, and grew smaller. He jumped once and his whiskers perked up, but he did not run away. I whistled loudly in the hope that it would bring him to his senses, make him realize that he was free. He only turned around and sluggishly, as though suddenly aged and shrunken, moved toward the hutch. On his way he stopped for a while, stood up, and looked back once again with his ears pricked; then he passed the rabbits gazing at him and jumped into the cage. I closed the door, though it was unnecessary. He now carried the cage in himself; it bound his brain and heart and paralyzed his muscles. Freedom, which had set him apart from other resigned, drowsy rabbits, left him like the wind-driven fragrance evaporating from crushed, dried clover.*

---

*From *The Painted Bird*, by Jerzy Kosinski. 1976 Complete and revised edition. Copyright © 1965, 1976, by Jerzy N. Kosinski. Reprinted by permission of Houghton Mifflin Company.

Foreword

In recent years we have seen a flood of books and articles on biomedical ethics. By comparison, very little attention has been devoted to ethical issues in nursing. This book is a welcome addition to the literature of biomedical ethics as it relates to health professionals other than physicians.

Two points need to be made about the relations between biomedical ethics and the ethics of nursing practice. First, nursing ethics is continuous with other ethics; the same moral principles apply to nurses as to other health professionals, including physicians. Second, nursing ethics is different. Even though the same principles apply, what they imply for the conduct of any health care professional will depend in part on the structure of the health care system and on the various roles within it. For example, even if we hold that the patient has a right to the truth about his or her condition, we still have to ask *who* among the various agents has the obligation to disclose the truth. Thus our roles (such as nursing) are important for determining our moral responsibility—for determining to whom and for what we are responsible.

The issue of moral responsibility is central in nursing. In the past 25 years, as codes of nursing ethics indicate, nurses have redefined the issue of to whom they are responsible. Earlier codes held that the nurse's primary responsibility was to the physician; recent codes hold that the nurse's primary responsibility is to the client. The presumption is no longer that the nurse will obey the physician but that the nurse will respect the client's rights. These alterations in the codes reflect important changes in the self-consciousness of the nursing profession. But they also signal unresolved tensions, many of which involve moral disputes, among nurses themselves and between nurses and other health professionals.

In this book Professor Fromer approaches these moral disputes from her own experience and familiarity with the literature of biomedical ethics. With clarity and insight she writes "to help nurses identify the moral and ethical issues, to raise questions, and to propose possible avenues of inquiry." She seeks to open debate and engage nurses and others in examining their moral responsibilities within health care.

James F. Childress, Ph.D.
University of Virginia

vii

Preface

The impetus to write a book on bioethics for professional nurses sprang from my experiences with and observations of nurses in a variety of settings and from an increasing interest in philosophy and ethical theory. Although nurses are now doing more and are involved in many more kinds of independent activities than ever before, it does not seem to me that they are *thinking* more about the broad ethical issues that are so completely and intimately intertwined with delivery of health care.

Life is becoming more complex with each passing day, and the health care system is keeping up with, even far outstripping, the pace of life's increasing complexity. More people are involved in the delivery of health care, and there are more and more options for choice, both for the providers of health care and for the consumers of that care. No longer is there only one prescribed way to treat a health problem. There are usually several treatment modalities (and the choice of no treatment) for each problem; deciding the best and most effective one often creates an ethical dilemma. Nurses are becoming involved in helping clients make these kinds of choices, and in order to be of the greatest service to the client they must have a thorough understanding of the ethical issues involved.

Acquisition and accumulation of human knowledge are growing by leaps and bounds, as are technologic advances in the delivery of health care. Scientists are doing research of the most frightening and awe-inspiring kind: they are examining both the very nature of life and the quality of that life. How much can we intervene in the nature of life and death before that nature is irrevocably changed, and how will humanity be affected by those changes?

It seems that our ability to handle, both psychologically and ethically, the technology we use everyday has lagged behind the development of the technology itself. We have at our fingertips the means with which to manipulate human life and health, but the consequences of that manipulation are so grave that we shy away even from thinking about them. That is what this book is about: to help nurses and other health professionals identify moral and ethical issues, to raise questions, and to propose possible avenues of inquiry. There will be no answers given here. Nurses must come to their own conclusions about what is right and wrong, about what should and should not be done for and to a client. It is, of course, the client and his family who must ultimately make decisions about health care, but it is the nurse with whom he will be speaking and from whom he will be seeking guidance.

The ethical and moral nature of our lives is changing; our values and sense of what is important are vastly different today than they were 50 or even 20 years ago. This does not necessarily mean that "the good old days" were better, but they *were* simpler. Health professionals, especially those who make health policy decisions, appear to be lost in a sea of endless debate and indecision about what to do when presented with a variety of ethical choices. It is time for nurses to enter the discussions and to have a voice in decisions. Nurses, if they are to be responsible members of the health care team, can no longer be content to sit on the sidelines of moral responsibility. No book about health care ethics can provide answers, but it should be able to give some cohesive form to the questions.

Ethics is a system of moral principles, rules of conduct about a particular class of human actions or a particular group of people. It is also that branch of philosophy dealing with values relating to human conduct in respect to whether certain actions are right or wrong and whether the motives and ends of such actions are good or bad.

In formulating a moral policy a person or group examines ethical principles, weighs available facts, and then makes a decision about what should be done in any given situation. The process is basically the same for any human ethical decision, no matter how large or far-reaching its consequences. Whether the decision is to call in sick from work and go skiing instead or to disconnect a "dead" person's life-support system, the *process* of making the decision is the same: the facts, persons, and principles involved in the situation must be assessed and the consequences of the action evaluated.

This book is divided into chapters about various substantive health care issues that create serious moral problems. Regardless of the area of human endeavor, certain ethical problems are basic; for example, conflicts between technology and ethics, that is, between the pursuit of knowledge for its own sake and the consequences of research. It is in the nature of research that one discovery leads to another and opens up new avenues of inquiry. When one gains new knowledge, it is natural to want to put it to use. Most of today's ethical issues in health care concern the use to which knowledge is put, not simply the fact that the knowledge exists and is available for use.

Another issue is the potential or even probable conflicts that arise from the different values of health care professionals and the client, the person who must make the decision about care. The values of the client himself are, of course, the most important ones to be considered. Subtle or not so subtle forms of coercion, however, can be applied to the client so that his needs become secondary to the needs and goals of the care providers. This kind of situation occurs countless numbers of times a day, and the health professional can and should be instrumental in ensuring that it is the *client's* value system that determines the course of action.

The issue of human rights—personal, civil, and those that are international in scope—has been brought often to the public's attention in the past several years. Nowhere is this issue more important than in delivery of health care. Almost every agency and institution providing health care and human services has developed a normative concept of human rights. A formal policy declaration may exist, or there may be simple unwritten standards of the way business is conducted. Whatever the degree of formal structure, each person who is in any way involved in the provision of care must be involved in the formation of the concept of human rights. Basic to delineation of rights is the value of humanity, the value of the life of a single individual or life in the aggregate—human nature as we understand it. This issue must be thoroughly examined as we continue to feel the impact of technology and as we face the issue of the needs, rights, and values of an individual in contrast to those of society in general or even a segment of society.

This book is written for nurses as well as other health professionals both for the reasons stated at the outset and for another important reason. It has been my observation that nursing students enter school with a spirit of altruism, kindness, humanity, sensitivity, and a feeling for the dignity of human beings. They often have a definite, albeit naive, sense of right and wrong and seem to be genuinely concerned with the moral and ethical consequences of their actions. Somewhere along the line after graduation these concerns and values become lost or at least are repressed enough that they are no longer present at a conscious level in professional functioning. Many nurses have been described as uncaring, insensitive, and hardened to the needs of their clients. Often they do not seem to care about the social and ethical ramifications of professional practice. A number of factors seem responsible for this deteriorating sensitivity:

1. Nurses are exposed continually and intensively to massive doses of human suffering. That they seem to become inured to suffering may result from never having been taught how to deal with it realistically and effectively. It becomes easier to ignore a person's pain than to acknowledge it and face the fact that the nurse may have only limited resources to alleviate the pain.

2. Health care delivery is inexorably moving toward becoming a scientific technology and away from being a human art. It concentrates on disease rather than on people, and on machines rather than on souls. Health professionals cannot help but be caught up in this scientific and technologic fervor, which does not provide a favorable climate for ethical introspection.

3. The curricula of many baccalaureate nursing programs place heavy emphasis on the physical senses while minimizing the importance of the humanities as required courses. There are almost no programs in the United States that require nursing students to study ethics or philosophy. (Those schools that do are almost all sponsored by religious institutions.) This stress on the quantitative delivery of health care sets the stage for the eventual diminution in importance of a sense of ethics.

4. The nature of the work that nurses do in hospitals, in community health agencies, and in private practice leaves them little if any time to think about human values. A hospital nurse who is run ragged by attending to the physical needs of ten or more clients is frequently too harassed and exhausted to think of the ethical considerations of what she is doing. A community health nurse who spends all day racing from one client's home to another's—with a few hours at a crowded clinic in addition—is not going to have much time or energy for quiet reflection.

The purpose of this book is to look at the qualities and components of ethical issues. The morals and ethics of society in general are changing; health care ethics merely reflects and absorbs this change. Philosophic, moral, and ethical questions, when debated by rational and humane people, rarely lead to answers. Instead, new kinds of questions are asked, and new problems and issues are presented. It is not sufficient for nurses to place all moral and ethical responsibility in the hands of physicians, who have traditionally held it. What will be discussed here is *human* responsibility and the functions of nurses as human beings while they provide health care.

Productive ethical discussion and inquiry can take place only when there is disagreement about what ought to be done. Total agreement with what has always been done or with what another person thinks ought to be done never leads to advancement of thought.

Margot Joan Fromer

Contents

1

Professional accountability

RIGHTS

Before one discusses who is accountable to whom in the delivery of health care, it seems wise to look at what is involved in the idea of accountability. The basic issue concerns health, but when one looks at ethics in relation to health, it is imperative also to examine the issue of rights. The question of whether health is a right or a privilege is so old and so often asked that it runs the risk of being a cliché. What exactly is a right? We think we know, especially when it comes to ourselves, as in these statements: "I have a right to paint my house any color I want." "I have a right to know what you wrote in the chart about me." "You have no right to tell *me* what to do." A right is usually defined as a just claim or title or something that is due one according to just claim, legal guarantees, moral principles, and so on, or a moral, ethical, or legal principle considered an underlying cause of truth, justice, morality, or ethics. These appear to be reasonably clear-cut definitions, and one could even begin to form ethical concepts based on them, but the next logical step in defining rights is to ask how they are derived. They are not simply there; they did not come with the original creation package described in Genesis. They *do* exist, but they must have an origin: they were devised and refined over the years.

Several views exist about the origin and subsequent development of human rights. One view is that they derive from natural law, that they are created by God, the Creator of all natural things, and that they are as much a part of nature as human beings themselves. This view is somewhat simplistic in that it leaves no room for a hierarchy, that is, some rights taking precedence over other rights. Because of this there can be no way to determine the outcome of a conflict based on different rights. Rights, if they are all similar because they all derive from one God, cannot be assigned priorities and cannot be *used* to solve ethical dilemmas about the application of rights to life situations.

Some philosophers deny or put aside the idea that natural rights exist. Others believe that rights are assigned by the state, that is, by human beings in the form of governmental systems, although they do not deny the possibility of the existence of natural rights. This is a precarious way to assign and ensure rights. If rights are created and protected by persons, then they can be equally destroyed or not protected. Our own century provides dozens of examples of flagrant and murderous

1

governmental disregard for the rights of its citizens: slavery in many parts of the world, Stalinism in Russia, the oppressive life-style of the People's Republic of China, apartheid in South Africa, and most monstrous of all, the murder of 6 million Jews and 2 million other non-Aryans in Nazi Germany. Rights that are based on laws made by people are subject to the capriciousness of the humanity of those very people.

The legal view of rights gives a person power to control a situation, as with civil rights that permit citizens freedom from governmental interference in certain areas; personal freedom leads to the power to control one's own life within a set of given limitations. This view implies that if there are rights, there are obligations. For instance, if the United States government grants me the right to move freely from state to state, then the government is obligated not to erect barriers to prevent my freedom of movement. Legal rights do not exist without legal obligations.

Except in limited instances, of public health, no written guarantees of a right to health exist. However, if we assume that health or health care is a right rather than a privilege, then we must also assume that obligations are involved. If health care is demanded as a right, are certain people in society obligated to provide it for others? Who is obligated to provide what and for whom? The claim of a demanded right to health is not enforceable because it is not a legal right; therefore it would seem that no obligation exists. But we *feel* obligated to provide health care for ourselves and others, and most health professionals feel that health care is a right. Thus in the matter of health care, a view other than the legal one motivates the provision of that care as a right.

The view of rights as a matter of personal values will be discussed more fully later in this chapter in terms of the development of a professional value system. A personal concept of rights has much to do with one's ethical development, with the way one conducts one's life, with the decisions one makes, and with one's concept of right and wrong and of good and evil. This is the essence of ethics and morality. Personal rights are based on a sense of justice and fairness and the universality of principles such as autonomy, beneficence, and nonmaleficence.

Option rights and welfare rights

When the discussion of the view or origin of rights becomes too muddled or confusing, we can try to define rights by distinguishing between the two major kinds: option rights and welfare rights. Option rights involve ideas of freedom and choice, that is, are based on the right to live one's life exactly as one chooses *within* a set of prescribed boundaries. For example, I may dress as I please as long as I remain dressed in public, and I may swing my arm with my fist clenched so long as it does not come too close to your nose. As Golding[1] puts it, the individual is a kind of sovereign within a certain sphere and may act as he pleases. The boundaries of the sphere are sometimes clear-cut, as in the number of garments one is legally prohibited from removing in public. But at times the boundary is shadowy and indistinct, as in the statement, "I have a right to paint my house any color I want." Your neighbors would surely agree as long as you paint it in a way that it blends harmoniously with the rest of the neighborhood. But what if you paint it bright pink with purple dots and yellow stripes and execute a modern art mural on the whole length of your driveway? Your neighbors are, of course, furious. Have you stepped over the boundary and infringed on their right to live in the kind of environment they had selected, a street filled with houses painted muted greens and browns? This is where the discussion of option rights heats up and becomes interesting. What rights are guaranteed? Do rights overlap? Which ones take priority over others? According to Golding option rights

should not be taken as implying a general principle to the effect that one has the right to do as one pleases as long as no one else is harmed. The validity of this principle is a contested point in normative ethical theory and social and political philosophy. Whatever its validity, the principle does not follow from the concept of option rights as such. As far as the concept itself is concerned, the possibility is left open (1) that there may be things a person has no right to do even if others are not harmed and, contrariwise (2), that there may be some things that a person has a right to do even if others are likely to be harmed. In a free society the risk is taken that an individual might do things that have harmful consequences to himself and others. Nevertheless, option rights, and the spheres of freedom that correspond to them, must be limited in various respects; it would be self-defeating if everyone in a society had the right to do whatever he pleased.*

Option rights involve not only one's personal freedom but also some degree of control over others. If I have the right to do as I please, given those boundaries, then you are obligated not to interfere with that right. Thus I have some control over your actions. But you have a right to inform me when my actions take me out of *my* sphere of sovereignty and into yours. And if I refuse to desist from what I am doing, you have a right to stop me. Thus you have some control over me. The matter of priorities and values in option rights is the basis for a great deal of our legal system, our concepts of morals and ethics, and the development of our own personal value systems. Go to civil court and observe at random any suit, such as two giant corporations locked in an antitrust fight or two men arguing over who dented the other's automobile fender; the basis for the suit and the premise of all the arguments are option rights.

Welfare rights are the legal entitlement to some good or benefit, such as a free public education or a certain safety standard in highway or elevator construction. A claim is a request or demand for those rights; conflict ensues when people lay claim to rights that do not exist in law but that *do* exist in the moral value system of those claiming the right. Sometimes when a sufficient number of people claim a welfare right that does not exist, if these people are stubborn and tenacious in their demand, a new welfare right will be created by law. Examples of welfare rights that resulted from just such demands are the laws against being sold into slavery, child labor laws, Federal Aviation Agency (FAA) regulations about air traffic control, and quite possibly the passage of the Equal Rights Amendment to the United States Constitution that will prohibit discrimination based on sex.

I have distinguished between option rights and welfare rights in an effort to

---

*Golding, Martin P.: The concept of rights. In Bandman, Elsie L., and Bandman, Bertram, editors: Bioethics and human rights, Boston, 1978, Little, Brown & Co., pp. 44-45.

further define the origin and function of rights. These rights are intertwined even though they are defined differently. For instance, are some welfare rights mandatory, that is, are we obligated to take advantage of them? If some welfare rights are not mandatory, do they then become option rights because we have a choice to avail ourselves of them or not? A tuition-free public education until one reaches the age of 16 is a mandatory welfare right. But one does not have to send a child to a public school; a private or parochial school can be substituted. Thus a free public education is a welfare right, but an education (neither free nor public) is a *mandatory* welfare right. Even this, one of the most basic of all American welfare rights, is not agreed to by everyone. The Amish people in central Pennsylvania have for years fought bitter court battles to remove their children from organized established schools and to educate them at home or not at all if they choose.

What are the conditions for having rights, and why do societies involve themselves in the complexities and conflicts of assigning priorities to rights? The concept of freedom, which is subscribed to by all democracies, is tied to the concept of rights. One cannot be free if one has no rights. The right to be free from interference by others, including government, is the right to one's own domain: privacy, body, religion, property, and any other sphere in which an individual operates. Freedom is also the right *not* to exercise one's rights, no matter how foolish that may seem to others. In contrast to this idea, Feinberg describes Nowheresville, a world without rights:

> There will, of course, be delegated authorities in the imaginary world, empowered to give commands to their underlings and to punish them for disobedience. But the commands are all given in the name of right-monopoly who in turn are the only persons to whom obligations are owed. Hence, even intermediate superiors do not have claim-rights against their subordinates but only legal *powers* to create obligations in the subordinate *to* the monopolistic right-holders, and also the legal *privilege* to impose penalties in the name of that monopoly.*

What Feinberg is describing in Nowheresville is a society in which obedience is expected to flow from subordinates to superiors, the latter being the only ones to whom rights are owed. People who exist between the subordinates and superiors serve as expediters for exacting obligations from the subordinates and rights owed to superiors. It is a completely totalitarian system.

If no legal guarantee of health exists in either federal or state law, how can the concept of rights be applied to health care? Laws *do* exist concerning public health and safety. For instance, Public Law 91-572 (1971), the Family Planning Services and Population Research Act, authorized $30 million each for research and services in family planning. One could avail oneself of the results of the research and use the family planning services, and one could even say that the right to the services is a welfare right, but it is not a right to health. This might seem incongruent: if one could control the size of one's family, one would seem to be healthier. True, but the public law still does not guarantee anything. If one feels healthier because

---

*Feinberg, Joel: The nature and value of rights. In Bandman, Elsie L., and Bandman, Bertram, editors: Bioethics and human rights, Boston, 1978, Little, Brown & Co., p. 24.

of a control over reproductive capacities, one is benefitted by the law and that may have been the law's purpose, but it still does not imply or guarantee a right to health. Another example: Public Law 89-749, the Comprehensive Health Planning and Public Health Service Amendments (1966), sometimes called the Partnership for Health Act, mandated consumer participation in health planning services. Again, no right to health is implied, only the right to plan those programs and services that would ultimately result in better health. Better health care is a benefit of the law, not a right.

It is logical to look at some option rights in terms of how they might be applied to health care. If one of my option rights is the freedom of control over my own body, then I should be the only one who determines if and when it should be poked, prodded, x-rayed, medicated, or cut open. My brain is party of my body, and one of my option rights is not to have that part of my body deceived, tricked, or coerced in any way: the right to informed consent. If my option right is the freedom of control over my body, then health care professionals are *obligated* to help me maintain that control. So far that seems simple and agreeable. But what about the professionals' moral obligation to care for me, to improve my health, to bring to fruition whatever rights are due me? Here we run into conflict. If I am given a certain right, for instance to have a health procedure explained to me, then I also have the right to exercise that right: someone must explain the procedure. In fulfilling that obligation, how far is the health professional required to go? How much explanation is sufficient to fulfill my right?

The granting of rights automatically implies corresponding duties and responsibilities; one cannot exist without the other. Which rights involve corresponding obligations, and to what extent is one responsible for or obligated to protect the rights and freedoms of others? The following basic questions can serve as a guide, although the answers can by no means be considered definitive:

1. Is the right practical, and can it be acted on? For example, is the health care client claiming a right that is possible to be claimed, or is he requesting a surgeon to be clairvoyant in predicting exactly how long he can be expected to live? The surgeon obviously cannot do this.
2. Can the right be considered impartial in its application, or is the claimant demanding rights either that are not accorded to anyone else or that are different from or better than those of anyone else?
3. Is the right important? This involves standards and values in determining what is and what is not important, but there should be some consensus that the claimed right has sufficient value to make others obligated to act on it. So many people and organizations are today claiming specialized rights that the patience of those obligated to fulfill them runs the risk of being strained.
4. Are resources available to make it practical to claim a right? If they are available, are people obligated to allocate them in a manner claimed as a right? Again, in the matter of health care, suppose it were considered a right that every American have an adequate, well-balanced diet. Resources are certainly available, but does each citizen have the right to be fed or must he take some of the responsibility for himself? Who is obligated to do what?

The right to health care is a concept that is gaining acceptance in the United States; it is a premise of this book. I believe that everyone has the right to be as healthy as he *wants* to be and as current knowledge and expertise *permit* him to be. This view is shared by the vast majority of health professionals. Some Americans have access to health care, but some, in varying degrees, do not.

The advocates of the concept [the right to health care] are no doubt motivated by good intentions: they wish to correct certain inequalities in the distribution of health services in American society. That such inequalities exist is not in dispute. What is in dispute, however, is how to distinguish between inequalities and inequities and how to determine which governmental policies are best suited to the securing of good medical care for the maximum number of persons.*

Another difficulty that Szasz postulates about the right to health care is the confusion between rights and claims and between protection from injury and the provision of goods and services. He uses an example of the person with diabetes: the diabetic has less than optimum health and in an effort to regain it, which he sees as his right, requires medical attention and certain drugs. Here the diabetic comes into conflict with the rights of others: the physician's right to sell his services when and to whom he chooses and the right of the pharmaceutical company to sell or not sell the drugs it owns. The rights of the physician and pharmaceutical manufacturer are actual rights, protected by law, but the rights of the diabetic are only alleged rights, not legally protected. This is an excellent example of the lack of the right to health and health care.[2]

Szasz sees only two methods to ensure or protect citizens' rights to health care. The state may coerce physicians and other health professionals to serve clients (he refers to them as state-owned slaves), or economic, moral, and political circumstances can be created that are favorable to a plentiful supply of health care such that individuals can then care for themselves. The former solution solves a human problem by recourse to an all-powerful state but in so doing creates another problem: the subjection of the interests of one group to those of another, a hallmark of collectivism and communism. The latter solution depends on individual initiative and voluntary association, thus providing the rights necessary for the provision of health care without providing the right to health care itself. These are characteristics of individualism and capitalism.[2]

THOSE TO WHOM PROFESSIONALS ARE ACCOUNTABLE

Again we begin with a definition and a description. The following are characteristics of a professional:

1. The profession is worked at full time and is the professional's principal source of income.
2. The professional sees his work as a commitment to a calling. It is more than just a job, and the energy he devotes to it extends beyond the hours of actual work.

*Szasz, Thomas: The theology of medicine, Baton Rouge, 1977, Louisiana State University Press, p. 101.

3. The profession and professional are set apart from the laity by certain signs and symbols that are readily identifiable.
4. Professionals are organized with their peers for professional reasons, that is, for reasons that transcend money and other tangible benefits.
5. The profesional possesses useful knowledge and skills based on an education of exceptional duration and difficulty.
6. Professionals exhibit a service orientation that goes beyond financial motivation.
7. The professional proceeds in his work by his own judgment; he is autonomous.

Because professionals are responsible almost entirely to themselves for the proper use of their knowledge and skills, it is incumbent on them that they guard and protect the interest of the client and do whatever is necessary to earn the client's trust. A balance between loyalty to the client and loyalty to the professional community must exist. This balance is always precarious and is affected by a number of factors. If a professional works with a group of colleagues and is salaried— for example, a physician working for a health maintenance organization (HMO)— the collegial control is stronger than if the professional works alone in a fee-for-service setting. Those professionals who work in close proximity to colleagues are more likely to keep abreast of professional developments than those who work in more isolated environments. Those professionals who interact frequently with their colleagues usually have greater loyalty to their colleagues than to their clients, especially in terms of how the value of the association is perceived. The relationships of physicians to their colleagues and to nonpaying clients, for example, show this contrast. If a professional works for an agency, with its attendant collegial scrutiny, the agency may impose controls that can either enhance or inhibit the professional's responsiveness to clients. When a professional's autonomy increases, usually when he works with fewer colleagues, his responsiveness to clients is a function of the extent to which the professional and client share expectations about the benefits to be derived from the relationship. As professional autonomy decreases, responsiveness to clients becomes a function of how the bureaucracy for which the professional works shares expectations with clients.

The socialization of professionals is a major factor in the way in which the professional views his role, his responsibilities, and his relationships with colleagues and clients. Socialization can be seen as one or a combination of any of the following:

1. The process by which a person learns the culture and mores of a group so he can function in it
2. The narrowing of an individual's inborn behavioral potentials to a certain specified range
3. The learning of social roles and attitudes of a particular group

People are socialized by both formal training and the actual performance of a profession, although the influences of the latter are stronger and longer lasting than the former.

Simpson[3] studied the socialization process in a group of 95 baccalaureate nursing students and found that they began their studies motivated primarily by the humanitarian concerns of alleviating suffering and helping people. The first phase of the socialization process quickly changed this emphasis to the mastery of tasks and skills and the acquisition of knowledge. Students temporarily abandoned the role of helper. The second phase in the process occurred when students moved from the classroom to a clinical setting, and again the students' perception of themselves changed. Instead of the client being seen as the most significant other in their professional environment, that role was transferred to co-workers: physicians, fellow students, and registered nurses. They began to evaluate and judge their own performance by the standards set by colleagues, not by the perceived standards of clients. They began to acquire the norms of the professional group. The third phase of the process, as seen by Simpson, involved an intensification of the second phase. The degree to which this takes place depends on the extent of work relationships with colleagues rather than outsiders and the extent to which the student is insulated from pressures from outsiders. The socialization process is complete when the values of the profession are fully integrated into the values of the person.

Considerable debate exists about whether the complete internalization of professional values is ultimately good, that is, beneficial to the client. If one accepts and believes all the values of one's colleagues, how much mental energy is left for inquiry, questioning, doubt, and challenge? Without some iconoclasts within its ranks to question and challenge existing beliefs, a profession is in grave danger of becoming brittle and unproductive, an anachronism, and in the case of health professions, a public menace. If one internalizes values without first subjecting them to intellectual scrutiny, of what benefit are those values to the professional?

Motivation for the ethical behavior of professionals does not usually arise from a fear of punishment but rather in the fact that a formal code of behavior exists (as it does in virtually all professions) and the practitioner is expected to adhere to the code. An ethical code, as applied to professionals, is a collective statement about the group's expectations, a standard of behavior. In instances when the code is made public, clients then join colleagues as judges of professional behavior. Each profession expects certain role behaviors as norms; professional values are implicit in these norms, and the professional is expected to strive toward a set of ideals. It is implicit in service professions that the role player, the professional, should exert a maximum degree of performance. The practitioner, as he becomes enmeshed in the socialization process, is expected to make the transition from the ethical theory he learned as a student to ethical practice with the awareness that he alone is responsible for his behavior.

Ethical rules and penalties

Ancient Romans believed that the primary rule of the physician was to do no harm: *Primum non nocere* (First, do no harm), a noble goal but one filled with complexities and questions. Who is to be protected from harm, what constitutes harm, and what are the consequences if harm is done? A discussion of responsibility and accountability must be expanded to include all health professionals because we are all a product of some kind of educational training and are therefore responsible.

One could make a case for dividing accountability, particularly as it pertains to nursing, into three more or less equal sectors: to the self, to the client, and to the employing institution. The view that the nurse is primarily responsible to herself stems from means-ends behavior; that is, if she takes an action, then she must be aware of and responsible for that action and must defend it. This view could be considered ethically correct if the nurse's actions involved no other people, if she had no potential for doing mischief or causing harm. But she does do things to or for a client who is at least partially dependent on her choice of actions and who has placed his trust in her ability to carry them out correctly and appropriately. Thus she also has a moral responsibility to her client. She enters the profession knowing that her actions have a potential for harm, and the socialization process increases her perception of the consequences of her actions. She sees her own behavior as part of the larger health care system. Therefore the circle of means-ends behavior should be expanded to include the client.

Many believe that the nurse is also accountable to the institution for which she works. By paying her salary and giving her the opportunity to practice her professional skills, the institution is putting trust in the nurse. Is she obligated not to misplace that trust when it comes in conflict with her own or her client's values? Is she obligated to behave in a way the institution wants her to because it has "bought" her services?

When does the concept of doing harm enter the picture of accountability? Is it always possible to do good without doing harm? What if the doing of good involves the necessary doing of harm? If a nurse in a burn unit inflicts pain on a client when she debrides dead tissue, she must hurt him to eventually help him. If a psychotherapist wishes to help a client understand and change some negative behavior, the client might find it painful to look at past experiences he would prefer to keep hidden. Perhaps the avoidance of harm, a negative action, is not a sound or practical basis for making moral judgments about health care. A more positive view is examining the conflicts between good actions, the harm they might cause, and the eventual benefit that might result. Choosing between two or more positive actions, or even deciding if an action *is* positive, is a more difficult moral task than is differentiating between beneficial and harmful actions.

Health professionals are also accountable to society at large. Societal power is complex in establishing rules and consequent penalties. Generally whatever group is in control of a society or system has power to make the rules and expects to be the recipient of accountability. This may not be the way things should be, but very often it is the way things are. Those who have the power to control a system and to make ethical rules usually came to power by following the rules made by others. Power is often the reward for obedience to existing power. Those who spend years following certain ethical rules become socialized into the way of life represented by those rules and are not likely to suddenly change their values and become iconoclasts when they achieve their own positions of power. Thus ethical rules remain more or less fixed, and the same group or class of people continue to have input into the formulation of modes of ethical conduct.

The way this system works can be seen in the relationship of nurses and nursing to the health care delivery system as a whole. Nurses are notably absent from the roster of power; their socialization process, if it continues as it is now, will keep them outside the power structure or on the very fringes. Nurses are victims of the paternalism of the health care system, mainly because of the distribution of the sexes: 99% of nurses are women, and 93% of physicians are men. Other members of the health care power structure—hospital administrators, health insurance executives, and a few academics—are almost all men. We do not need to belabor the point that the physician-nurse relationship is a superior-inferior one. We can even acknowledge that the curricula of many if not most baccalaureate schools of nursing state that they emphasize nurses' professional responsibility and accountability (implicit in the concept of being accountable and responsible is the need to make one's own moral decisions based on personal and professional standards and values). What is troubling is that all these good *intentions* will be for naught if the socialization process, which occurs most strongly after graduation from nursing school, remains as it is. If nurses continue to believe that they cannot and should not make their own moral decisions, they will not. If they continue to bend to the will of others, they will never be able to stand up straight. If they continue to see themselves as inferior members of the health care system, they will not be able to grow and accept moral responsibility for themselves.

Purtilo sums up the issue of who should be accountable:

Any person, group, or institution, with the power to effect change in other persons, groups, or institutions, can be asked to justify their actions. In this sense the account is a protection for the weak (out-group, minority, vulnerable, oppressed). Its goal is to prevent or diminish oppression and exploitation and to facilitate just action.*

We return to the subject of rights. Part of the reason for behaving in a morally correct or good way is to protect people's option and welfare rights. Those who are strong, healthy, and protected by society (the rich, powerful, and educated) have little trouble knowing what their rights are and laying claim to them. Those who are weak, ill, poor, uneducated, and disenfranchised are the ones to whom health professionals owe a special moral obligation. If we do not voluntarily protect the rights of these people, it is likely they will be abrogated. If professional accountability does not carry with it the implication of reward or punishment, the system is unlikely to be effective. This reward or punishment may be in the form of official or unofficial professional sanctions, legal apparatus, or the approbation of one's colleagues, but it must be built into the socialization process so that all members of the profession are aware that it exists and are affected by it. Without it the recipients of health care would be forced to depend entirely on the personal ethics of those providing care, and history has shown this to be insufficient.

---

*Purtilo, Ruth B.: Essays for professional helpers: some psychosocial and ethical considerations, Thorofare, N. J., 1975, Charles B. Slack, Inc., p. 16.

Why is one professionally accountable?

For what purpose can professional accountability be required either by the profession or by oneself? One reason is to evaluate new professional practices and to reassess existing ones. Any new health care procedure or technique involves such far-reaching complexity that one is never certain of all the eventual consequences. Ethical ramifications need to be explored and discussed before definitive action is taken. Existing professional practices must be continually examined to avoid the "we do it this way because we've always done it this way" syndrome and because repetition of any action leads to a decrease in the amount of thinking about the rationale behind the action.

Professional accountability also exists to maintain goals and standards, as measured by peer review, audits of medical and nursing records, reevaluation of employment contracts, inspection and relicensing of care-giving institutions, and other forms of professionals controlling the behavior and actions of other professionals. Another form of accountability is a guideline for professional action, which usually results in a code of ethics. Public policy and codes of ethics will be discussed in greater detail in Chapter 9 on human experimentation.

The most important reason for the existence of professional accountability is the provision or enhancement of self-reflection, ethical thought, and personal growth. Whether one is accountable to the client, the institution, or society at large, one is always, definitely, and finally accountable to oneself, and one must function in a way that reflects and harmonizes with one's beliefs. A religious view proposes accountability, in this life or in a possible next one, to God. One might feel responsible for upholding a social or political cause. And some people feel responsible to the memory of a loved one who has died. All these feelings involve *personal* responsibility: the consequences of immoral acts will involve inward suffering even if no discernible harm has been done to another person. When the peer review, the application of codes of ethics, and collegial criticism are all over, one must ask *oneself* whether an action was morally justified and whether a mistake was "honest" or was based on carelessness, thoughtlessness, or poor professional judgment.

If a person is accountable to certain rules of behavior, then his own behavior is predictable, at least in particular spheres of activity. This predictability makes colleagues view each other as reliable and in effect *causes* reliability. Sensitive, thinking, and caring people in the health care system will then go beyond their own reliability and predictability to discover *why* they behave as they do and will reassess their values concerning beliefs and actions.

If the realm of ethics is not finite, if it is constantly expanding, contracting, and changing shape, and if there are few immutable laws, how can one human being pass judgment on any other or on himself? When the question is asked in this way in reference to a profession that seeks to be nonjudgmental, one would expect the answer to be that we *cannot* pass judgment on each other. But we can, we must, and indeed we do. To live without moral judgments is to live in a moral vacuum and to court anarchy or totalitarianism. Most of us are sufficiently astute students of history to know that this is not a desirable way of life. We require moral structure and direction; without them we feel at loose ends and insecure. The issue is not whether moral judgments should be made—they are being made and will continue to be. It is, rather, a question of who makes the judgments and on what bases. We as nurses pay lip service to the notion that we are captains of our own moral ships, and in our personal lives we may very well be, but in professional relationships with other people delivering health care, we are only passengers on that ship, not even occupying first-class cabins.

DEVELOPMENT OF A PROFESSIONAL VALUE SYSTEM

In a discussion of values and ethical bases for practice, we must define *what* we value. For most health professionals the foundation of all such discussions rests on the quality of human life. Life itself is a purely biologic function, but we are concerned with what differentiates human life from all others. What is a human being, a person? Is a person different from a human being? Does having human form mean that one is a person? Fletcher[4] made an attempt to define personhood by listing positive and negative human criteria. The following are the positive:

1. *Minimal intelligence*. An individual whose score on a standard Stanford-Binet intelligence test falls below 20 cannot be considered a person. Fletcher thought that a score between 20 and 40 put one in a category of questionable personhood. Many people disagree with the severity of Fletcher's criterion of intelligence, pointing to the thousands of profoundly mentally retarded individuals who would thus be denied personhood.

2. *Self-awareness*. An individual lacks this quality in a state of incorrigible unconsciousness, the coma of oblivion from which there is no reasonable hope of recovery and that is indicative of irreversible damage to the neocortex of the brain.

3. *Self-control*. An individual must not be totally subject to the will of others (except by force) but must have conscious control of his own actions and exhibit means-ends behavior. The temporary loss of control because of illness or accident does not, of course, jeopardize one's personhood; the condition must be permanent.

4. *A sense of time*. This is meant to be clock time, not time in the metaphysical sense. To be a person, one must be aware of the passage of time. This criterion also refers to a permanent loss of awareness, not to those who are asleep or temporarily unconscious.

5. *A sense of futurity*. One must be aware of time yet to come. The concept of personhood implies goals, strivings, and yearnings, and these cannot exist in the human mind if it has no idea that a future exists.

6. *A sense of the past*. This involves the person as a product of his culture, learned behavior, and linkage with past events as a result of conscious recall. This criterion differentiates a person who has learned a fact because of his cognitive ability from a dog who has learned a trick because of conditioning.

7. *The ability to relate to others*. Fletcher makes no judgments about the *quality* of one's relationships—only that they should exist. To be a person, one needs to be aware of the personhood of others and to relate to others on a human level. Some animals do indeed live in social systems (even lower species such as ants and

bees), but they relate to each other on an instinctual level rather than a conscious, cognitive one.

8. Concern for others. This does not necessarily mean altruistic or charitable concern but refers more to the concern for the personhood or humanity of others.

9. Communication. A person is not totally isolated from other human beings and thus must be able to make his thoughts and needs known. Whether he chooses to or not is his own business, but a person must be *able* to communicate.

10. Control of existence. All people are subject to physical and psychic determinants of their behavior, but within these limits a person sets his own course in life; he can control his functions, mobility, and behavior. To be totally subject to the whims of nature is not to be a person.

11. Curiosity. Human beings want to know things; to be totally indifferent to the world is not to be human. What one *does* with the curiosity is not important; the criterion is to be curious.

12. Change and changeability. Mere biologic growth and physical change are not indicative of personhood. What matters is the ability to change one's mind: proof of the ability to think.

13. Balance of rationality and feeling. Fletcher believes that a person is neither a coldly rational machine nor simply a creature of feeling and intuition. He makes no distinction about the proportion of rationality to feeling, only that some sort of balance exists. This is one of his most subjective criteria.

14. Idiosyncrasy. To be a person is to be recognizable as a distinct individual, to have an identity, to be different from all other human beings.

15. Neocortical function. This is the criterion on which all the others are based, the cardinal indicator. No matter how much life exists in a *body*, to be noncerebral means to be not a person.

Fletcher also listed negative human criteria:

1. A person is not non- or anti-artificial. If an individual is humanly reproduced, that is, a product of a human ovum and sperm, he is a human being. The conception may not be entirely natural, as with in vitro fertilization (the test tube baby), but the individual is nonetheless a person.

2. A person is not essentially parental. Having reproduced is not necessary for personhood.

3. A person is not essentially sexual. Engaging in sexual activity and feelings of sexuality are not essential to being considered a person.

4. A person has no natural rights. Fletcher believes that the notion of human nature has given rise to the idea that people have natural rights to which they are automatically entitled as if these rights were absolute and eternal. Rights are granted by social systems and are not a requirement of personhood.

5. A person is not necessarily a worshipper. Belief in God or any supernatural reality is not a requirement of personhood. In this sense spirituality is like sexuality, commonly felt but not essential to be considered a person.

Two years after publication of these criteria and after much collegial reaction, Fletcher[5] narrowed them to four different traits that are not mutually exclusive: neocortical function, self-consciousness, relational ability, and happiness, the last included in a not altogether serious vein. The ultimate question, of course, concerns which of these traits is a precondition for the others. One view states that subjectivity or self-awareness distinguishes human beings from other life forms; the emergence of consciousness creates personhood. This view eliminates fetuses and perhaps even neonates and young infants from personhood, which will be upsetting to many. Another view is that the quality of human life depends on the quality of human relationships, and thus an individual who has no relational ability has no claim to be considered a person. Distinction is made between the ability to relate to others and the choice to do so. A hermit who prefers solitude of mind and body must still be considered a person, although if he should decide to increase the quantity of his social interaction, the quality of those relationships might be diminished by long absence from them.

Happiness is an elusive phenomenon so subject to changes in tone and amount that is almost impossible to use it as a criterion for humanhood. An imbecile or someone who is profoundly retarded may appear to be happy or euphoric, but if he meets none of the other criteria it is doubtful, according to Fletcher, that he could be a person. When I stroke my cat and rub her cheek, she purrs and thumps her tail with happiness, but she is not a person.

Fletcher maintains that neocortical functioning is the one requisite on which the others are based; it is therefore a precondition for the others and the essence of personhood. One can argue about the quality and amount of the other traits and can even debate their existence as necessary criteria for personhood, but without a neocortex or its minimal function an individual simply is not *there* and thus cannot be considered a person. This view, as stated by Fletcher, is shared by many but not by everyone. The debate about who is a person becomes particularly heated when it concerns abortion and euthanasia.

Process by which values are developed

A value can be considered a perspective or a way of looking at something. Values are subjective; they are purely personal or cultural or, more commonly, a combination of both. Simon and Clark have established a set of criteria for the process of consciously acquiring values. Values must be freely chosen from among alternatives; the outcome of each alternative must be thoughtfully considered, and those chosen should be prized and cherished; one must make values known to others; and values should be integrated into one's life-style and should precipitate action if necessary.[6]

Values are developed and incorporated into one's life by the process of socialization. This process occurs in much the same way as the professional socialization described earlier, but values socialization is more complex and long-lasting. Values clarification is a phrase encountered frequently in the philosophy and conceptual framework of baccalaureate nursing programs. What exactly is meant by values clarification, and is it and should it be within the province of nursing educators? The clarification or development (for the purpose here the terms are synonymous) of values is the process of an individual choosing a set of standards, an ethical or moral guide on which he bases all his actions. It is a process of choice in which a person learns about himself, the world around him, and his relationship to that world. A person's set of values is one of the characteristics by which he is known or described by others and by which he describes himself. Values imply a certain steadiness of character and are an anchor in a world that changes rapidly and is often violent and confusing. They can be a shelter, a haven of personal behavior when one is confused and perplexed by the values of others.

We develop values as a result of the behavior and attitudes of parents, the cultural and religious environments in which we were raised, the kinds of reading and thinking we have done, the quality of our sensitivity, the influence of teachers and significant social relationships, the experiences we have had, the ways in which we were treated during our early years, the ways we learned to respond to stimuli, our individual intelligence, and our relationship to spiritual matters and to God. In fact, little in our experiential realm does not affect the development of values. We make choices, we incorporate these choices into the way we live, and finally we are called on to act on our values. This action does not necessarily involve high drama or a momentous decision, although these are not precluded. It is much more likely to involve small, routine acts: the way we treat our friends and associates, things we do for leisure, how we calculate our income tax, the care we take of our bodies, and how we choose to earn a living.

Professional values are a reflection and expansion of personal values. When we enter nursing or any other profession we do not suddenly begin to develop values, nor do we change them to meet new life circumstances and experiences. What happens is that we *adapt* existing values to professional experiences and expectations. We may broaden the horizons of our thinking as we encounter situations that are new and perhaps unique to a particular occupational role, but we do not change our basic value systems, ethical beliefs, or even our general outlook on life. Neither does this mean that we are fixed, rigid, or immutable, unless, of course, we do not value change or emotional and intellectual growth. Most nursing students begin their professional socialization in late adolescence or early adulthood when they already have a clearly developed sense of values, but their range of experience is still so limited that there is yet much room for growth in applying values to new and constantly changing situations. The issue of the intertwining of personal and professional values is so complex and so subject to a variety of interpretations that an example is needed to illustrate it.

Melanie grew up in an upper-class home. Her family had had money for several generations, and although neither parent needed to work both had a strong need to be useful and consequently held full-time jobs. The family was white, Protestant, and very insulated in its way of life. Melanie grew up and went to school with people who were like her, and if she thought about the rest of the world it was in terms of "them" as opposed to "us," the people with whom she felt comfortable. In the course of her education she learned about poverty, oppression, misery, degradation, humiliation, and other life tragedies. She watched television newscasts and read the papers and thus knew about human brutality, war, famine, the slaughter of innocents, and even genocide. Melanie knew all this, but it did not *touch* her; those things happened to "them." She firmly believed that if she were polite and pleasant to everyone and worked hard, she would be fulfilled. She also believed this to be true about everyone else, including "them." When she thought about it at all, which was rare, Melanie really believed that if people applied themselves to a task and worked at it diligently, they would achieve their goal. She was bright, had a rational and logical turn of mind, and was, as her mother described her, "kind to people less fortunate than she."

She chose nursing out of a somewhat vague need to help people, survived her initial squeamishness at having to deal with things that were physically repugnant to her, and did well in her courses. When she encountered people in physical pain, she was quick to provide relief in the form of medication. Her essential kindness and good manners made her an excellent listener, and her logical mind helped her solve nursing problems in a creative, innovative way. She liked the hospital with its atmosphere of purpose and direction; most of the people seemed to work hard, and the hospital had identifiable goals. She could easily integrate the hospital workers' values into her own personal ones.

Then in her junior year Melanie took a course in community health nursing and her world was turned upside down. She was exposed to people and situations she had never experienced and finally came into personal contact with "them." The people whose tragedies had formerly only flashed by on the 6 o'clock news were now telling her their stories while she sat gingerly in their kitchens. Her good manners helped her not betray her feelings, but inwardly she was in turmoil because her values were in conflict with those of her clients. She had been sufficiently socialized into the profession to believe that everyone has a certain amount of dignity and worth (this was also consistent with her own sense of goodness, kindness, and fair play), but her clients demonstrated none of the self-reliance, independent hard work, and goal-directed behavior she held dear. Melanie's first impulse was to dismiss them as unimportant and unworthy of her professional help. She wanted simply to walk away, because she did not know how to incorporate the community health experience into her view of things. But students do not have the luxury of dismissing what they cannot handle. Because of her basic kindness and sensitivity she allowed herself to be drawn into their lives, at least peripherally. Her sensitivity allowed her to be sufficiently open and receptive that she could understand some of the circumstances that caused them to lead the lives they did. She could not feel their pain, and her own experiences gave her no ability to grasp the magnitude and the sheerly basic nature of their problems. She could feel sympathy but not empathy.

Melanie still believed that work and determination could lead to success, and she was able to use these values in persuading some of her clients to think about improvements in their health. She was even able to convince a young woman to use contraception by painting an imaginary picture of a more desirable life without unwanted children than with them. She was able to use her own values to help some of her clients, and she was able to incorporate these new experiences into her own value system. She was even able to expand her values so that "they" no longer seemed so alien and strange. But Melanie never *changed* what she believed.

Perhaps nursing education should look again at the goal of values clarification, and instead of thinking how students will develop new values it might be educationally more sound to examine a variety of health care issues and ethical dilemmas to see how established values can be used to solve ethical problems.

Nursing educators frequently caution students not to make value judgments about the lives and behavior of their clients. The term *value judgment* is a hazy one that is usually invoked when what is meant is the judgment of someone's behavior, not values. We caution students when assessing clients' problems not to use the words *good, bad, sufficient, doing well,* and the like because those terms reflect our own values. We are not quite certain, however, why we feel our own values should be left out of professional practice or even if they *can* and should be. It is unlikely that anyone can completely separate personal and professional values and doubtful that they *should* be separated. A more practical goal, in terms of teaching values clarification in schools of nursing, is to help students integrate personal values into the existing structure of professional values and those of their clients. It may be that the student will find so much incongruence that she could not continue in nursing, but more likely she, her clients, *and* the profession will grow and mature during the process. The process of integration of values necessitates reevaluation and introspection, which almost always lead to intellectual and emotional growth.

Kohlberg[7] has described six stages of moral development in children and adults, divided into three levels.

I. At the preconventional level one is responsible to society's rules of right and wrong but responds to these concepts in terms of the physical or hedonistic consequences of action as a result of the physical power of those who enforce the rules.

1. Punishment and obedience orientation. The physical consequences of an action determine whether it is seen as good or bad, regardless of the human value of the action. Avoidance of punishment and deference to power are values in their own right without regard to the underlying moral order supported by the authority.

2. Instrumental relativist orientation. Right action is that which satisfies one's own needs and occasionally the needs of others. Elements of fairness are present but always in a pragmatic form ("You scratch my back and I'll scratch yours") of reciprocity. Loyalty, gratitude, and justice are absent.

II. At the conventional level one maintains the expectations of himself or his immediate group (family, country, and so on) without regard for the consequences. There is conformity and loyalty to the existing social order, and the person is involved in maintaining, supporting, and justifying those responsible for the social order.

3. Interpersonal concordance. Good behavior is that which pleases or helps others; it is frequently judged by intent. There is conformity to stereotypical or natural behavior, and one earns approval by being nice.

4. Law and order orientation. Right behavior is the maintenance of authority, fixed rules, and the social order for their own sake.

III. At the post-conventional, autonomous, or principled level there is a clear effort to define moral values and principles that have validity apart from existing authority and apart from one's identification with groups in authority.

5. Social-contract legalistic orientation. Right action is usually defined in terms of general individual rights and standards that are agreed to by the whole society. There is an awareness of the relativisim of personal values and emphasis on a procedure for reaching consensus. Laws exist but can be changed to meet social utility.

6. Universal ethical-principle orientation. Right action is defined by self-chosen ethical principles based on comprehensiveness, universality, and consistency. The principles are abstract (as with the golden rule) rather than concrete moral rules (as with the Ten Commandments). They are universal principles of justice, reciprocity, equality of human rights, and respect for dignity.

According to Kohlberg these stages are sequential: an individual must achieve one before he can go on to the next.

Legal implications

One may discuss values and professional accountability forever; it is interesting, informative, and stimulating. But sooner or later abstract concepts and principles must be applied to real situations, and nurses, being pragmatic people, will want to know where various abstract moral principles fit into their scheme of daily activities. It is appropriate to look at some legal implications of morality to fit those principles into the realm of nursing activity.

"A person who is not responsible for causing the harm he did ought not to be punished for it."[8] This principle is a foundation of our moral and legal systems and has strong implications for professional accountability. A defendant pleading not guilty to a criminal charge because of temporary or permanent insanity, self-defense, accident, mistaken identity, and so on frequently is relieved of legal responsibility for his act; the implication is that he is also relieved of moral responsibility. Bedau[8] has given some examples of recent cases in which defendants presented novel excuses hoping to be absolved of criminal guilt. All the following examples have parallels in the area of professional accountability.

In Miami, Forida, Ronald Zamora, age 15, murdered an elderly woman in the course of a burglary in her home. Zamora's lawyer did not deny that the murder occurred, but he claimed that the boy was so influenced by violence on television that he was no longer certain if he was participating in a television show or realtiy. He had watched violence on television 6 to 8 hours a day for 10 years and was suffering from what his attorney called "television intoxication." The jury was unimpressed and found Zamora guilty of first-degree murder.

It may not seem likely that television intoxication could be seen as a parallel to a professional health care situation, but such a situation comes immediately to mind. There is not a nurse or physician in the country who has not worked to the point of physical and mental exhaustion. Residents in hospitals do it routinely, and so do nurses who are asked to work a double shift or who have worked around the clock because of some accident or crisis. The feeling of total exhaustion affects people differently, but many report a feeling of unreality or of not being completely "there" even when ostensibly awake. At this point of exhaustion physcial and mental reactions slow, and reality becomes fuzzy around the edges. If a health professional makes an error during this time—and chances are increased that he will—and harms a client, is he professionally, morally, and legally accountable? Can he say that he was forced by circumstances (lack of sleep from a busy "on call" night, from working overtime because hospital administration requested it, or from doing a double shift because both nurses on the next shift called in sick) to work and perform potentially harmful acts even though he knew his performance level was lower than it would have been if he were completely alert? Can he plead not guilty by reason of fatigue imposed by others, or should he have refused to do the assigned work because his professional ability was temporarily impaired, thus causing him to be a hazard to clients?

Thousands of excuses for errors are made each day. "If you had wheeled the right patient into the operating room, I wouldn't have amputated the wrong person's leg. It's your fault." "Well, he *told* me his name was Smith. How was I supposed to know he was so sedated he didn't even know his own name? It's not my fault." "I told you I wasn't familiar with all these new drugs. You shouldn't have assigned me to this unit. It's your fault." This list could go on forever; we are all aware of the number of errors made in health care institutions. But can we blame others for our own mistakes, even if another person's complicity was clearly involved? Yes, the operating room personnel should wheel the correct person into the designated room, but the surgeon has a responsibility to know whose leg he is cutting off. If more than one person is responsible for the care of a client, whose ultimate responsibility is it, and who is accountable when something goes wrong?

In Camden, New Jersey, Roxanne Gay stabbed to death her husband, a professional football player, in his sleep because he beat her severely and frequently. She claimed that she killed him to protect herself from the beatings. She was judged insane and acquitted but was committed to a state hospital. Francine Hughes of Lansing, Michigan, poured gasoline on her husband's bed and set it ablaze. She justified her act by saying that after a divorce her husband moved back into her home and resumed beating her. She was acquitted for the same reason, temporary insanity. Both women were in no *immediate* physical danger when they killed their husbands; they committed the murders because they feared and knew that what had happened in the past (being beaten) would again occur in the future. The man's death seemed the only certain way to stop the beatings. The ethical issue is whether the women could have taken some definitive preventive action during a period of relative safety between beatings.

Again, a parallel can be drawn to the safety of clients. Can a nurse who sees dangerous things happening to clients and who has participated in dangerous situations (severe understaffing or witnessing a professional colleague's incompetence or cruelty) be held responsible if the same situation occurs again and she had not made an effort to prevent it a second or third time? For example, a nurse on the evening shift is expected to work with so few other staff that should an emergency arise, the clients' safety would be in jeopardy. Let us assume that she has requested more help, but hospital administration has not complied with her request. She continues to work in the understaffed situation, and finally a crisis occurs in which a client dies because there are not enough staff to provide the appropriate help. Who is responsible—the staff nurse because she knew what could and probably would happen, the nursing supervisor because she did not put enough pressure on the administration and was also aware of the danger, or the hospital administration because it chose to ignore a repeated request from the nurse who could be considered an expert in that situation? The ethical issue is similar to that of the women who murdered their husbands. What could the hospital and its employees have done to ensure the safety of clients before the crisis occurred? What could have been done in the intervening safe period?

To protect the rights of the innocent and of the falsely accused, the law bends over backward to examine every excuse, mitigating cirucumstance, and possible justification of a person accused of a crime. This state of affairs has resulted from the democratic need to protect the rights of every individual, but in our zeal to ensure these rights have we overlooked the safety and well-being of the majority and have we created so many legal loopholes that an incredible variety of criminally irresponsible behavior can slip through? In the hugeness and complexity of the health care system, have we not created the same ease of abdicating moral responsibility for professional behavior?

Many of the legal implications of professional accountability have to do with protecting clients' rights. We have seen that there is no right to health or health care but that all human beings, whether health care clients or not, have the right to be protected against the intrusion of their personal and physical privacy by another person. Any text about nursing and the law will enumerate those acts that are permitted, those that are not, and many of the legal ramifications involved. What we are more concerned with here is how professionals are accountable and responsible to each other in protecting clients' rights.

> Consideration of the integrity of the rights of patients is only as secure as the commitment of those who have the authority to protect them; this responsibility rests chiefly with the nurse and the physician. Their subtle recognition of the rights of patients can permeate the climate in which health care is delivered.*

Theologic implications

Theology is the study of God and divine happenings. It is ironic to note that in the end and always God remains a mystery, the reason for doing things unfathomable and forever unknowable. Yet we continue to speculate about God without ever coming to definitive conclusions. God chooses to remain aloof, chooses to be unknowable, and has demonstrated no signs of changing this state of affairs. Theology is fascinating on an intellectual or theoretical level, but outside of speculation about what God might do next or what plans there might be for the future of the universe, it seems pointless to debate God's reasons for actions. One either accepts the existence of God or does not. If one believes that God exists, then one must

---

*Murchison, Irene, et al.: Legal accountability in the nursing process, St. Louis, 1978, The C. V. Mosby Co., p. 103.

decide what role a divine presence plays in daily activities. This can range from the view that God watches and controls every human action to the almost opposite view that God gave us all free will and then withdrew from control. Views on the presence and activity of God range between these two extremes, and once one has settled on a view, at least for the time being, there seems to be little purpose in further debate.

A more profitable exercise is the debate over health professionals' view of the sanctity of human life, which is an integral part of the question of divinity in everyday life. This issue is basic to professional accountability. Belief in the sanctity of life is the reason why health care exists and the reason why we are all concerned with the improvement of that care and its provision to all who want it. It is reasonable to assume that all health care professionals believe in preserving and protecting human life. It is *not* reasonable to assume that everyone agrees *what* human life should be preserved and protected and what should not. This, I think, should be the basis of a discussion of the theologic implications of professional accountability.

As one becomes more ill and weak, one's hold on life becomes more tenuous. Illness leads to weakness, which leads to dependence on those who provide care.

> In general, the more dependent a person is on another, the greater will be his need to aggrandize his helper, the more dependent he will be on him. The result is that the weak person easily becomes doubly endangered: first by his weakness and, second, by his dependence on a protector who may choose to harm him.*

The essential element of Szasz's comment above is the last phrase: health care workers do have significant power to cause harm, and this power is completely within their choosing. Standing between the client and the health care worker's power are the conscience and professional scruples of the worker and the sense of accountability and responsibility that the worker feels toward the client, himself, and his profession. Closely related to these protections is what the health care worker feels about the sanctity of life and the protection of the life of the client.

One could look at the theologic implications of health care ethics and professional accountability in terms of what ought to be or what God wants us to do. Again, we cannot know what God wants unless we believe the fundamentalist view that this is clearly stated in the Bible. Biblical teaching, however, leaves almost unlimited room for speculation and interpretation, so we can form principles for health care only on the basis of ethical principles in general, which may have nothing or everything to do with theology, depending on one's point of view.

Purtillo[9] has described three general positions that one could take in defining the relationship between professional (health care) ethics and theologic (or philosphic) ethics:

1. Professional ethics and philosophic/theologic ethics are mutually exclusive. Ethics that are related to the delivery of health care are so specific and specialized that they cannot be drawn from the realm of general philosophic ethics. This posi-

---

*Szasz, Thomas: The theology of medicine, Baton Rouge, 1977, Louisiana State University Press, p. 2.

tion maintains that the health care system has so many exclusive qualities that it should remain outside the domain of general society.

2. Professional ethics and philosophic/theologic ethics are the same. This position is held only by a few who believe that ethics should be studied only in abstract and conceptual terms and should not be applied to the practical problems of any profession.

3. Professional ethics and philosophic/theologic ethics have many characteristics in common and are intricately related. This is the most widely held view. The challenge comes in exploring how they are related and what principles are foundations for others.

Psychologic implications

Psychology can state that something happens, and it can even explain why it happens or why people behave as they do. But it cannot determine whether an event or behavior is right or wrong, that is left to ethicists and moralists. Psychology explains what is; ethics expains what ought to be. When a professional allows his own values to play such a significant part in the professional-client relationship that the behavior of the client is affected, psychologic implications of ethics are involved. Readers, particularly nurses, may react negatively to this situation. They will remember all they have learned about nonjudgmental behavior and will agree that the professional's values should not influence the client. But is this always practical or even desirable? It may not be practical because it is impossible to leave one's values home when one goes to work. It may not be desirable because the health professional may hold values that may be beneficial for the client also.

For example, a community health nurse works in a district of a large metropolitan area that consists mostly of poor people. Many clients in her case load are adolescent mothers. Girls 11 or 12 years old who become pregnant are not uncommon though most are 15, 16, or 17. Almost all have quit school, and practically none are married. The pattern is depressingly familiar: young women, who know practically nothing about conception control and the physiology of sex and reproduction, have sex, get pregnant, have the babies, continue to live at home with their parents (usually only a mother), refuse to use contraception for a variety of reasons, have sex, and repeat the cycle several more times until they are convinced by some clinic physician to be sterilized. The nurse can *believe*, in a moral and ethical sense, that she has no right to impose her own values about sex and reproduction on her clients. But she sees that little good can come from perpetuating these conditions. The educational level of the community will remain low, and the economy will suffer because fewer people are working and more tax money is spent supporting these mothers and children, who for the most part are unwanted and therefore run a higher risk of being abused. The mothers are young and are considered to run a higher risk of having antepartal complications, and the infants are more likely to be of low birth weight and to be mentally and physically retarded.

The nurse sees all this, but at what point does she intervene in their lives to try to stop or change the cycle? She can provide health care in the form of counseling and referral to appropriate clinics and agencies, but is it morally permissible to impose on her clients her values concerning education, the size and spacing of families, and employment? Would they be better off if they adopted her values, which reflect the middle-class majority, or could she be considered elitist for wanting a better life for her clients? How far should she personally, and the health care system as a whole, go in imposing its will on clients to improve their lives by influencing a change in their behavior? It is a moral dilemma, one that health care professionals will face more frequently as the delivery of care moves out of institutions for the acutely ill and into the community.

Society *can* compel people to change their reproductive behavior, but should it? How far should we carry our desire to help and to alleviate suffering if it means interfering in the private behavior of other people, and in what behaviors is it ethically permissible to intervene? Even in the areas of specific sexual behavior we are faced with dilemmas. Is it any more or less morally permissible to try to stop young women from having intercourse without using conception control than it is to try to stop homosexual men from having intercourse with each other? Both are acts of private behavior, both involve sexual activities that some people find morally reprehensible, and both involve society to some degree, although not in the same way. Which, if either, behavior should we seek to change?

Philosophic derivations

The study of philosophy involves an examination of essential truths and principles of existence. It is usually divided into three branches: metaphysics, epistemology, and ethics. Ethics deals with questions of human conduct, the right or wrong of actions, the motives and ends of actions, and the formulation of principles for standards of conduct for groups of people. Health care ethics, also referred to as biomedical ethics or bioethics, refers to standards of behavior that are applied to the delivery of health care by individuals, agencies or institutions, and the system as a whole. Anyone who thinks seriously about these important questions can be considered a philosopher, but a few people throughout history have made philosophy their life's work and have written, often movingly and beautifully, about the subject.

Socrates believed that reason rather than emotion should determine our ethical decisions and that to do this we must have factual information about a situation and keep our minds free of emotion as we deliberate issues. Ethical dilemmas must be solved, according to Socrates, on the basis of what is *right*, not on the basis of what is generally accepted by other people or what the consequences of an action might be. Socrates acknowledged that two or more moral rules might be applied to the same situation; he felt that decisions could be made by determining which rules take precedence over which others. The Socratic method has survived for over 2000 years because of its flexibility; it can be used to excellent advantage in solving health care dilemmas.

A full-fledged discussion in moral philosophy develops when we pass beyond the stage in which we are directed only by traditional rules of conduct, which have limited application to complex ethical stiuations, and move to a stage where we think critically about an ethical dilemma in ways that allow us to use traditional rules as general principles coupled with ethical reasoning going beyond these traditional rules.*

Plato believed that one cannot lead a good or healthy life without grounding his actions in justice, which is based on the principle of never harming anyone. This presupposes that one knows what is just so that harm can be avoided. Plato got around this problem by developing the concept of fuctionalism: one who functions knows what he is doing and by knowing, will do no harm. Plato believed that knowledge is virtue, ignorance is vice, and knowledge underlies all virtuous and just actions. Plato's ethical system is almost impossible to apply to health care. We see evidence that knowledge does not necessarily lead to justice and even if we agreed with Plato the complexity of health care delivery almost ensures that absolute knowledge will be elusive when applied to ethical dilemmas.

Immanuel Kant postulated the form of the categorical imperative, a maxim that can be interpreted as universal law. The categorical imperative states that a person should be used as an end, never as a means, and certain unconditional moral commands must be obeyed and are necessary and obligatory under all circumstances. One must obey without looking at the consequences. Each person should be morally autonomous with no outside authority to tell him what to do. Kant's position is a fundamentalist approach and is difficult to apply to complex moral dilemmas, particularly those that face health professionals.

Jean-Paul Sartre and to some extent Friedrich Nietzsche espoused the existential view that moral decisions are to be made in the context of one's inner direction without dependence on established external moral principles. One must be responsible for one's own decisions and the consequences of those decisions without being pressured by others. Existentialism is basically an ethic of personal honesty, consciousness, and accountability; principles do count, but one must choose to follow them and then internalize them to solve ethical problems, particularly when time is a crucial factor. The use of internalized principles applied by an individual to a variety of circumstances is what many people think health care ethics is all about.

Throughout the book various ethical principles and rules will be discussed, such as utilitarianism, deontology, autonomy, beneficence, nonmaleficence, justice, and the like. They will be defined and applied to various ethical dilemmas and case situations. It is felt that these principles will be meaningful to the reader if they are used in the context of situations to which they apply.

Concept of personal choice

One can study philosophy, one can understand various ethical approaches, and one can say that he holds a certain set of beliefs. But the determination of action rests with personal choice. Choice is based on belief in and adherence to principles, but the choice to behave in certain ways always comes from inside oneself. Personal choice is the exercise of conscience, what we want to do because we feel a moral need to do it. We may do what we feel we *should* to avoid guilt, but in that

---

*Davis, Anne J., and Aroskar, Mila A.: Ethical dilemmas and nursing practice, New York, 1978, Appleton-Century-Crofts, p. 3.

avoidance of guilt we choose the correct action. Sometimes (some say always) the reasons for actions are not as important in a pragmatic sense as the actions themselves.

Guilt is the remorse or shame felt as the result of having done wrong or evil. If avoiding guilt causes us to do right or good, then this is a sufficient reason to take an action. Some say that the avoidance of guilt is morally neutral, that good does not necessarily occur if bad is not done: For example, if I am broke and need money and decide *not* to steal, am I doing good by not stealing because I do not want to face either my own guilt or more pragmatic consequences (criminal prosecution), or am I simply not doing evil? In this instance the choice not to steal could by seen as morally neutral. In health care ethics, however, situations are unlikely to be so clear-cut. If a nurse elects not to help a client obtain an abortion because the nurse's personal choice is the preservation of all life at all costs, she has indeed avoided her own guilt, but can it be said that she has done good? Her decision and behavior *may* be morally neutral if the client has access to other avenues of help and is not harmed by the nurse's refusal to give information. But if the client is delayed in finding help for so long that an abortion becomes impossible or risky, has the nurse's personal choice done good for the fetus or harm for the client—or both or neither? According to Gaylin,

there are two routes to good and unselfish behavior. We behave in socially approved manners even though it brings us in conflict with selfish interest or desire, first out of fear of punishment. . . . This is the mechanism dominated by guilty fear. Secondly, however, we internalize a model of goodness which may arise from a parent or an idealization of a parent, but once incorporated becomes a sense of ourselves—our better half, if you will. It is the way we would like to be. It is the person we feel we ought to be and it is the standard by which we measure ourselves. When we fail this internalized ideal, we feel we have betrayed ourself. We have done an injustice to that which we might have been and to that which we would like to be.*

When we exercise personal choice do we automatically disregard the will or wishes of others? Can we reconcile individual good (our own) and the common good? If we make a behavioral choice we believe to be good and correct or at least the lesser of two evils, and if that choice does harm to someone else, have we indeed made the correct choice? Does personal choice in ethical decision making ever have to bend to the will of others? Is it ever better to ignore the action we would prefer to take in favor of another action? How personal should personal choice be?

CRITICAL INFLUENCES ON ETHICAL DECISIONS
Agent

An agent is a person who performs an act, the one who makes the decision and carries it out or causes it to be carried out. In terms of health care the agent is usually a professional who has specific knowledge and skills and who, we must

---

*Gaylin, Willard: From Twain to Freud: an examination of conscience, Hastings Center Reports, 6(4):8. Reprinted with permission of The Hastings Center. © Institute of Society, Ethics and the Life Sciences, 360 Broadway, Hastings-on-Hudson, N.Y. 10706.

assume, has some amount of professional responsibility and accountability. The professional is accorded respect and certain privileges by the public and is in turn expected to behave in a certain way. He makes a commitment to the public good in a variety of ways, but since responsibility is in the hands of the agent, the public good may or may not be served—an agent is the instrument by which either good or evil can be done. The dominant force in the making of most health care decisions is the physician, and hence he is the agent with the most power. Nurses, social workers, and other health professionals are also agents, but their roles are different. They *do* make decisions that have profound effect on clients, but those effects are mostly in the psychoemotional domain. The physician agent has more power over life and death.

Certain characteristics can be expected of an agent who is responsible for making health care decisions and who is caring for clients who make their own decisions. The agent should be professionally qualified by a state license, an academic degree, completion of an apprenticeship, or examination by his colleagues. He is expected to have good moral character, a characteristic that is subject to all manner of interpretation and speculation. For the purposes here let us assume that good moral character is indicated by a sense of responsibility and accountability.

Circumstances and intent surrounding the issue

The circumstances and intent of an act and the agent who performs it can make the difference between morality and immorality. A tooth extraction is a good case in point. When a tooth is pulled because it is hopelessly diseased and when it is extracted in a dentist's office with sufficient local anesthesia, it is a morally neutral act. It could even be seen as an act of good if the dentist thinks the decay might cause a systemic infection. But the same extraction when performed without anesthesia by Nazis during World War II to remove the teeth of Jews and other non-Aryans for the gold or simply as form of torture is an act of moral evil. Circumstances and intent make the difference; the act remains the same.

The person upon whom the act is performed can also alter the circumstances and intent. An excellent case involve tubal ligation, or sterilization. For example, two acts of sterilization are performed, one on a middle-class married woman in her early 30s with two children, and the other on a lower-class 19-year-old unmarried woman with three children. Both women have signed a consent form, and both say they understand the implications of the operation. Even though both acts *may* be morally neutral, the circumstances of the two women are so different that the intent of the person performing the sterilization must at least be suspect and subject to further investigation.

The intent of the person performing the act can complicate the moral issue. When pain is the result of an act, one must ask if the intent was to cause pain or if the pain was secondary to an act designed to result in good. Is it morally correct to commit an act that will eventually cause good but will also cause pain, and is the resulting pain intentional or unintentional? If health professionals believed that the causing of pain was immoral in all circumstances, their hands would be tied; they could not perform surgery, debride a burn wound, or even do a blood test. Thus it cannot be that the *causing* of pain is immoral, but one does have to look at the intent behind the infliction of pain.

In his essay "A Map for Medical Ethics: Moral Justifications of Medical Interventions,"[2] Szasz states the three usual reasons for intervention in the face of disease. A person should have treatment

1. Because he has a disease—a disease-oriented justification for intervention
2. Because he will then be cured—a treatment-oriented justification for intervention
3. Because he seeks it and because it is available—a consent-oriented justification for intervention

Szasz does not believe that these justifications are sufficient. He sees discrepancies between the medical facts and the moral justifications for intervention:

1. Illness may not justify intervention if the client rejects it for personal or religious reasons. Intervention may be justified in the absence of disease as in abortion or vasectomy.
2. The cure (therapeutic effectiveness) may not justify intervention if the client rejects it, and some interventions *may* be justified in the absence of proved therapeutic effectiveness (electric shock treatments, for example).
3. Consent may not justify intervention, as with a physician administering morphine to an addict, and in some cases intervention may be justified in the absence of consent, most notably in emergency situations.

The intent and circumstances surrounding an act are intricately bound up with its morality. Szasz and many others believe that life is inherently a tragedy, that our fate is often involved with tragedy, and that the moral choices we are given and the way we act on those choices lead us to embrace or avoid tragedy.

The belief that we can have a medico-ethical and medico-legal system that combines the virtues, but not the wickedness, of justifying medical interventions by illness, treatment, and consent is, I submit, such a tragedy. It is, in other words, not a tragic fate we must bear, but a tragic folly we must avoid.*

Consequences of act affect issue as a whole

Some people feel (the school of philosophy known as utilitarianism) that the consequences of an act are or should be the only decisive factor in choosing to commit the act. If the act will have positive consequences, then a moral good has been done. If the reverse is true, then a moral evil has been done, no matter what the intent was. This view poses problems in the delivery of health care. If consequences are the only factor that determines morality, no risks can be taken, no experimentation done, no therapeutic intervention tried in the hope that good will result. No physician will be able to say, "Let's try this drug and see if it works better than the other." The drug may or may not be better, and if the consequences of the drug are not positive (although not necessarily negative), the physician could be said to have acted immorally. This could have far-reaching impli-

---

*Szasz, Thomas: The theology of medicine, Baton Rouge, 1977, Louisiana State University Press, p. 28.

cations for medical intervention. If a nurse says to a hospital client who is in pain, "Try lying on your side with your knees drawn up and see if you feel more comfortable," she is intending to relieve the client's pain. The new position may or may not be better than the previous one, but if the nurse were acting only within the framework of the utilitarian view, she would not be free to suggest an act that may not turn out positively.

Consequences must be considered, of course, when one decides whether to commit an act, but they cannot be the only factor, and in and of themselves they are not the only indicator of morality. Consequences must be viewed with the act itself, the intent, and the circumstances in detemining the ultimate outcome of an issue or question. Consequences that do not occur as planned or intended are not, however, to be confused with excuses and justifications for acts that turn out negatively because of some factor in the commission of the act. If a nurse administers a medication or a treatment and the client experiences an untoward effect, a negative consequence has occurred. The crucial question and factor involves not the consequence but the nature of the act. Was the act itself, and the attendant intent and circumstances, committed in a positive or negative way? This is the essence of the morality of the issue.

PROFESSIONAL COMMITMENT

One's commitment to a profession derives almost entirely from one's view of life and to a lesser extent from socialization into the profession. For the health professional, the life view can center on the value or sanctity of life. But a commitment to professional values may not always be consistent with one's life view or with the values of the profession itself. Even the profession may not always be consistent with its own stated commitment and beliefs. For example, nursing professes to believe in the rehabilitation of the chronically ill and disabled, to bring people to their highest possible level of functioning. Yet nursing administrators in hospitals and community health agencies frequently will not hire a nurse with health problems that might on a few occasions interfere with professional functioning, for instance, an epileptic or a "brittle" diabetic. Medicine professes to treat all people equally without regard for their social class or economic status. But try walking into a private physician's office and announcing that though you have no money and cannot pay for his services, you expect to be treated because of his professional commitment. Most physicians would send you down the street to the hospital outpatient department or the local clinic. This is not necessarily evil or immoral (the fee-for-service system is based on a profit motive and is recognized as an aspect of capitalism), but it is in conflict with the stated commitment of the medical profession.

Empathy and help

No health care professional begins education and training without the desire to help people. In some cases profit is a strong motive, but one could find easier and faster ways to earn a great deal of money than by becoming a physician with the profession's attendant trials and tribulations. We assume that all health care professionals have some degree of empathy with their clients and that they all want to help, but what is not clear is how far a professional is obligated to go in giving help and empathy. Each client-professional relationship entails a bond of trust and faith. The client must trust that the professional will give enough time, care, and expertise for him to get well or at least have his condition alleviated to the maximum extent. The professional must trust that the client will not make demands that he cannot fulfill. How much is enough? How much time is a professional required to spend with a client to relieve pain and anxiety? How much of the professional's time is his own and how much belongs to the client? Eight hours a day? What if 8 hours is insufficient to fulfill a basic professional commitment? Should another professional of equal competence take over? Then are we not abdicating *our* responsibility to another? And what of the client's role in making demands on the professional's time and energy? Is he obligated to realize that the professional has limitations, or is he entitled to all the professional's ability simply because he is the client?

Duty. Duty is a concept that has lost popularity in recent years because it conjures up military and even monastic images, but duty must play a role in professional commitment and is part of the desire to help and serve clients. Several views of duty can be applied to the provision of health care. The utilitarian view, in which a desirable consequence is the ultimate goal, is that we have a duty to bring about that consequence; the means to its completion are secondary to the consequence itself. The goal is to achieve the maximization of pleasure (good) and the minimization of pain (evil) for the greatest number of people. This view causes problems in the delivery of health care when the demand for health care (good) far outstrips the ability to provide it. If eveyone cannot be guaranteed a good consequence, where lies the duty of the provider of care in deciding how goals should be reached and what the consequences should be?

The Kantian view of duty, that of the categorical imperative, states that consequences are relatively unimportant but that action is obligatory because of moral duty and any act performed from a sense of duty is morally worthy and thus cannot cause harm. This view could be dangerous if applied to health care. A sense of duty is too nebulous and too open to interpretation to be accepted as carte blanche for the performance of any act. Suppose a person felt morally obligated by a sense of duty to prevent all people with a certain hereditary disease, for example, Tay-Sachs disease, from reproducing. Everyone agrees that there is nothing positive about Tay-Sachs disease: the children always die rather horribly, and there is no cure. The world would surely be improved if Tay-Sachs disease did not exist, and if all people who are carriers of the disease were prevented from reproducing, eventually it would disappear. Is the person who feels duty-bound to eradicate Tay-Sachs disease obligated or even permitted to do his duty in any way he sees fit, regardless of the means or the consequences? In the Socratic view some moral rules take precedence over others; in this instance the duty to maintain an ethical and trustworthy relationship with one's clients is more important than the duty to eradicate a certain disease.

Another view of duty states that we are obligated to develop certain attitudes and then act on them. One of those attitudes is the willingness to "go the distance" in doing whatever is necessary to help clients—that as health professionals we are not subject to the usual boundaries of other workers or other professions. If an architect can go home at 5:00 before the building is designed, probably no one will be harmed, but the health professional cannot go home until the needs of the client are met. We would like to embrace this altruistic view, but it is not usually practical or even humanly possible. It does, however, result in the most conflict. Where do we stop (or at least rest from) giving, how much of our emotional selves must we give to clients, how much pain must we subject ourselves to in order to alleviate the pain of others, how many hours do we work, and how much do we sublimate our own needs to meet the needs of clients?

Competence

It is not sufficient that a professional is committed to his clients or to his profession: he must also be competent to practice. Competence is difficult to measure except in very limited and defined ways. One may pass examinations given by colleagues (state licensure examination, oral comprehensive examinations, defense of a dissertation, final examination of a particular course, and so on), but these measure only minimal knowledge in a given area. Passing an examination does not mean that the professional is competent to function in any situation in which he may suddenly find himself. I once heard a story told in a nightclub by a raconteur. A man who was having pains in his stomach sought the help and advice of a physician. Alone in the physician's office he looked at all the diplomas and certificates on the wall. The physician had had a distinguished career, and his wall was covered with impressively framed documents. Then the physician walked in, saw the man examining the documents, and asked, "Are you impressed?" The client looked at him and said, "Tell me, Doc, when you were in medical school, what grade did you get in stomachs?" It is an amusing story, but it illustrates that although examinations have been passed and kudos awarded, one wants to know if the practitioner is competent to do what he is doing.

Beyond the passage of certain basic examinations that usually measure minimal ability and are given at the beginning of a professional career, how can one be certain of being competent, and how can one recognize competence in others? How many errors can a professional make before he is considered too incompetent to practice? What mechanisms exist for the assurance of professional competence?

Professional standards. The goal of establishing professional standards is the provision of the highest possible quality of care for clients.

Quality assurance can be defined as activities performed to determine the extent to which a phenomenon fulfills certain values and activities performed to assess changes in practice that will fulfill the highest or a predetermined level of values. A quality assurance program is a process designed to determine the extent to which a practice achieves selected objectives based on specified values.*

---

*Lang, Norma M.: The overview of quality assurance. In Davidson, Sharon VanSell: PSRO: utilization and audit in patient care, St. Louis, 1976, The C. V. Mosby Co., p. 5.

With Lang's definition as a guideline several areas can be delineated to measure or examine the competence of health professionals.

1. Each profession needs to establish standards of *practice*. To have passed an examination establishing minimal levels of knowledge is not sufficient. A way to periodically evaluate practice needs to be instituted. This is threatening to some, particularly those who know they will not measure up, but it is a system designed either to weed out incompetent individuals or to ensure that they will improve their professional expertise and skills.

2. Continuing education should be mandatory for relicensure. Nursing is one of the professions currently engaged in a battle over mandatory continuing education. Although it will not *guarantee* that minimal standards are maintained, it is a first step in that direction and several states have already taken this step.

3. A profession must demonstrate that it can regulate itself. Self-regulation distinguishes professions from occupations that need to be regulated by government agencies or public scrutiny. This is not to say that the public should not be aware of the way in which a profession regulates itself. There should be public awareness, but the regulation itself should come from within the profession. This has been accomplished recently by the establishment of Professional Standards Review Organizations (PSRO), most notably within medicine.

4. There should be an audit of services rendered. This has usually been accomplished by reviewing written records to determine if the objectives of care stated at the outset were met and to what degree. An audit is a valuable tool to determine care that was recorded, but it is not usually an accurate measure of how well the goals were achieved and in what manner the care was given. To say that a procedure was done does not necessarily mean that it was done completely or professionally.

5. The utilization review is a popular method that can succeed in determining *how* facilities are being used and in some measure whether they are being used for the intended purpose. The utilization review has been used almost exclusively to measure the effectiveness of institutions such as hospitals and nursing homes, but the concept could be applied to professional *people* as well.

6. The ombudsman is one of the most effective ways of keeping standards of practice high.

All these methods of standardizing professional behavior to some degree and ensuring that those standards remain high rest on one basic premise: that the individual professional is responsible for his own behavior and is accountable to himself, his colleagues, and the client.

SUMMARY

This chapter deals with professional accountability, responsibility, and rights, especially as they pertain to health care.

Option rights involve the ideas of freedom and choice in the way one lives, and welfare rights are legal entitlement to some good or benefit and are usually bestowed by government. Option rights and welfare rights are different but intertwined, and it is frequently difficult to distinguish between the two, but no legal right to health care exists. Most health professionals agree there is a *moral* right to health care, but aside from isolated public laws that are designed mostly to protect public safety, the right to health care is not guaranteed by either federal or state law. Granting rights automatically implies corresponding duties and responsibilities, and the determination of which rights involve which responsibilities creates ethical dilemmas.

Characteristics of a profession are defined, as is the socialization process of professionals. It becomes clear that this process has a far greater impact on the way a professional functions and the kinds of attitudes he espouses than does formal education.

Professional accountability can be divided into four more or less equal components: self, client, employing institution, and society. Disagreement will always exist about the way the professional is accountable to all four. The professional's position of being able to do both good and harm and the separation of the two are often a source of ethical dilemmas.

Nurses are socialized not only into the profession of nursing but also into the health care system as a whole, which is organized on the same base and with the same values as society in general. This means that nurses are devalued, are not in positions of power, and are not part of the ethical decision-making process.

There are several reasons why a professional should be held accountable: to evaluate new practices and reassess existing ones; to provide for or enhance self-reflection, ethical thought, and personal growth; and to determine on what bases moral judgments will be made and who will make them.

In the course of the development of a professional value system it must be determined what is valued. For most health professionals the basis for any discussion of values is the value of life itself. Fletcher's criteria for personhood are the ones most commonly used, although many people disagree with them. In reevaluating his own thoughts Fletcher came to think that the one characteristic basic to all others is the presence of neocortical functioning, without which biologic life may exist but personhood does not. Health professionals are concerned with the quality as well as the sanctity of life. It is unlikely that human beings will ever reach agreement about what is an acceptable quality of life.

A value can be considered a perspective or a way of looking at something. It many be personal or societal but is more likely a combination of both. The development of values is the process by which an individual chooses a set of standards by which to behave or a moral guide by which to live or both. Values are developed in a variety of ways and involve practically every stimulus we have experienced. Professional values are a reflection and expansion of personal values.

There are implications to the exercise of professional values. For example, what is the legal responsibility for causing harm, and how far does one's moral responsibility go in the protection of clients' safety? The degree of professional expertise is a component here, and most courts have agreed that a professional is responsible for knowing and acting within his own limits. Problems arise when the professional is subject to the will of others (usually an employer) in determining what tasks he will perform and what his work schedule will be.

Theology is a fuzzy area when one is discussing values and accountability. Fundamental to the issue is the choice of belief in the existence of God. The sanctity of life is related to the question of a divine presence, and it is probably more practical for health professionals to concern themselves with this issue.

Psychology describes and explains reasons for events; ethics deals with the right or wrong quality of those events. One important psychologic implication of professional values is the influence that the health professional can have on the client's values and behavior, which may or may not be a desirable state of affairs.

The positions of a few well-known philosophers are described as they relate to health care ethics and the modern health care system. Inherent in any philosophic approach is the concept of personal choice, which is the exercise of conscience to take a particular action because of a perceived moral obligation. Guilt is the remorse or shame felt as a result of having chosen a wrong, evil, or immoral action. The knowledge of whether an action is good or bad is the basis of values, and the action taken on that knowledge is the exercise of choice.

Every ethical decision consists of several critical factors. An agent is the person who performs the act, who makes the decision and carries it out. The circumstances surrounding an act and the intent of the agent(s) help determine the morality of the act or decision. Some feel that regardless of the intent or circumstances the ultimate good or bad nature of an act is determined only by the act's consequences.

Commitment to one's profession derives almost entirely from personal and professional values and to some extent from socialization into the profession. Commitment takes many forms, including empathy with the pain and suffering of clients, the desire to help, a sense of duty or obligation, and professional competence. It is usually not enough merely to *feel* committed to one's profession; one has to demonstrate it by actions. Development of and adherence to professional standards are one tangible way, as is demonstration of professional accountability and responsibility.

REFERENCES

1 Golding, Martin P: The concept of rights. In Bandman, Elsie L., Bioethics and human rights, Boston, 1978, and Bandman, Bertram, editors: Little, Brown & Co.

2. Szasz, Thomas: The theology of medicine, Baton Rouge, 1977, Louisiana State University Press.

3. Simpson, Ida H.: Patterns of socialization into profession: the case of student nurses, Sociological inquiry, pp.47-54, Winter 1967.

4. Fletcher, Joseph: Medicine and the nature of man. In Veatch, Robert M., et al. editors: The teaching of medical ethics: proceedings of a conference sponsored by the Institute of Society, Ethics and the Life Sciences and Columbia University College of Physicians and Surgeons, New York, June 1-3, 1972, pp. 52-57.

5. Fletcher, Joseph F.: Four indicators of humanhood—the enquiry matures, Hastings Center Reports 4(6):5, December 1974.

6. Steele, Shirley M., and Harmon, Vera M.: Values clarification in Nursing, New York, 1979, Appleton-Century-Crofts.

7. Kohlberg, L., et al.: Moral stage scoring manual, Cambridge, Mass., 1975, Harvard Graduate School of Education.

8. Bedau, Hugo Adam: Rough justice: the limits of novel defenses, Hastings Center Reports 8(6):8, December 1978.

9. Purtilo, Ruth B.,: Essays for professional helpers: some psychosocial and ethical consideration, Thorofare, N.J., 1975, Charles B.Slack, Inc.

BIBLIOGRAPHY

Bandman, Bertram: Option rights and subsistence rights. in Bandman, Elsie L., and Bandman, Bertram, editors: Bioethics and human rights, Boston, 1978, Little, Brown & Co.

Bedau, Hugo Adam: Rough justice: the limits of novel defenses, Hastings Center Reports 8(6):8-11, December 1978.

Bensman, Joseph: Dollars and sense: ideology, ethics, and the meaning of work in profit and nonprofit organizations, New York, 1967, Macmillan Publishing Co., Inc.

Burt, Robert A.: The limits of law in regulating health care decisions, Hastings Center Reports 7(6):29-32, December 1977.

Churchill, Larry R.: The ethicist in professional education, Hastings Center Reports 8(6):13-15, December, 1978.

Combs, Arthur, W.: Florida studies in the helping professions, Gainesville, 1969, University of Florida Press.

Davidson, Sharon VanSell: PSRO: utilization and audit in patient care, St. Louis, 1976, The C. V. Mosby Co.

Davis, Anne J., and Aroskar, Mila A.: Ethical dilemmas and nursing practice, New York, 1978, Appleton-Century-Crofts.

Feinberg, Joel: The nature and value of rights. In Bandman, Elsie L., and Bandman, Bertram, editors: Bioethics and human rights, Boston, 1978, Little, Brown & Co.

Fletcher, Joseph F.: Four indicators of humanhood—the enquiry matures, Hastings Center Reports. 4(6):4-7, December 1974.

Fletcher, Joseph: Medicine and the nature of man. In Veatch, Robert M., et al., editors: The teaching of medical ethics: proceedings of a conference sponsored by the Institute of Society, Ethics and the Life Sciences and Columbia University College of Physicians and Surgeons, New York, June 1-3, 1972.

Fromer, Margot Joan: Community health care and the nursing process, St. Louis, 1979, The C. V. Mosby Co.

Gamer, Mary: The ideology of professionalism, Nursing Outlook, pp. 108-111, February 1979.

Gaylin, Willard: From Twain to Freud: and examination of conscience, Hastings Center Reports 6(4): 5-8, August 1976.

Golding, Martin P.: The concept of rights: a historical sketch. In Bandman, Elsie L., and Bandman, Bertram, editors: Bioethics and human rights, Boston, 1978, Little, Brown & Co.

Halmos, Paul: The personal service society, New York, 1970, Schocken Books, Inc.

Harding, Sandra: Can nurses act ethically? In Smith, Sherry, and Monteira, Louis, editors: Clincial dilemmas: ethical issues in nursing, New York, 1980, Holt, Reinhart & Winston.

Kaufman, Andrew L.: Law and ethics, Hastings Center Reports (Special Supplement) 7(6):7-8, December 1977.

Kohlberg, L., et al.: Moral stage scoring manual, Cambridge, Mass. 1975, Harvard Graduate School of Education.

Lang, Norma M.: The overview of quality assurance. In Davidson, Sharon VanSell: PSRO: utilization and audit in patient care, St. Louis, 1976, The C. V. Mosby Co.,

Marshall, T. H.: Class, citizenship, and social development, New York, 1965, Anchor Books.

May, Judity V.: Professionals and clients: a constitutional struggle, Beverly Hills, 1976, Sage Publications.

Meyer, Genevieve R.: Tenderness and technique: nursing values in transition, Los Angeles, 1960, Institute of Industrial Relations, University of California at Los Angeles.

Murchison, Irene, et al.: Legal accountability in the nursing process, St. Louis, 1978, The C. V. Mosby Co.

Pavalko, Ronald M.: Sociology of occupations and profession, Itasca, Ill., 1971, F. E. Peacock Publishers, Inc.

Purtilo, Ruth B.: Essays for professional helpers: some psycho-social and ethical considerations, Thorofare, N.J., 1975, Charles B. Slack, Inc.

Ramsey, Paul: The nature of medical ethics. In Veatch, Robert M., et al, editors: The teaching of medical ethics: proceedings of a conference sponsored by the Institute of Society, ethics and the life sciences and Columbia University College of Physicians and Surgeons, New York, June 1-3, 1972.

Rehr, Helen: Ethical dilemmas in health care, New York, 1978, PRODIST (Neale Watson Academic Publications, Inc.).

Simpson, Ida H.: Patterns of socialization into professions: the case of student nurses, Sociological Inquiry, Winter 1967, pp. 47-54.

Steele, Shirley M., and Harmon, Vera M.: Values clarification in nursing, New York, 1979, Appleton-Century-Crofts.

Szasz, Thomas: The theology of medicine, Baton Rouge, 1977, Louisiana State University Press.

Walzer, Michael: Teaching morality, The New Republic, June 10, 1978, pp. 12-14.

Wertz, Richard W., editor: Readings on ethical and social issues in biomedicine, Englewood Cliffs, N.J., 1973, Prentice-Hall, Inc.

2

Justice and allocation in health care

Any health professional or lay person who picks up a newspaper or magazine must realize that health care is in an almost impossible economic situation. Costs have escalated so rapidly that a person without health insurance or a prepaid health plan cannot possibly pay for any but the most minor or routine health care. Part of the problem is that the health care system is *designed* to provide care as expensively as possible. Other businesses attempt to provide goods and services economically, but two basic factors make economy impossible in the present health care systems. (1) Health care is essentially a sellers' market, that is, the consumer has limited freedom in the matter of which health services he will purchase. The consumer does not comparison shop for a cholycystectomy as he would for a refrigerator or telephone laboratories to get the best bargain on blood tests. (2) The fact that most health care is paid for by government and private health insurance companies has removed all effective cost controls and price limits.

Because consumers do not directly pay out of their own pockets, prices can escalate indefinitely. When clients ask the price of a procedure, health care providers commonly respond, "Why do you care? Your insurance is paying for it." Third-party payments are so prevalent that only 6% of hospital care and 39% of physicians' fees are paid out of the client's pocket.[1] The market rule of supply and demand, which tends to partially contain inflation, does not exist in health care; therefore prices can keep going up with no end in sight. Factors that tend to encourage spiraling inflation include the following:

1. More hospital beds are built than there are people to fill them; thus hospitals must charge more to cover the cost of empty beds producing no revenue.
2. The nature of medical practice has become more sophisticated, thus generating more hospital business and use of high technology.
3. When it legislated Medicare and Medicaid, Congress closed its eyes to cost controls. Blue Cross/Blue Shield with its system of reimbursing physicians encourages them to charge higher and higher fees.
4. High technology is poorly utilized in that too much equipment, such as CAT (computerized axial tomography) scanners, exists for the number of people who require its use. The competition among hospitals to have as much sophisticated equipment as possible adds to inflation.
5. Hospitals are inherently expensive places that maintain only partially used facilities (an emergency room must be fully staffed and operational at all

35

times, even though it is used only sporadically) and have a high ratio of personnel to consumers. Aggressive employee unions have contributed enormously to hospital costs.

6. Physicians feel they have a right to charge high fees to compensate for long years of expensive medical training. The median annual income of a physician in the United States today is $65,000.[1]

7. The technology of routine health care, even for those who never go near a CAT scanner, escalates costs. A machine that can analyze 20 different blood chemistries at once is a remarkable achievement, but the technologic sophistication must be paid for by consumers.

8. Many tests and procedures done are not medically justified, and some are even unnecessary. The increase in malpractice suits has led physicians to order many more diagnostic tests than are indicated.

Various suggestions have been made to solve the problem, including mandatory government cost controls, reformation of private insurance practices, tighter control on Medicare and Medicaid payment policies, and HMOs. These methods all are partly workable and partly impractical, and they will all affect the amount and kind of care provided to consumers. The appropriate first step in solving the cost problem is to examine the allocation system now in effect, that is, who receives care and what quality of care is given to which people.

THEORIES OF JUSTICE

"Allocation of scarce resources" has become a catch phrase among health policy planners. It conjures up images of some giant health provider dealing out services to consumers the way a Las Vegas dealer allocates cards in a game of blackjack. Each player is entitled to a certain number of cards but must request more if he needs them. Specific rules govern card games; allocating health resources is not so simple. Justice is the principle that ought to be used but rarely is in allocating resources.

Justice is sometimes seen as intuition: we feel that something is unfair because it does not correspond to what we have come to believe is fair or just. It is difficult, however, to precisely define principles of justice. Many people equate justice with fairness. Others view it as one's deserts; that is, justice has been served when a person has been given what he is owed or what he deserves. What a person feels he deserves is usually based on a moral claim that is acknowledged by at least a majority of society. By the same token a person should be punished only if he deserves to be punished. There are several different types of justice, all of which can be applied to allocation of health resources.

With comparative justice "what one person deserves is determined by balancing the competing claims of other persons against his claims."[2,p.169] This kind of justice is frequently used when several people want the same thing (for example, a heart or kidney for transplant) and a determination must be made about which of them is to receive it.

Distributive justice involves the conditions of scarcity when there is competition for benefits; it differs from comparative justice in that what a claimant deserves may not be taken into account. Distributive justice tends to be broader in scope and usually involves large-scale provision of health care. If there were enough of everything to go around, there would be no need for distributive justice.

Principles of justice of any kind would not be necessary if society were composed of people who are inherently fair and unselfish enough to create a just society. But interests conflict, and people are naturally eager to meet their own needs. Some may be harmed during the course of solving conflicting interests. Rules of justice are needed to balance conflicting claims that occur in society; these rules are often reflected in law, which is not always just. Laws can be disobeyed on the basis of moral principles, an action known as civil disobedience. Two of the most famous practitioners of civil disobedience were Mahatma Gandhi in India, who protested the unjust colonialism of the British, and Martin Luther King, Jr., in the United States, who encouraged blacks to disobey peacefully those laws that were discriminatory toward blacks. Civil disobedience is a potent political expression that could be used to great advantage by consumers of health care if they could be organized into a sufficiently cohesive group to make their pressure felt.

Formal justice, attributed to Aristotle, is based on the concept that

equals ought to be treated equally and unequals unequally. This elementary principle is referred to as the principle of formal justice, or sometimes as the principle of formal equality. It is *formal* because it states no particular respects in which equals ought to be treated the same. It only says that no matter what respects are under consideration, if persons are equal in those respects, then they must be treated equally. More fully stated in negative form, the principle says that no person should be treated unequally despite all differences with other persons, unless it has been shown that there is a difference between them relevant to the treatment at stake.*

For example, if two people have deteriorating kidneys and treatment is to be provided only on the basis of the illness, then that person whose kidney has deteriorated more should have greater access to a donor kidney if physical illness is the only respect with which they are to be treated. This use of formal justice would be sufficient if the conditions are unequal. If the conditions are equal in both people, then the concept of comparative justice should be applied: which of the two people has a greater claim to the one available kidney, and on what bases will comparison be made?

Formal justice is one of those principles with which everyone can agree (except those with a particularly dictatorial outlook), but its lack of pragmatism causes problems. All people are not equal in all respects, although we might wish this were not true. Some people are smarter than others, some contribute more to society than others, some are more moral than others, and some deserve more than others. This is a fact of life, and again most people will agree in principle. The problem comes in deciding which inequalities matter in which areas of allocating benefits. In a court of law a person's past behavior should not matter in relation to the particular crime of which he is accused. His behavior does matter, however, to

---

*Beauchamp, Tom L., and Childress, James F.: Principles of biomedical ethics, New York, 1979, Oxford University Press, p. 171.

some members of the jury who in the absence of hard evidence may base their verdict on the feeling that the defendant *could* have committed the crime because of the kind of person he appears to be. And when passing sentence a judge takes into account the kind of life a person has led.

In terms of health care, the contribution a person has made to society may determine the kind and amount of care he receives. Those people who are not poor are seen as making a greater contribution and thus receive private care with its attendent comforts. Those who are poor receive public care, which is not as comfortable and which is frequently provided without sensitivity and sometimes with a lack of competence. For example, prison physicians and those on the staff of public institutions such as state mental hospitals are sometimes far less competent than those who are affiliated with private medical centers. For a variety of reasons prisoners and mental patients are seen as undeserving of excellent health care. Sometimes inequalitites in character or life-style can be justified as reasons for providing unequal care, but more often they cannot. That a person has no job and is on welfare does not *necessarily* mean he should go to the back door for treatment. It could be argued, however, particularly by utilitarians, that if he is a deliberately slothful person, has never made an effort to contribute to society, and is a criminal to boot, he has not added to society's good and thus should not reap the same benefits from that society as those who have contributed more. A deontologist would point out that society has a duty or obligation to provide health care regardless of who is receiving the care. The rules of equality should take precedence over considerations of deserts.

In a system of material justice properties are defined on the basis of how societal burdens and benefits are distributed. These properties are generally defined as (1) to each person an equal share, (2) to each person according to individual need, (3) to each person according to individual effort, (4) to each person according to contribution to society, and (5) to each person according to merit.[2,p.173] Most societies use a combination of several of these properties when distributing burdens and benefits. For example, admission to higher education is based on merit and equal access to a share of that education. Continuation of higher education is based almost solely on merit. Health care should be distributed only on the basis of equal share, but it is more likely a result of contribution to society, merit, and individual effort.

It may seem appropriate to use all properties and principles when distributing societal burdens and benefits, but in almost all instances priorities must be assigned because benefits are limited. This creates conflict. Theories of distributive justice attempt to resolve the conflict. An egalitarian would insist on equal access to anything a rational person might want, a utopian state of affairs. Marxists distribute benefits on the basis of need, but an arbiter is required to determine degree of need. The libertarian emphasizes contribution and merit, but those who have contributed little through no fault of their own are eliminated, for example, those who are physically disabled or politically disenfranchised. Any theory of justice rests on the quality of its moral argument, especially as it is veiwed in relation to societal mores. For example, a person who espoused Marxist theory in the South 100 years ago, when slavery was no longer legal but was greatly mourned by white planters, would have been laughed out of town. An egalitarian approach would not be treated seriously in a country like India or Saudi Arabia where society is based on a well-defined class system.

The concept of equal treatment for equal need depends on how need is defined. An adolescent who needs a new dress for the prom is expressing a kind of need different from that of a man who needs a job to feed his family. Need can be viewed in terms of harm: a basic human need is one that will result in harm if it is not met. A minimum standard of health care is a need; a private hospital room is not. Protein is a need; pork chops are not. The system of formal justice requires that everyone's basic needs be met if we are to live in a decent society. The American health care system does not now meet all basic needs, but the situation could be improved if resources were allocated differently and if principles of justice were applied more fairly. For example, everyone who required a kidney transplant could receive one if no cadaver were buried with its kidneys. It seems only just and fair that a living person has a greater claim to a kidney than a dead one regardless of the person's wishes before dying. As another example, if all physicians and nurses for a specified period in their career were required to provide health care for those who had less access to mainstream health delivery, access to care would become more equal.

Moral principles determine what relevant properties apply in particular situations when justice is being distributed. Some properties are relevant in some situations, but others are not. All must be supported by moral principles. Some properties can be established simply by creating rules to which a majority agree; for example, a scholarship should be awarded to a needy person who demonstrates the most potential for academic success. Granting a full professorship to a person because he is the brother of the president of the university is an instance of applying irrelevant properties to the reward and is therefore unjust. Even the application of principles can complicate matters, as a recent spate of "reverse discrimination" suits has proved. Giving a particular opportunity to a black or member of any other minority simply because he is in a minority and has historically been denied opportunity is not necessarily based just on relevant properties if it discriminates against a white or member of any other majority who is more qualified for the opportunity. Even the Supreme Court is in conflict over these principles of justice.

A classic example involving relevant properties is given by Beauchamp and Childress.[2,pp.275-276] A 40-year-old widow has glomerulonephritis and most likely will not survive for more than 4 to 6 months without a kidney transplant. She has four children, ages 11 to 14, and wants a transplant so that she can live to raise them. The woman's brother refuses to donate or be tissue typed, and her sister is willing to donate but is not eligible because she is a diabetic. There is, however, a 35-year-old mentally retarded brother who has been institutionalized since the age of 8. He is histocompatible but is so severely retarded that he cannot understand any of the risks involved in nephrectomy. He recognizes none of his family and has not seen them in years. The 14-year-old daughter wants to donate a kidney to her mother and appears to have a clear idea of the risks involved, but she is not nearly as good a match as the retarded brother. The woman's brother and sister (the sister is the legal guardian of the retarded brother) both feel that the mentally retarded brother should have his kidney removed to save his sister. A majority of the physicians, nurses, and social workers surveyed thought that a court order should be sought to take the mentally retarded brother's kidney. This is an issue of selection criteria between two potential donors, one willing but most likely highly influenced by emotionality and other unknowing and ignorant of what is to happen. "This case shows that when rather concrete policies must be formulated, abstract principles of justice provide only rough general guidelines, and further moral argument is needed to fix the specific relevant properties on the basis of which an actual choice can be made."[2,p.177]

Classes or groups of people are sometimes the object of justice or injustice, but unless commonalities of that particular group are relevant to the distribution of justice or the choice to be made, justice has not been served. For example, women were exempt from the draft. The fact of gender was not relevant to the characteristics of a good soldier; therefore woman held an unfair advantage while men were asked to bear the entire military burden. Justice was not served. Another example is the use of prisoners in human experimentation. Should prisoners as a class be exempt from serving as subjects because their situation is inherently coercive, should they as a class be compelled to serve to atone for their crime, or should they not be treated as a separate class when research subjects are chosen? Is the fact that they are prisoners *relevant* to their role as research subjects? If that question cannot be answered with assurance, then treating priosners as a separate class in this regard would be unjust. Some people are grouped together in classes and are victims of injustice or beneficiaries of justice because of circumstances over which they have no control or for which they are not responsible. Examples that come immediately to mind are discrimination on the basis of race, sex, or religion.

Justice or injustice in health care is sometimes subtle and sometimes blatant. An example is treating people differently in regard to informed consent because of their intelligence. A health professional explaining a moderately complex procedure to an intelligent, alert person who asks probing questions will probably spend more time with that person and give clearer, more precise information than he would with a person who needs several explanations in increasingly simple language and who even then seems to have difficulty understanding. Consent in the latter case may not be as informed as in the former. The treatment of the less intelligent person is unjust because he cannot be held responsible for the difference between himself and the more intelligent person.

Discrimination between classes of people is morally justified only if properties of the groups are the moral responsibility of the group members or if they are the sort of properties that can be overcome. Education can be used as an example. Everyone in the United States has an opportunity for a free public education through high school. If an employer requires a job applicant to be a high school graduate and can prove it is necessary for the job, he would not be acting unjustly if he refused to interview anyone who had not graduated from high school. Let us take the distinction a step further and imagine that all the high school graduates who applied for the job were white and all the nongraduates black. Because educational opportunity is available to everyone, blacks could not be necessarily considered to have been treated unjustly on the basis of race because race was not a relevant property to distribution of justice in this case. Those who did not graduate from high school have properties that they had an opportunity to overcome and for which they are responsible.

Rawls[3] believes that the fundamental concept of justice is fairness, although he discounts the idea that justice and fairness are the same. He postulates that justice is a virtue or practice of social institutions to formulate restrictions in assigning positions, offices, powers, liabilities, rights, and duties. The meaning of justice varies depending on whether it is applied to practices in general, to particular actions, or to persons. Justice is only one quality of a good society and "is essentially the elimination of arbitrary distinctions and the establishment, within the structure of a practice, of a proper balance between competing claims."[3p.164] This is similar to the definition of comparative justice described previously. Rawls refines his concept of justice into two basic principles: (1) each person participating in a practice has an equal right to a liberty that is extended to all who participate in the practice, and (2) inequalities, unless they work out to everyone's advantage, are arbitrary and unjust. Justice therefore is a complex of three ideas: liberty, equality, and reward for services contributed to the common good. This can be described as Rawls' social contract theme concerning how criteria are selected to result in the greatest degree of justice or what material principles of justice should be used in a given situation.

He believes that social and economic inequalities can be justified when the greatest benefit leads to the greatest disadvantage. For example, if the person with the most money in a society can be seen as being at a great disadvantage (for example, paying the most taxes) *because* of the money, then inequality of riches can be justified. Inequalities are also justified if they are open to all with equal opportunity.

Rawls also looks at justice as a compromise between persons of roughly equal power who would prevail over each other if they could but who because of the equality of forces between them and for the sake of peace and security treat each other justly because it is the prudent thing to do. This conjures up an image of two equally matched gladiators who do not fight to the death because in so doing they would both die. So they circle each other cautiously and give each other room to move *only* because it is to their mutual benefit to do so.

Rawls proposes a system of justice in which society is structured as though one's position in it is assigned by one's enemy. For example, if you are Minister of Housing in a brand-new society, it would be unwise for you to authorize building or maintaining housing that *you* would not be satisfied to live in. This could effectively eliminate envy, and because procedural justice would exist, all principles of justice would be strengthened. Justice as fairness, according to Rawls, is a primitive moral notion because it implies that the concept of morality is mutually imposed by all participants in an activity who are competing or cooperating with one another. In this way justice can be seen as merely a set of rules to ensure fairness and to prevent some people from taking unfair advantage over others. "A practice will strike the parties as fair if none feels that, by participating in it, they or any of the others are taken advantage of, or forced to give in to claims, which they do not regard as legitimate."[3,p.170]

Rawls' theories of justice, which have been widely quoted and discussed, can be applied to health policy. "Social primary goods" (as distinguished from "natural primary goods" such as intelligence, vigor, and good health) are bestowed by those having power and authority in society and are affected by the social structure. The health care system is a part of the social structure that plays a role in distribution of social goods and that should depend on principles of justice. Health care is frequently a function of the distribution of income, a social primary good that is based to a large extent on principles of justice. Rawls' social contract theme can be used to determine which material principles apply in the distribution of health care benefits that will reflect liberty, equality, and reward for services contributing to the common good. Several questions regarding justice must be raised when health care policy is established. How important are the services to the people using them? How do they compare with other goods or services, such as income or personal freedom, when health services are scarce and must be distributed on a basis that precludes absolute equality? How would rational people want the services distributed? How extensive should health services be, and how far should the general priority of and commitment to health care be extended when compared to other societal needs and priorities? When if ever should health services be sacrificed to meet other priorities? By what mechanism should health services be distributed?

The usual choices in distributing services are (1) free and competitive marketing, the basic distribution process in effect in the United States today; (2) a lottery; (3) some sort of rationing; or (4) government direction and control such as what national health insurance would provide. These questions and solutions will be addressed in the section on allocation.

Justice, particularly as it is concerned with distribution of societal benefits, is a component in the exercise of power. Power can be defined as the capacity of an actor to change specified future events by using a particular action. This process can be divided into components of ascending order: influence, authority, and power. Influence is highly personal, charismatic, and individual. It generally involves the relationship between two people or between one individual and a group. Authority is institutionalized and derives from societal status or communal behavior. The structure of society permits some people to have authority over others, either legally or by governmental fiat. It is implied that principles of justice will be used to exert influence and authority. This is not necessarily the case when power is involved. Power is what is left over or leaks through societal structure. It is the ability to command resources and to use them for control. Justice may be a part of power, as in a military structure, or it may be completely absent, as in dictatorial power. The health care system is concerned with influence (convincing an individual to engage in activities that will lead to improved health), authority (the way the system itself is run), and power (distribution of benefits or coercive measures used to treat certain people in certain ways).

Rights and obligations

Rights are usually defined as claims that individuals or groups make on other individuals or groups. Legal rights are those that are justified by legal principles and have been agreed to by society as rights that can be claimed by every citizen, such as the right to a trial by jury. Moral rights are those that can be claimed by moral principles, such as the right to autonomy. Moral rights and legal rights are often the same or similar, such as the right to practice one's religion without government interference as long as in so doing no harm comes to others. Moral rights and legal rights can conflict, such as certain aspects of the right to privacy.

Rights involve duties and obligations (which are not necessarily the same but for the purpose of this discussion will be treated as synonymous). A logical correlation between the two can be expressed this way: if X has a right, then Y has an obligation to provide or assure X's right. A moral correlation can be stated: if X has a right, then X also has an obligation to Y, if Y provides X's rights. The moral correlation involves justice, but the logical correlation does not. The "doctrine of logical correlativity of rights and obligations holds that it is possible to start from a right and infer a correlative obligation, and vice versa. It indicates that we can secure the same moral content from either standpoint, that of the right or of the obligation."[2,p.49]

Mill differentiated between duties of perfect obligation and those of imperfect obligation. In duties of perfect obligation a correlative right resides in some person, such as the duty of justice. Duties of imperfect obligation do not give birth to any right, such as the duty of charity. Everyone has a right to justice, but no one has a right to charity.

Rights can also be classified as positive and negative rights. A positive right is a right to another person's positive actions; that is, if one person has a positive right, another person has a duty to *do* something. A negative right is a right to another person's omission or forebearance; that is, if one person has a negative right, another person has a duty to *refrain* from doing something.

If health or health care is viewed as a positive right, then someone in society has a positive obligation to provide those services that will improve or maintain health. If health or health care is a negative right, then society has an obligation to stop doing those things that are known to undermine health, such as polluting the air or using known carcinogens to preserve packaged food. In terms of health care we might express rights as follows: X has a right to Y from Z. X is everyone or every individual in a society who claims a right; Y is health care, and Z is the provider of that care. Does Z, as a person designated by society and personal choice, have a corresponding obligation to X to provide Y for all members of society? What exactly is the content of the Y that Z is obligated to do? How far does Z's obligation extend, and does X have a corresponding obligation to provide Y for himself? Viewing health as positive right makes no sense because health cannot be guaranteed no matter to what extent Z goes to fulfill the obligation. Viewing health as a negative right is logical because Z can take actions not to interfere with X's health, although one would need to determine exactly what actions interfere with health. Does refraining from doing something always result in good health? If a person refrains from going into the polluted atmosphere of crowded cities, or even if society refrains from polluting the air, one still cannot be certain that healthy lungs will result. It makes more sense to talk about health *care* as a positive or negative right than it does to be concerned with health itself. Even so, it is difficult to know what kind of actions must be taken by Z to provide Y (health care) for X. How much and what kind of care is necessary to ensure that all the Xs of society have equal access to that care and receive a minimum level of care?

Fried[4] proposes an argument that may seem reactionary and unjust to many. He maintains that

1. A right to health care does not imply a right to equal access, that whatever is available to one should be available to all.
2. "Equal access" is a dangerous slogan and could become a reality only by means of intolerable government controls or unreasonable expense.
3. "Some of the major sources of the exaggerated demands for equality are the pretentions, inflated claims, inefficiencies, and guild-like, monopolistic practices of the health professions."[4,p.452]
4. The right to a decent standard of care for all is not to be equated with the best available care.

These are strong, accusatory, even undemocratic statements, but Fried defends his arguments. He states that the right to health care has no historic basis, most probably because it was not until recently that society had the technologic means to deliver health care; thus there was little use to guarantee what could not be provided. Society provides few other amenities to the poor (and those that it does provide are given grudgingly); therefore health care should not be singled out as a special right. The poor have as little access to health care as they do to other social benefits, such as a superior education, decent housing, and the like; Fried sees no reason why this should change proportionately.

Fried defines rights as claims of entitlement, those claims that people *must* have and not those they prefer to have or it would be nice to have. He stresses that rights should not be confused with the concept of equality, especially as it pertains to health care. He explains this with an analogy of the right to freedom of speech. Everyone is equal in having the freedom to speak his mind on whatever subject he chooses; equality, however, does not extend to the right to access to public airwaves, to speak eloquently, or to be admired or applauded. Equality of the right stops once the person speaks; *how* he does it is not a matter of equality of rights.

Since health care is absurdly expensive, we cannot afford to provide everyone with an equal quality of care without going so far above budgetary allowances for health care that some sort of halt would have to be called. Different standards of care based on the cost of a particular kind of care or treatment have to be instituted for different societal groups. Relatively cheap care, such as immunization for communicable disease or fluoridation of water, can be provided equally to everyone. Expensive care, such as an artificial heart or a kidney transplant, can not. Fried states that "as long as our society considers that inequalities of wealth and income are morally acceptable—acceptable in the sense that the system that produces these inequalities is in itself not morally suspect—it is anomalous to carve out a sector like health care and say that *there* equality must reign."[4,p.459]

Fried asks if health care is different from housing, food, and education. We are satisfied that everyone should have a safe, decent place to live, but we see nothing morally wrong with some people living in a 50-room house set on 100 acres of woodland. His analogy is not precise, however, because people do not die or suffer pain from living in a row house in South Philadelphia or attending public school, but they *may* die if they cannot receive a donor kidney or are refused a CAT scan because the treatment is too expensive. Fried suggests that minimum care should be regarded as a societal right and be provided equally. The problem, of course, is where to draw the line between minimum care and all the rest. Do we give everyone infant immunization, a preschool physical examination, and an option on major surgery once in his lifetime, and beyond that minimum he is on his own?

Fried believes that defining a decent minimum is basically a political process. Many people believe that the answer to the problem of oversupply and disproportionately high income of physicians is government regulation, such as a physician draft to redistribute provision of care or an income ceiling. The physicians' guild system is one of the tightest that exist; they have succeeded in convincing the public that their expensive and arcane services can be performed by no one else. Fried wants to debunk this myth and maintains that less well trained and "less pretentious" persons can perform many functions that physicians hold dear. Fried would also dilute some of the physicians' power by removing many of the decisions they now make in areas such as hospitalization, drug prescription by brand or generic name, and diagnostic tests. As the system stands today, consumers have no choice in these matters. Nor do they have a real choice between a fee-for-service system and prepaid group plans because little cost difference exists between the two. Reducing the cost of health care delivery by bureaucratic control would be useless unless the restrictive practices of those who control the provision of care can be loosened. Fried proposes that each person be assured a certain amount of money to purchase health services as he chooses, therefore placing more power in the hands of the consumer. This idea is similar to Milton Friedman's concept of a negative income tax or guaranteed minimum income that has been repeated by various economists from time to time. Considering the nature of our economic system and continuing inflation, an individual's buying power for health care would soon become as impotent as is his buying power for steak and cheese.

It can be stated without much argument that people need health care, but existence of a need does not necessarily imply a corresponding *right*. The position that there is a right to health care or equal access to health services has become politically expedient. One has to be for equal access to health care in much the same way as one has to be for civil rights or for conservation of energy. A politician who does not pay lip service to these concepts will find himself voted out of office by the many special interest groups that exert political influence. But health care must be provided at someone's expense unless the consumer pays directly for care, as presently is done by less than 5% of the American population. Those who cannot pay for their own care but demand it as a right are in effect demanding the charitable services of others. Either government will pay for the services with tax money, or health professionals must voluntarily donate their services. *Someone* must pay. Do people have a right to make demands that imply corresponding obligations in others? What about the rights of those who are obligated to provide the service—can they demand rights in return? If A, who has a mouthful of dental caries, demands that B fix his teeth because he believes that healthy teeth are his right, can B in return demand that A limit his sugar intake and brush his teeth twice a day? Does B have the right to say, "I'll fix your teeth this time, but if I see you drinking soda and eating candy, don't expect me to fill any more cavities"? Does a right to health care, if it exists, also imply an obligation to do those things that will protect and maintain one's own health? If a person smokes cigarettes, does he voluntarily give up some of his rights to health care? Can the system lower a person's health care allotment by denying a certain percentage of rights for each 5 kg of excess weight? If rights automatically imply obligations, then it would seem that the right to health care is not absolute. The consumer must be obligated in some way if he demands the right.

Health is surely not a positive right, and according to many neither is health care. Good health does not obligate someone to do something. But health could be considered a negative right; that is, it is incumbent on others not to do things that will jeopardize an individual's health. Consequently we see lawsuits brought against companies that pollute air and water and that expose their employees to toxic chemicals. Government regulatory agencies, such as the U.S. Public Health Service and the Nuclear Regulatory Commission have been established to protect public health and safety. Sparer[5] suggests that the *legal* right to medical care (he distinguishes medical care from health care, the latter being broader in scope) exists only under two conditions: (1) when a definable duty exists on the part of care providers to give care to particular persons or to persons in general and (2) when persons who are beneficiaries of the duty have a legal remedy they can use to enforce performance of that duty and to collect damages if the duty is not performed.

Without these two conditions one can request care, point out the moral obligations to provide it, and even offer to buy it, but one does not have a legal right to demand it. In the United States today there is no legal right to medical care unless a contract has been established, such as a prepaid health plan or the agreement that exists between a hospital and client when the client has been admitted for care. A hospital may voluntarily agree to care for an individual, but *must* it? Common law indicates that no individual or institution is legally obligated to provide care, even in an emergency, although individual cases demonstrate exceptions. In *Wilmington General Hospital v. Manlove*[6] the Supreme Court of Delaware found that because an ill person relied on a well-established custom of a hospital providing emergency care, the hospital is consequently obligated to provide that care. The case was not sufficiently broad to provide legal precedent because proof of damages depends on whether a person could have gotten to another emergency facility quickly enough to have avoided further harm. Lawsuits frequently depend on precise proof of damages. But how can it be proved that a hemorrhaging individual was damaged by having to drive an extra 10 minutes to a hospital that would provide care, unless he was so severely damaged that his life was in jeopardy and absolute proof of this existed? How long does a person have to spend looking for another emergency facility before he can claim damages? Some states have adopted statutes that require certain designated general hospitals to provide emergency care, although clients are not relieved of their obligation to pay for that care.

The Hill-Burton program of 1946 required that any hospital built even in part with Hill-Burton funds is obligated to set aside a certain number of beds and outpatient services for clients who cannot pay. The provision requires that free services be provided up to 10% of the size of the Hill-Burton grant or 3% of the hospital's total operating costs. This provision was largely ignored until a number of lawsuits were brought, but even these have had no lasting effect. A person can be denied admission to a hospital for many reasons other than his inability to pay, and therefore the hospital can meet the Hill-Burton requirement in any number of roundabout ways without providing service to indigent clients who can *prove* a legal right to care but who do not always receive it. Particular groups of people have legal rights to be treated at certain kinds of hospitals, such as Veterans Administration hospitals, or at hospitals that are supported by public tax money, such as state mental hospitals. This can be seen as a right to an earned reward (providing military service to the country) or a benefit derived from paying taxes rather than as a right to health care.

A legal right to care derives from a legal contract that is expressed or implied. The legal contract one makes with a physician or hospital does not differ significantly from the legal contract one makes with a house painter or gardener. One has a right to fulfillment of the terms of a contract but not to health care itself, because a physician or hospital is not obligated to enter the contract in the first place. Even Medicare and Medicaid do not establish a legal right to health care. "Like private insurance, they create rights to payment for care if the applicant is eligible for the program."[5,p.42]

The availability of health care in any society depends almost entirely on the supply of services desired or demanded, and that supply depends on individuals to provide it. No government can control the supply of care unless it has regulatory power over those individuals who are trained and educated to provide care. Therefore individuals cannot claim a right to health care except in certain defined situations.

Mill says that the idea of a right resides in an injured person: violation of the right is substantiated by existence of the injury. Rights are possessions acquired by nature (for example, liberty), work (property), inventiveness (a work of art), or inheritance (property or money), that is, things a person *has*. In this sense there is no right to health or health care because it is not something a person has. In contrast, a person can claim a right, but that does not mean he has the right to *have* the right. A student can claim he did superior work on a term paper and thus demand the right to receive an A, but the claim is in conflict with the right: the latter belongs to the student only by proof of superior work. Claims and rights can be viewed as two entirely different concepts.

THEORIES OF ALLOCATION

Health resources increasingly are becoming scarcer and more expensive while the population is increasing and inflation shrinking health care dollars. These phenomena create a conflict that is economic, ethical, and political. Every aspect of care is in short supply: blood, trained technicians, organs for transplant, research facilities, and money. The basic problem of resource allocation is how to distribute available resources to those who need them in the most equitable and economically feasible manner. Because demand for resources exceeds supply, some people will receive less than others. Deciding who will receive what and on what basis decisions will be made requires the wisdom of Solomon, the leadership of Moses, and the generosity of spirit of Jesus. Since these three are not here to tackle the task, it must be left to economists, ethicists, and politicians.

The economic problem is how to distribute the resources as efficiently as possible in view of the fact that the amount of money available to pay for them is finite. The ethical problem is one of justice: by what means can everyone be treated as fairly as possible? The political problem involves keeping everyone as content as possible, given the enormity of the situation. Allocation can be divided into two levels. Macroallocation is concerned with decisions about how much money and other resources shall be expended by society for health compared to that for other societal needs such as education and defense and about how the resources should be distributed. Microallocation is concerned with decisions made by individual health care providers or institutions about who shall receive whatever resources are available. These two levels will be discussed in detail later in the chapter.

Choices have to be made. A humane society provides moral underpinnings to decisions that may result in death or unimproved health. The first and most dramatic issue involves who shall live and who shall not. For example, 10 years of kidney dialysis at home costs about $65,000 at 1970 prices and the cost of a kidney transplant (if a kidney is available) is about $15,000 for the surgery and thereafter about $500 a year for follow-up costs. The total cost of a heart transplant is estimated at $50,000.[7] Who among us is worth that much money?

The allocation problem was most dramatically brought to the public mind in 1963 when a selection committee was established by Dr. Belding H. Scribner at the University of Washington Swedish Hospital in Seattle to determine the social worthiness of clients to receive kidney dialysis. It was the prototype of many such committees and used the following selection criteria: medical acceptability (likelihood of surviving the physical rigors of dialysis), psychologic adaptability to being attached to a machine two or three times a week forever, and receptivity to serving as a research subject (undoubtedly more than a little subtle coercion was used).

The original Swedish Hospital committee was composed of seven people: a lawyer, a clergyman, a homemaker, a banker, a labor leader, and two physicians. Their identities were kept secret to protect them from public pressure, because they did in fact become a "death committee." They had to choose 10 out of 30 applicants to be placed on dialysis. They were advised to eliminate children and those over age 45 as poor medical risks. The committee requested the following information about the applicants: age, sex, marital status, number of dependents, occupation, income, net economic worth, emotional stability, past performance, future potential, and names of people who would serve as references. One's immediate reaction to this list might well be horror. Aside from the information about emotional stability (one wonders what criteria were used to determine stability), past performance, and future potential, no other piece of information the committee requested should have any moral bearing on whether a person deserves to be admitted to dialysis. Some think that even these criteria should not have been admissable.

The decision-making process was capricious and judgmental, to say the least. In the instance of a chemist and an accountant competing with three other people for two places, the debate took place on economic grounds: should they be ruled out because they both had considerable net worth (presumably their families would not suffer financially if they died) or admitted because they had the best education and therefore the greatest potential for service to society?

Concerning a small businessman with three children, a surgeon on the committee was impressed with the fact that "this man is active in church work," which was for him "an indication of character and moral strength." Or, countered the lawyer, "help him to endure a lingering death." Whereupon a minister spoke: "Perhaps one man is more active in church work than another because he belongs to a more active church." Both these men having made ample provision for their families, their deaths will not force their families to become a burden on society. But that would be to penalize the very people who have been most provident.*

The Seattle selection program seemed to favor people who had many children, were not too wealthy, went to church regularly, and were not artistic. That the criteria they used measured only a narrow idea of social worthiness seemed to matter little to the committee members. We are shocked perhaps by the capriciousness and self-righteousness of these committee members, especially if our lifestyle is different from the Seattle standard (one critic remarked that the Pacific Northwest is no place for a Henry David Thoreau with bad kidneys), but the point is that *some* set of criteria must be used in allocating scarce health resources. In the section to follow on microallocation other methods will be discussed.

The Seattle selection committee has ceased functioning, and there are generally enough dialysis machines in the United States today to provide care for almost everyone seeking it. The allocation problem, however, particularly as it relates to social worth, still exists. And Americans are now if anything more conservative in their attitudes about who deserves access to scarce resources than they were when the Seattle committee was in full swing.

Ramsey[7,pp.249-252] reports a 1967-68 study[8] of kidney dialysis centers across the

---

*Ramsey, Paul: The patient as person, New Haven, 1970, Yale University Press, p. 241.

country made by the School of Public Health of the University of California at Los Angeles under the sponsorship of the Kidney Disease Control Program. About 80 centers responded to the survey. In response to a question about selection of clients for dialysis, the following criteria were reported, listed here in rank order: medical suitability and absence of other disabling disease, age, psychiatric evaluation and potential for vocational rehabilitation, social welfare evaluation of the person and his family, willingness to cooperate, intelligence, financial resources, and practical considerations such as living distance from the dialysis center and suitability for home dialysis. Some of the centers were specific in determining criteria for social worthiness and others were not, but all mentioned that it was impossible to remove all personal bias from the selection procedure. In the sample of 688 people on dialysis there were only 169 women, although kidney disease is not significantly more prevalent in men than women and one might assume as well that all other factors were equal. Thus one might assume that in 1967 and 1968 women were considered by some to have less social worth than men. If a woman's worth is based *primarily* on her sex rather than on her qualities as a human being, she would indeed lose points in the selection process.

Paradigm of allocation

Human blood can be viewed as a paradigm of all allocation dilemmas. It is in constant need and is constantly in short supply. It can be given only by human beings and is desperately needed by other human beings to save life. An artifical heart or kidney transplant may be a more dramatic example of the allocation problem, but blood is needed by more people than all artifical organs and high technology combined. It is a major allocation dilemma because there is no substitute on earth for human blood.

Demand far outstrips supply for several reasons: sophisticated surgical techniques require massive transfusions (for example, open heart surgery requires about 60 units of blood per operation), more sophisticated or routine surgery is being performed now than ever before, and increasing violence in the street and on the highway increases the number of trauma victims demanding blood. Supplies of blood are limited for several reasons: only about half the population is medically eligible to give blood and of these only a fraction is willing to donate voluntarily, limits are set on the number of times a year a person can donate, blood is perishable and must be discarded after a certain length of time, and certain diseases like serum hepatitis cannot be detected in a blood sample and thus a careful history must be taken to screen out possible carriers.

One of the moral dilemmas in the supply and demand for blood is the voluntary nature of the donation. A person lying bleeding in an emergency room is dependent for his very life on the generosity of others and their willingness to spend an hour in a blood center, to be stuck with a needle, and perhaps to feel slightly woozy for an hour afterwards. The number of people who are willing to do this is miniscule compared to the number of people who *ought* to do it.

It is my belief that blood donation should be mandatory, with appropriate exemptions for health or religious reasons. Those who disagree will point out that a charitable act loses its characteristic of charity if it becomes mandatory. But blood donation should not be considered charity any more than taxes are considered a charitable donation to government. The two things given most frequently in the name of charity are money and time, and the supply of both is finite. Time once spent is gone forever. Money once spent is also gone; it can be recouped, but some amount of personal effort is involved. But blood once given is remade by the body in a few days with no effort or consciousness of the inner process. For this reason blood donation cannot be considered an act of true charity.

People complain bitterly about paying taxes, but those same people benefit from the societal goods that taxation provides. In addition to saving human lives directly, blood is used in various research projects that ultimately contribute to improved health. Societal benefits are reason enough to require people to donate blood on a regular basis, just as they pay taxes on a regular basis. Richard Mc-Cormick believes that participation in human experimentation is something we ought to do if we subscribe to certain human values such as good health. Blood donation also is something we *ought* to do. If everyone has a right to life, then a corresponding obligation is to do that which preserves life, and donating blood is one of those things.

Another objection to mandatory blood donation might be based on the fact that blood banks now exist that are designed to collect and distribute blood on a membership basis. Most blood banks require members to donate a unit of blood at specific intervals (usually not more than once or twice a year); this guarantees as much blood as the member needs in an emergency. A member may, however, substitute a specified amount of money when it is his turn to donate. Thus the blood bank gambles that more members will give blood than money and that more members will donate than will become involved in accidents or have surgery. Is this ethical? Is justice served when I can receive as much blood as I need simply because I wrote a check for $25 or $50 while my neighbor has been donating blood twice a year for 20 years? In the event we are both injured in the same accident and enough blood is available for only one of us, who should receive it? The humane and just response is that my neighbor should. Mandatory blood donation would make us equally worthy beneficiaries of blood in an emergency, and a moral choice would not have to be made. One of the advantages of mandatory blood donation is that it would reduce shortages of blood. There would, however, continue to be instances in which blood was in short supply and moral choices still had to be made. Those choices may be even more difficult when everyone has donated an equal amount of blood and some people have a greater need to receive blood than others.

Any system of allocation of blood short of mandatory donation will be unjust in some way. Paid donors, such as alcoholics and drug addicts who sell blood to support their addiction, cannot always be trusted to reveal diseases transmitted by blood; they need the money too badly to be bothered with the niceties of honesty. To sell blood on the free market like any other consumer commodity would not only raise the price to an impossible level but would also encourage enough fraudulent practices to throw consumers into a justified panic. "Blood for sale" would automatically cause the death of those who could not afford it, even as now the poor have less access to health services than the nonpoor. They are not totally without access, but they most assuredly receive care that is inferior in both kind and amount. The unpaid voluntary donor now gives blood of his own free will to an anonymous recipient. He is thanked politely by the blood bank but otherwise receives no real recognition. Should we have to depend indefinitely on his largesse—and his whim? It is a gamble society should not have to take, particularly in view of the fact that less than 10% of blood comes from these voluntary sources. The rest is sold by other individuals or given by prisoners who cannot be said to be true volunteers.[9] This makes the consumer of blood—everyone—dangerously exploited. He has to pay a high price and has no control over the quality of the product. He cannot specify donated or purchased blood and risks serious disease or even death from the blood that is supposed to be saving his life. For this he is asked to be supremely grateful. Mandatory donation would avoid these problems and solve the ethical dilemma of allocation as well.

Blood is collected in five basic ways: (1) by the Red Cross, which depends on voluntary donors, (2) by nonprofit community blood banks, also dependent on volunteers, (3) by hospital blood banks, (4) by commercial blood banks that operate on the free market, and (5) by commercial blood banks operated by pharmaceutical companies. About a third of all blood comes from paid donors, and about half from people who are "exchanging blood for blood." The latter are those blood bank members who donate for "insurance" for the day they might need blood, those who donate for friends, and those who work off a cash charge levied by hospitals for blood already received (for example, a person who received 3 units of blood during surgery can either pay or donate 3 units at intervals after he has recovered). About 5% of all blood comes from "captive" voluntary donors (that is, prisoners and servicemen), and the remaining 10% comes from true volunteers.[10]

In Great Britain all collection and allocation of blood is accomplished by a branch of the National Health Service. No fee is paid to donors, hospitals do not pay the health service, and recipients of blood are not charged. Blood donation is not mandatory, and no unpleasant pressure results from refusing to pay back blood received. There is no commercial aspect whatsoever to the collection and allocation of blood.

Several comparisons can be made of the British and American systems. About the same amount of blood is collected per capita in each country, although much more American blood is wasted (conversion to plasma after the period of safe storage of whole blood has elapsed is usually counted as waste) because of inefficiencies that occur between collection and transfusion. Blood is wasted in the United States also because more unnecessary surgery is performed; this results in more cancelled surgery because sufficient blood is not available. One could hypothesize a resultant increase in death resulting from hemorrhage, but no statistics are available to prove how many people bleed to death as the direct result of the unavailability of blood.

The quality of blood used for tranfusions in Great Britain is better than that in America. Serum hepatitis causes one death in every 150 transfusions in the United

States; in Great Britain the death rate is negligible.[10] Hepatitis contracted as a disease through transfusion is more common than death from hepatitis. This difference results from the fact that blood is not commericially marketed in Great Britain. The risk of hepatitis from plasma is even greater than that from whole blood because plasma is often pooled from many donors; one donor with hepatitis may infect 100 recipients of plasma.

Blood is expensive and of poor quality in the United States even though people are paid to donate, whereas the opposite is true in Great Britain. Some feel that the commercialization of blood is an exercise in self-defeat because people's natural altruistic impulses are extinguished. The realization that one *can* be paid for what others voluntarily donate is too great a temptation for many people. "The existence of a market sector thus contaminates the voluntary system. The attitude óf personal caring disappears; perhaps this accounts for the greater waste in the American system."[10p.1702] If more blood is wasted in the United States, where it is not free, than in Great Britain, where it is, then the use or misuse of blood must depend on factors other than monetary consideration. Purchased blood is more likely to be contaminated by disease than is blood given voluntarily. Therefore blood handlers and technicians perhaps feel that waste is not immoral because "it's no good anyway." A blood bank technician would be less likely to waste blood he was certain was safe than blood he strongly suspected was contaminated. Since there is no way to be certain, good blood is thrown away with the bad and shortages result. The British system works because it uses a market allocation system in which all people must make autonomous choices that will ultimately benefit themselves. Self-interest becomes self-sacrifice, and the sacrifice is seen to be less than the benefit. Spending 2 hours a year donating blood more than compensates for eliminating much of the risk of bleeding to death.

Improving allocation

If we can agree that the delivery and allocation of health care are unjust and inefficient, what are the characteristics of an improved system? A decrease in the individual entrepreneurship of physicians, hospitals, and other providers of health care would lessen the aura of health care as a market commodity available to high bidders. The "anything you can do I can do better" philosophy of health care institutions now fuels the spirit of competition and drives up prices (competition in a buyers' market usually holds prices down, but consumers of health care do not create an ordinary buyers' market) Administrators who planned health care delivery based on what is needed by consumers rather than on what is wanted by providers could create a more equitable system. It is impractical to suggest that all health care services be provided free of charge, but the present system must be altered. Prepaid health plans are not a financial answer but merely an alternative to private insurance. Only those who are employed can pay the maintenance fees, just as only those employed can afford private insurance. National health insurance has been suggested as a solution, but government is a notoriously poor administrator as evidenced by the bureaucratic confusion that now accompanies Medicare and Medicaid. National health insurance, except for what is called catastrophic coverage, would be prohibitively expensive; some believe it would create an unmanageable strain on the economy.

Another characteristic of a workable system is that anyone who needed care could receive it through the operation of a fair payment system. For example, for a person who requires open heart surgery but cannot afford it, the present system charges the entire cost of the surgery to others (the hospital, taxpayers, private charities, and so on). These economics cannot be supported indefinitely; a new method of allocating and paying for health care must be devised.

Macroallocation

Macroallocation is the process that deals with the societal problem of determining what percentage of total resources should be used for health care and what the priorities should be in distributing that care. Society must decide how to arrange its priorities among defense, education, space exploration, energy conservation, maintenance of national historic landmarks, funding of research in the humanities, health care, agricultural research, and all the thousands of other societal benefits we have come to expect and feel we cannot live without. Is health care more or less important than NASA's Viking program? If they are equally important, will they receive equal funding?

Once an amount of money has been allocated for health care, what portion will be spent on cancer research, what portion on preventing heart disease, and what portion on immunization programs for infants and children? Is neonatal research more important than respiratory disease control?

The Department of Health and Human Services has the largest budget of any government agency, larger even than that of the defense department. Research is increasingly being funded by federal tax money as well as by larger amounts from private foundations. People are beginning to recognize that "this large expenditure of funds cannot be based solely on economic considerations untempered by principles of justice in public policy."[2,p.189] Abstract principles when applied to practical reality, however, often create conflicts. The first involves government: should it be in the health allocation business or should allocation of all health goods and services be left to the open market? In the paradigm of blood discussed previously, the National Health Service in Great Britain was seen to be an equitable and efficient administrator in the matter of collection and distribution of blood, but in the United States the federal government has made a bureaucratic mess of the health services it presently administers. Should private individuals or government determine allocation of health goods and services and their market value?

The second conflict comes in determining the right priorities in the distribution of all societal goods and benefits. Using the principle of justice does not always work. Comparative justice balances the competing claims of persons; for example, how does a society determine whether a national defense project in the form of newer missiles is more or less deserving of public funds than invention of a totally implantable artificial heart? Each requires millions of dollars of research money, and each will eventually save lives. Is the decision made on the number of lives ultimately to be saved in relation to the amount of money spent, or is it made on the basis of how *necessary* the benefit is to the quality of citizens' lives? It is almost impossible to determine relevant properties when comparing such vastly different societal benefits.

A third conflict involves the best ways to protect life and health or to prevent death and disease. Should prevention or cure receive greater funding? What other societal goods have an effect on health? The space program has spawned thousands of technologies that have greatly added to the quality of health and have provided procedures used to prevent and detect disease. Should more money be put into alleviating the suffering of those who are already ill, or should more be spent on preventing disease? The latter is more economically and societally beneficial, but how will we feel as a society if we devote less than full energy and resources to treating the ill? Which health problems deserve the highest priority—ones that kill the greatest number of people, such as heart disease and cancer, or ones that involve a more reasonable hope for success, such as diabetes or arthritis? Or perhaps should it be those problems from which people tend to suffer for long periods of time, such as chronic respiratory disease and the range of neuromuscular ailments? Should allocation concern itself more with high technology, such as developing improved kidney dialysis machines and an artificial heart, or should money be spent on mass education about health and prevention of disease, such as vigorous anti-smoking campaigns and mass screening programs?

Beauchamp and Childress[2] present an example of an allocation conflict that involves different types of health problems. Dr. Alan Sanders, Director of the National Institute of Arthritis, Metabolism, and Digestive Diseases, tried to pressure the Director of Budget Planning at the National Institutes of Health to increase the budget for research on arthritis. He argued that $3^{1}/_{2}$ million people in the United States suffer from arthritis severely enough to limit activity, and that there are almost 4 million hospital days and 57 million days of bed disability attributable to arthritis. Dr. Sanders claimed that no one takes arthritis seriously because it causes virtually no deaths. The government ignores it even though it results in the country's second largest number of people with limitation of activity. The suffering from arthritis is enormous, but budget planners were using formulas for allocation of research funds that predicted number of days of life that could be saved in relation to the amount of money allocated. With this formula, arthritis would receive almost no funding. Sanders compared the amount of arthritis funding with that of heart disease. Both health problems produced approximately the same number of persons with limitation of activity, but the budget for heart disease was 20 times the size of that for arthritis. He thought that the heart disease budget was so much larger because the high death rate from heart disease makes it so much more dramatic than arthritis. The Director of Budget Planning was faced with a dilemma: how to allocate research funds between a disease that produces some disability but is the leading cause of death and a disease that is the second greatest debilitator but causes no death. He perceived the following options in deciding how to allocate funds:

1. Use a cost/benefit ratio to maximize the number of days of life added per dollar invested.

2. Use cost/benefit analysis to calculate the number of dollars lost from work.
3. Use cost/benefit analysis to calculate both the cost of the disease and the potential research.
4. Survey people to ask how they would like their money to be spent and then calculate the average apportionment.
5. Allocate funds in proportion to the number of people suffering from the disease, regardless of the cost of treatment and research and the number of deaths.
6. Ask experts in each of the two diseases when and where a breakthrough is most likely to occur and allocate funds according to those estimates.
7. Let politicians decide.

All the options (except possibly the last) have elements of justice and injustice as well as feasibility and impracticality. Any health care administrator who has to make a decision based on any one or a combination of these options will have to consider the nature of the problem before deciding on what basis it can be solved. All these options are currently being used to make decisions about the allocation of health care.

Another conflict is that different allocation strategies may compromise various societal values and principles that should be acknowledged when devising public policy. For example, one of the values of society is the freedom of choice of life-style involving eating, drinking, and smoking as an individual chooses. However, certain life-styles are known to predispose people to certain diseases, such as lung cancer, heart disease, and liver damage, all of which carry a high fatality rate and enormous cost to society. They are also preventable to some degree and could be considered "self-chosen" diseases. Should the allocation of funds for these diseases be decreased to permit an increase for those over which people have no control and which cannot be said to have been brought on by themselves? How would this policy conflict with the value of freedom of choice, and how could it be administered? People who do not smoke contract lung cancer, and not every case of cirrhosis of the liver results from alcoholism. If the allocation of funds for these is decreased, will not blameless people be unjustly punished? Can we really slam the health care door in the face of a heavy smoker? By the same token, should people who engage in fewer risky behaviors be forced to pay the burden of those who are not so cautious? Beauchamp and Childress think that national health insurance will increase pressure to limit the individual's liberty to engage in risky behavior because it will be seen as unfair to increase the burden of everyone else. The problem with penalizing people for risky behavior concerns where to draw the line. For example, can we say to a skier with a broken leg, "You'll have to pay for your own fracture reduction because you knew that skiing may cause broken bones"? What about a person who trips over a roller skate—do we tell him he should have been watching where he was going? Should everyone with a communicable disease be quizzed about whom he has been kissing lately? Drawing lines in the allocation of health resources is as complex a dilemma as determining the personhood of a fetus or deciding when to turn off the respirator.

Principles of justice can be used to defend several positions on formulating public policy regarding macroallocation. Some argue that the current market system is unjust because those people who are least able to defend themselves against disease (the poor, elderly, and uneducated) are the ones who receive the least health care. Rawls' principles of justice would prevent such a situation. Increasing preventive health care for society's disenfranchised "will place new burdens and restrictions on the controlling social classes, who have thus far resisted such measures. This resistance is said to be rooted in a free-market conception of justice that emphasizes individual responsibility and personal merit—especially responsibility for one's health."[2p.191] The principle of need is emphasized strongly by those who wish to take allocation out of the free market, but need is subject to a variety of interpretations and opinions. One might believe that an adolescent pregnant with her second or third child has a greater need of birth control information than a wealthy businessman with chronic arthritis has need of splints and other devices to prevent permanent deformity. On what basis is the comparison of need made: worth to society, eventual cost to society, immediate cost, ultimate personal gain? There is no way to make an entirely just comparison. Not everyone agrees that need is the most just or the most fundamentally basic principle by which to distribute health services. Another basis might be the ways that services will be used. For example, the allocation of a few orthopedic devices to the businessman might be ultimately beneficial to society because the man will use them to free himself of disability so that he can return to a productive life. The devices could be seen as worthier of allocation than spending hours of time (which costs more than the appliances) teaching the adolescent about birth control techniques that might fall on deaf ears with the result of more children to be supported by public funds. Need may not be the only acceptable or just criterion for allocation.

An interesting idea in allocation is the right to a "decent minimum" proposed by Fried, which "raises the theoretical and practical problem of whether one can consistently, fairly, and unambiguously structure a public policy which recognizes a right to have primary human needs for health care met, but without thereby incorporating a right to exotic and intolerably expensive forms of treatment."[11p.349] Is the goal of equal access to health care for every person in the United States, irrespective of income and geographic location, a reasonable and practical one? If one believes in the concept of agape which is the unselfish love of one person for another, the diffuse Christian definition of brotherly love, then each human being has to be regarded as equally valuable, equally potentially productive, and therefore equally worth of access to health care. It is difficult, of course, to put this belief into practice.

Microallocation

The essential question of microallocation concerns who shall live when not all can live, which is also the title of an essay[12] in which Childress discusses the distribution of scarce resources on a person-to-person basis. He uses the analogy of the famous lifeboat case, *United States v. Holmes* (1842),[13] in which a ship struck an iceberg and sank. The crew and half the passengers escaped in two boats. One was a longboat that was overcrowded and began to leak and founder in high seas. In an attempt to save the boat the crew threw overboard 14 men, and two sisters jumped after their brothers to join them in death. The crew's criteria for determining who should be sacrificed were "not to part man and wife, and not to throw over any women." Several hours later those on the boat were rescued and returned to Philadelphia. The rest of the crew disappeared one by one, but Holmes was indicted, tried, and convicted on a charge of unlawful homicide. The judge contended that lots should have been drawn because no other procedure would have been consistent with principles of humanity and justice. The counsel for the defense maintained that the sailors had chosen a priniciple of selection necessary in that kind of emergency. Edmond Cahn in *The Moral Decision* argues that some men should have sacrificed themselves to save the others and that if an insufficient number chose to do so, all should have waited and died together. He believed that no one should save himself by killing another. The act of self-sacrifice, however, is unlikely to occur often, and when it does not, the moral dilemma of who should be saved and who sacrificed remains. *Holmes* cannot be used as a direct analogy to microallocation because the act of killing one may not necessarily be morally equal to the act of letting one die, although in some instances no moral difference exists.

What moral criteria should be used in microallocation, and who should make the decisions? Medical criteria can eliminate those whose health would not improve as a result of a particular treatment or procedure (for example, a person who has diabetes and hepatic shutdown more likely would not benefit from renal dialysis). That is the easy part, although considerable debate exists among physicians about who can best benefit from particular procedures. Childress discusses the difficulties that arise in using social worth as a criterion for selection. Most criteria focus on the individual's potential for future social contribution, although this cannot necessarily be predicted from past performance or behavior. Another problem involves quantifying or ranking social criteria. How are needs of the body, spirit, and mind compared? Does Edward Teller get the kidney machine or does Reinhold Neibuhr? Does a social scientist receive the artifical heart or does a microbiologist? Even if an individual's social worth *could* be quantified and ranked (perhaps by public opinion polls), values and perceptions of justice change over time. Childress also points out that it is impossible to predict the social climate a few years hence and determine which persons will indeed fulfill their anticipated potential. Reducing a person to his social role for purposes of allocation is a utilitarian approach that blunts the importance of other human characteristics.

Childress proposes a form of random selection, either natural (first come, first served) or artificial (a lottery), to determine whose life should be saved if not everyone's can be saved. Critics see random selection as irrational, irresponsible, or even inhuman ("What if a derelict was selected and a Supreme Court Justice left to die?"), but Childress defends this system on several grounds. Making the selection on the narrow basis of illness and social worth would eventually take precedence over the broader basis of humanness, but randomness preserves human dignity and provides equality of opportunity.

The individual's personal and transcendent dignity, which on the utilitarian approach would be submerged in his social role and function, can be protected and witnessed to by a recognition of his equal right to be saved. Such a right is best preserved by procedures which establish equality of opportunity. Thus selection by chance more closely approximates the requirements established by human dignity than does utilitarian calculation. It is not infallibly just, but it is preferable to the alternatives of letting all die or saving only those who have the greatest social responsibilities and potential contribution.*

Random selection is also preferable to a dependency on the relationship of trust between the physician and client because trust depends on a respect for dignity that is based on differing values that cannot be guaranteed in life-and-death situations. Randomn selection is even preferable to mutually agreeable criteria that people determine for themselves, because people are self-interested (self-interest includes one's immediate family), are not basically motivated by altruism, and are ignorant of their own potential and could not rank themselves in comparison to everyone else. Another reason to favor random selection is that the psychologic stress from rejection would be less severe if it were based on pure chance rather than on lack of social worth. There would be fewer losers tempted to take revenge on the system that rejected them.

The "first come, first served" principle might be a practical way of applying random selection in situations in which people fall ill a few at a time, and a lottery would be the most practical method when one needs to allot health care to large numbers of people at the same time. The former is far more common than the latter, which occurs almost exclusively on the battlefield or in monumental disasters, in which case a triage system would precede the lottery. An interesting result of random selection might be the gradual disappearance of health care scarcities. If the system were faithfully adhered to, politicians and the powers that be in the health establishment might become so worried that they would lose out on a health benefit that they would allocate sufficient resources so that they and their families would not have to trust to luck. One might hear the cry in Congressional cloakrooms: "Damn the torpedoes! Full speed ahead—with the artificial heart."

In any system there must be exceptions. Childress narrowly circumscribes the situations in which exceptions would be allowed. A person would be exempt from the lottery only when society could not function without him in a given situation, when the danger of having to do without a particular person is too great to be risked (for example, the President in a grave national emergency). The exception would be rare and would be determined by a lay committee, not a panel of physicians.

The lottery system for saving some lives when not all can be saved is probably the most nearly perfect in terms of justice because it avoids an arbitrary determination of personal worth. It is almost impossible to fault it on a theoretical basis, but it is also unlikable and frightening. As I was reading the details of *United States v. Holmes*, I thought of myself in that lifeboat participating in the casting of lots.

---

*Childress, James F.: Who shall live when not all can live? Soundings 53(4):350, 1979.

Just *reading* about it precipitated prickles of anxiety, and I found myself deciding to put up a struggle if I were chosen to be cast overboard. Moreover, if all scarce health resources were allocated by lottery, the scheming, plotting, graft, and fraud that would result would make what happened with the military draft look like a beginners' course in political manipulation. If draft exemptions were sold for thousands of dollars, particularly at the height of the Vietnam war, the mind reels at the thought of what could happen when society realized that only a few places were available at the dialysis center or that only a certain number of artificial hearts could be manufactured. Opportunities for evil would be limitless. A scenario: as a person who is lucky enough to be chosen parks his car at the dialysis center, he is shot by a marksman hired by the person with the next lottery number. Because the system would have to be administered by human beings who have moral weaknesses similar to everyone's, those people who were in charge of drawing lots could be weakened by bribes, pleas, and every other imaginable kind of coercion. A lottery is a thoroughly fair and uncorrupt selection system, but life in the United States today is unfair and highly corrupt. It is my belief that no matter how morally correct a lottery is, and it is probably the fairest system to have been devised, it could not be put into practice in the kind of society we have arranged for ourselves.

If selection based on social worth is an unfair and unjust method of microallocation, and if the lottery is fair and just but unworkable, what system could be used? Everyone is familiar with the principle of triage on the battlefield or in a civil disaster: the most hopelessly wounded people are set aside untreated if it is determined that nothing can be done for them. The highest priority is given to those who can be restored to function as quickly as possible so that they can be recruited to help minister to the moderately wounded and to be useful in restoring order. The triage concept could be applied to the microallocation of scarce resources. For example, if only a certain number of dialysis machines are available, those who have the best medical chance of recovery, regardless of their social worth, would be chosen. It is possible with only minimal difficulty to place people in rank order on the basis of how much potential they demonstrate for responding to a particular treatment, and on those rare occasions when a tie occurs, lots could be drawn. This system would eliminate the unfairness of choosing according to social worth and would be more practical than a lottery, although it could be said that it contains elements of medical elitism or "health Darwinism." In some instances the very sick probably would not be given a chance to survive, and it might indeed seem cruel to give someone dying of kidney failure only supportive or palliative care. Although some people will need to be sacrificed, this system is less cruel perhaps than a lottery that would permit someone with end-stage disease who can barely function to use a dialysis machine while another person who has an excellent chance of recovery would be left to die. Although there are generally enough dialysis machines, other forms of costly lifesaving treatment are more scarce. The problems of microallocation still exist and can be expected to increase as more sophisticated and costly technology becomes available.

Another alternative is to permit *no one* access to life saving treatment until everyone has equal access. When Cahn maintained in discussing *United States v. Holmes* that a person cannot morally save himself by killing another, he implied that all those in the longboat should have drowned together. This goes against the grain of almost everyone's sense of self-preservation and probably could not be morally justified. It would likely decrease or totally eliminate all forms of medical research because there would be no purpose in developing new drugs or forms of treatment if they could not be used on at least a segment of the population.

Cahn imports the righteousness of mankind's ultimate covenant directly and unrefracted into the arena of legal decision and established societal practices and expectations. The dimensions of that crucial moral situation seem to him utterly incommensurate with the arrangement the judge (in *United States v. Holmes*) suggested: "the crisis involves stakes too high for gambling and responsibilities too deep for destiny." From what Cahn understands to be the absolute requirements of righteousness when men face such options, he is driven to conclude that none can "be saved separately from the others" and that "if none sacrifice themselves of free will to spare the others, they must all wait and die together.*

Ramsey does not believe that justice should demand this of people or that this is the kind of justice that should be exacted by law. The nature of human beings is not to commit mass suicide except in the most extreme or bizarre circumstances. Two mass suicides in which over 900 people died occurred almost exactly 2000 years apart. In 73 A.D. a group of 960 Jewish zealots killed themselves on top of Masada on the Dead Sea where they had fortified themselves after the Roman general Titus had conquered Jerusalem and expelled the Jewish survivors from the city. The war of harrassment lasted 3 years, but finally the Jews were surrounded and faced death or being sold into slavery. Eleazar ben Yair, leader of the band of zealots, wrote that "a death of glory was preferable to a life of infamy, and that the most magnanimous resolution would be to disdain the idea of surviving the loss of their liberty."[14p.12] Some see this act of mass suicide as large-scale martyrdom, and some see it as cowardly or merely foolish. It was entirely different in character from the mass suicide of 931 members of the People's Temple in Guyana in 1978. Those people faced slavery from within, that is, slavery devised by themselves or by their leader Jim Jones. There have been smaller examples of mass suicide throughout history, but it is unusual and not a practical or moral solution to the microallocation problem.

Rescher[15] discusses allocation of exotic lifesaving therapy (ELT) in terms of selection criteria that must be simple enough to be intelligible and plausible enough that they do not involve so many subtle ramifications that the average person could not understand them. The criteria must be justifiable in that most people would *believe* them to be justified, and they must be rationally defensible. Most important, the criteria must be fair in that they treat like cases equally and leave no room for influence or favoritism.

In devising a system to meet as many of these requirements as possible, Rescher lists three sorts of considerations that must be dealt with: the constituency factor, the progress-of-science factor, and the prospect-of-success factor. The con-

---

*Ramsey, Paul: The patient as person, New Haven, 1970, Yale University Press, p. 261.

stituency factor is concerned with determining what groups of people would be eligible for ELT at any given institution. For example, the elderly would not be treated at an army hospital, nor would children be constituents of a Veterans Administration hospital. Eliminating nonconstituents (other arbitrary constituencies can be devised, such as refusing treatment in New York City to residents of Philadelphia) from ELT is a legitimate and fair justification of selection criteria. The progress-of-science factor takes into account the needs of medical research which will ultimately benefit many in the future. For example, if researchers need to know how an artificial heart will function in a person who also has respiratory disease, it would be justified to choose a person for ELT who has emphysema in addition to heart disease instead of a person who has only heart disease. The prospect-of-success factor is self-explanatory and is the reason why children and people over age 45 are now excluded from renal dialysis.

Once a selection has been made based on these considerations, one must enter the final selection stage, which Rescher divides into five more factors: (1) relative likelihood of success, (2) life expectancy, (3) family role, (4) potential future contributions, and (5) past services rendered. The factor of relative likelihood of success is closely allied to the broader prospect-of-success factor, but in the final selection the choice is narrower because this selection is made individually rather than by eliminating blocs of people whose prospect of success could be evaluated by a cruder or more superficial method, such as age. A person who requires ELT only temporarily has a greater likelihood of success than a person who needs the treatment for the rest of his life. The factor of life expectancy is also self-explanatory: the longer one is likely to live, the higher should be his priority for ELT. The family role and importance of the individual to his family are considerations that should be given weight in the final selection, although aside from commenting that a mother of a minor child must take priority over a middle-aged bachelor, Rescher does not go into detail about what kinds of relationships are more important than others. The factor of potential future contributions concerns the pattern of services likely to be contributed by a person considering his age, talent, training, and past record of performance. This is the kind of social worth criterion that was discussed earlier as being unjust, but Rescher believes that a society that invests its scarce resources in a person is justified in examining probable return on the investment. He acknowledges that the standard is difficult to apply but does not think it should be eliminated for that reason. The evaluation on the basis of services rendered is actually a part of the preceding criterion in that its base is social worth. Rescher believes that society is obligated to reward people for services rendered, possibly because they might be expected to do so again in the future, and thus they should be given priority for ELT. Even if the individual himself could not be expected to render future service, the fact that he is rewarded for past activities could serve to spur others on to acts of social service, if for no other reason than thinking it might provide a kind of ELT insurance.

The position that social worth should be a criterion in microallocation is a utilitarian one. All human actions are judged in a variety of ways, and there is no escape from the judgment of fellow human beings. Why should this judgment not also be applied to the allocation of scarce resources? Rescher acknowledges that it is unpleasant to have to grapple with these issues, especially for people brought up with a "live and let live" attitude. Decisions must be made, however, and "failure to choose to save some is tantamount to sentencing all."[5p.182] Rescher agrees that there is no optimum system for selection and that imperfections are inherent in all systems, but he proposes a detailed procedure that combines scoring (social worth) with an element of chance. It would function as follows:

1. A first-phase group would be chosen on the basis of constituency, progress-of-science, and prospect-of-success factors. The number selected would be substantially larger than the number of people who could actually be accomodated with ELT.

2. A second-phase selection group would be chosen on the basis of a score achieved using criteria of the final selection stage previously described. This group is about a third or half again as large as the number of people who will be accomodated by ELT.

3. Final selection is made by random choice as long as there are no significant disparities among applicants.

Introduction of a lottery at the last stage of selection avoids a system in which all life-and-death choices are made by an imperfect system. Any selection system will have faults, but random choice gives people a chance to hurdle the built-in imperfections. Administrators of the selection system are relieved of having to make the final life-or-death choice, which is an awesome burden to have to carry.

Integral in any selection system of microallocation will be elements of unfairness and injustice. Even a lottery can be seen as unfair because all people are not equally deserving of exactly the same chance to be saved. The point is not that the system itself can be unjust but that the administrators of the system recognize the inherent unfairness and use rationality, humanity, and principles of justice to overcome imperfections as much as is humanly possible. We have to depend on human beings to dispense justice in the allocation of scarce health resources just as we have to depend on human beings to dispense legal justice. We are dependent on and beholden to each other.

SUMMARY

The health care system has become a sellers' market with costs escalating and administrative efficiency spiraling downward. Several factors encourage inflation, most of them related to personal greed and poor management. The result is an uneven distribution of all health resources and particularly those in short supply. The allocation of resources determines who receives how much care and what quality of care is given to particular groups of people. Because everyone cannot be treated equally by the health care system, theories of justice must be applied in developing allocation systems.

Comparative justice balances competing claims of persons. Distributive justice is broader in scope and refers to conditions of scarcity when competition for benefits exists. Comparative justice is more individualized than distributive justice.

Principles of justice would not be needed by any society if people behaved fairly to each other. Since they do not, these principles have been devised and are often applied to rules of law. According to formal justice, commonly applied in the courtroom (many believe it is not applied commonly enough), equals should be treated equally and unequals unequally. If persons are equal in the respects under consideration, then no other respects should intervene to create injustice. Material justice defines properties on the basis of burdens and benefits to be distributed. Properties relevant to distribution of justice depend on specific burdens and benefits and on standards of judgment. Classes or groups of people are beneficiaries of justice or injustice, but unless the common properties of a group are relevant to the societal benefit or burden in question, these properties should not be used to determine justice. Rawls believes that justice is a virtue or practice of societal institutions to formulate restrictions in assignment of societal rights, duties, and obligations. Justice is essentially elimination of arbitrary distinctions and establishment of a proper balance between competing claims. Justice and power are intertwined, particularly as degrees of authority fluctuate with changing societal mores.

Rights are defined as claims that individuals or groups make on other individuals or groups. Rights involve corresponding duties and obligations, although not always in equal proportions. A positive right involves another person's postive action to protect or maintain the right. A negative right is a right to another's omission or forebearance or the duty to refrain from interfering from the right.

The right to health or health care has been debated in terms of both rights and justice. Rational arguments can be made to support or deny a person's right to health care. A common view is that all people have a right to a decent minimum, although boundaries of that minimum are difficult to establish. Because rights also involve obligations on the part of the person claiming the right, the right to health care must be accompanied by certain behaviors that serve to protect and maintain one's own health.

Allocation of scarce resources must take place on a political, economic, and ethical level. The problem is basic: how to distribute available resources to those who need them in the most equitable way possible. Principles of justice should be used in any allocation system, but frequently the life-and-death nature of the problem defies even the most just and humane system. Blood donation and renal dialysis were used as paradigms of the allocation problem in which the difficulties could be easily seen.

Macroallocation deals with the problem of determining what percentage of total societal resources should be used for health care and what the priorities should be in distributing that care. It is concerned with deciding between health care and other programs such as those of national defense but also between competing health care programs such as immunization programs and development of an artificial heart. Conflicts arise out of societal values, personal behavior, and resources available.

Microallocation involves distribution of available resources to particular individuals or goups and is concerned with the question who shall live when not all can live. It poses some of the thorniest human dilemmas of all. Allocation can be made on the basis of medical criteria, social worth, random slection, or a combination of the three. Various proposals have been offered, but whatever system or group of systems is selected must be based on principles of rationality and justice.

REFERENCES

1. Health costs: what limit? Time **113**(22):60, May 28, 1979.
2. Beauchamp, Tom L., and Childress, James F.: Principles of biomedical ethics, New York, 1979, Oxford University Press.
3. Rawls, John: Justice as fairness, The Philosophical Review **67**:164-194, 1958.
4. Fried, Charles: An analysis of "equality" and "rights" in medical care. In Hunt, Robert, and Arras, John, editors: Ethical issues in modern medicine, Palo Alto, 1977, Mayfield Publishing Co.
5. Sparer, Edward V.: The legal right to health care: public policy and equal access, Hastings Center Report. **6**(5):39-47, October 1976.
6. 54 Del. 15, 174 A 2d 135 1961.
7. Ramsey, Paul: The patient as person, New Haven, 1970, Yale University Press.
8. Katz, Albert H., and Procter, Donald M.: Social-psychological characteristics of patients receiving hemodialysis treatment for chronic renal failure. Kidney Diagnosis Control Program, Contract No. PH-108-66-95, July 1969, U.S. Department of Health, Education, and Welfare.
9. Titmuss, Richard M.: Why give to strangers? Lancet, pp. 123-25, January 16, 1971.
10. Solow, Robert M.: Blood and thunder, Yale Law Journal **80**:1696-1711, 1971.
11. Beauchamp, Tom L., and Walters, Leroy: Contemporary issues in bioethics, Belmont, Calif., 1978, Wadsworth Publishing Co.
12. Childress, James F.: Who shall live when not all can live? Soundings **53**(4):339-355, Winter, 1979.
13. *U.S. v. Holmes* 26 Fed. Cas 360 (C.C.E.D. Pa. 1842).
14. Yadin, Yigael: Masada (Moshe Pearlman, translator), New York, 1966, Random House.
15. Rescher, Nicholas: The allocation of exotic medical life-saving therapy, Ethics (University of Chicago) Vol. **79**(3):173-186, April 1969.

BIBLIOGRAPHY

Beauchamp, Tom L., and Childress, James F.: Principles of biomedical ethics, New York, 1979, Oxford University Press.

Beauchamp, Tom L., and Walters, Leroy Belmont, Calif., 1978, Wadsworth Publishing Co.

Cahn, Edmond: The moral decision: right and wrong in the light of American law, Bloomington, 1955, Indiana University Press.

Chapman, Carleton B., and Talmadge, John M.: The evolution of the right-to-health concept in the United States. In Visscher, Maurice B., editor: Humanistic perspectives in medical ethics, Buffalo, 1972, Prometheus Books.

Childress, James F.: Who shall live when not all can live Soundings. **53**(4):339-355, 1970.

Feinberg, Joel: The nature and value of rights, Journal of Value Inquiry **4**(4):243-257, 1970.

Fried, Charles: An analysis of "Equality" and "rights" in medical care. In Hunt, Roberts, and Arras, John, editors: Ethical issues in modern medicine, Palo Alto, 1977, Mayfield Publishing Co.

Garfield, Sidney R.: The delivery of medical care. In Wertz, Richard W., editor: Readings on ethical and social issues in biomedicine, Englewood Cliffs, N.J., 1973, Prentice-Hall, Inc.

Health costs: what limit? Time **113**(22):60-68, May 28, 1979.

Illich, Ivan: Medical nemesis, New York, 1976, Random House, Inc.

Kass, Leon R.: The pursuit of health and the right to health, The Public Interest, No. 40, Summer 1975.

Kuskey, Garvan F.: Health care, human rights and government intervention. In Hunt, Robert, and Arras, John, editors: Ethical issues in modern medicine, Palo Alto, 1977, Mayfield Publishing Co.

Nelson, James B.: Human medicine: ethical perspectives on new medical issues, Minneapolis, 1973, Augsburg Publishing House.

Outka, Gene: Social justice and equal access to health care, Journal of Religious Ethics **2**(1):11-32, Spring 1974.

Ramsey, Paul: The patient as person, New Haven, 1970, Yale University Press.

Rawls, John: justice as fairness, The Philosophical Review **67**:164-194, 1958.

Rescher, Nicholas: The allocation of exotic medical lifesaving therapy, ethics (University of Chicago Press) **79**(3):173-186, April 1969.

Solow, Robert M.: Blood and thunder, Yale Law Journal **80**:1696-1711, 1971.

Sparer, Edward V.: The legal right to health care: public policy and equal access, Hastings Center Report. **6**(5):39-47, October 1976.

Szasz, Thomas S.: The right to health, Georgetown Law Journal **57**:734-751, 1969.

Telfer, Elizabeth: Justice, welfare and health care, Journal of Medical Ethics **2**:107-111, 1976.

Titmuss, Richard M.: The gift relationship from human blood to social policy, New York, 1971, Pantheon Books.

Titmuss, Richard M.: Why give to strangers? Lancet pp. 123-125, January 16, 1971.

3

Genetic manipulation

HISTORY AND DESCRIPTION

Clone is a new scientific buzzword. When comedians use it some in the audience titter a little nervously because they are not certain of its precise meaning. In Woody Allen's uproariously funny movie *Sleeper* a single human nose is placed on a gleaming steel table in a huge spotless operating room and scientists, breathing heavily, lean over and begin to "clone" it. The word is dropped into cocktail party conversations like olives into martinis, but scientific and ethical ramifications are rarely part of the chatter.

The process of cloning, or asexual reproduction (called asexual because only one parent is needed), is simple in theory but difficult in execution. Cloning is the exact duplication of any nonsex cell from any organism by stimulation of that single cell to begin mitosis and from there to grow into a complete organism. The clone is a genetic duplicate of its parent. Cloning is not to be confused with recombinant DNA, which is the transfer of genes from one life form to another for the purpose of altering that life form. Cloning works with life as it is, seeking only to make an exact duplicate of existing life.

The theory behind cloning is that every single cell in an organism has the same genetic equipment, like that of its first fertilized cell, to form the entire organism. In other words, each cell can give the same genetic instructions as every other cell to achieve specific functions and to grow in particular ways. Original research to prove the theory was performed with a technique called nuclear transplantation, in which the nucleus of an ordinary cell of a frog embryo was transplanted into an unfertilized frog egg from which the nucleus had been removed. It was thought the new environment would turn "genetic switches" on and cause the transplanted nucleus to begin to divide and grow. This work was done by Robert Briggs and Thomas King in 1951 at the National Institutes of Health.[1] The problems surrounding this seemingly simple transplant were enormous, and it took 2 years before the first frog embryo began to grow, but by the next year cloned frogs were hopping around the laboratories. The Briggs-King technique has now been used with other amphibians and a variety of plant life including asparagus and orchids. To date mammalian cloning has not been successful, possibly because the eggs of mammals are much smaller than amphibians' and are thus more difficult to manipulate. There is, however, no doubt that mammalian cloning with lower animals is in the immediate future, and from there it is a mere technologic jump to human cloning, a matter of improved technique rather than acquisition of new knowledge.

Cloning is based on three basic principles of nuclear equivalence: (1) any cell in an organism, not only a sex cell, may be made to reproduce the entire organism; (2) each cell carries a genetic blueprint for the entire organism; and (3) each cell, when it begins to specialize, uses only part of its potential.[1] For example, a muscle cell also has potential to become a kidney cell, but it does not because of the process of differentiation, which directs each undifferentiated cell to develop into what it will eventually become. Differentiation is not fully understood but is believed to be a part of the total genetic code that has yet to be broken.

Vegetable cloning is much simpler than that done with animals because no nuclear transplant is involved. Cells from the plant to be cloned are simply placed in a special growth medium where mitosis begins, and the plant develops into an adult. There is disagreement about vegetable cloning and its possible advantages over the traditional growing of crops by seeding. Using cloning techniques researchers at Rutgers University developed a new strain of asparagus that they believe will be more resistant to fungus and other diseases.[1] Still, large crops of cloned plants or vegetables would be all genetically identical and thus equally vulnerable to new strains of disease-producing organisms.

Several other possibilities for genetic intervention and manipulation now exist. Somatic cell alteration is the isolation and synthesis of genes. This has been accomplished with bacteria; altering human somatic cells is still at some unknown distance in the future. Synthesizing a human gene in a test tube and implanting it in a human cell would be a major step in the creation of "artificial" life. *If* a synthesized gene could be implanted into a single body cell, there is no way to know whether the natural cell would incorporate the genetic trait carried by the single synthesized gene into all the cells of the organism.[2] Introducing a foreign gene into a cell would be useful in controlling diseases that result from deficiency of an extracellular product, such as insulin in diabetes, but would have no effect on hereditary diseases caused by a defective gene.[2]

Germ cell alteration is similar to somatic cell alteration except that in the former the synthesized gene would be introduced into a cell in vitro. This would result in directed mutagenesis; that is, specific agents could bring about a specific alteration in the DNA. It could be used to reverse a current gene mutation or to create a new one.[2] This process is incredibly complex and has not yet been accomplished. To date all known mutagenic agents occur randomly, and their effects are generally negative. For a particular gene to be directed toward a specific place on the DNA strand, it would have to be attached to a molecule that could selectively recognize the destination. Without this tracking device germ cell alteration would be like telling an Amtrak train to find its way from Boston to Washington without providing an engineer, tracks, and signals. It would likely wander off into the Atlantic or end up in Cleveland. Germ cell alteration is still only theoretically possible.

A type of reversal of differentiation of somatic cells can be accomplished today in mammals. If an embryo is removed early from the uterus and its still undifferentiated cells are separated, each cell can be used to begin a new embryo. By this method large sets of genetically identical siblings could be produced. However, genetic structure would not be altered and would still be subject to random selection since fertilization by sexual reproduction would already have taken place. It would ensure uniformity of the offspring, but their genetic structure could not be predicted. All the odds of random genetic selection would remain the same; only larger quantities of the identical embryo would be produced. This is different from cloning in that reversal of differentiation involves sexual reproduction, whereas cloning is asexual.

The uses to which various forms of genetic manipulation could be put will be discussed in the next section. However, it seems appropriate at the outset to enumerate some dangers and possibilities of manipulating genetic structure. Gene transfer, according to Davis,[2] will not be the panacea that some anticipate, at least not in the foreseeable future. Certain monogenic defects might be eliminated, but most human diseases, hereditary or otherwise, do not depend on the structure and function of a single cell. The brain alone has 10 billion interdependent nerve cells, and altering a somatic or even a germ cell would likely have little effect on intellectual or emotional patterns. However, we cannot discount the possibility that the alteration of a few key genes could drastically change human nature. Therein lies the danger: not knowing what to expect. "While the improvement of cerebral function by polygenic transfer thus seems extremely unlikely, one cannot so readily exclude the technical possibility of impairing this function by a transfer of a monogenic defect."[2,p.1281] Davis[2] points to Nazi scientists and politicians in other countries and warns that technologic and scientific ability does not guarantee the beneficence of their intentions. If cell alteration becomes possible, it could be used for evil as well as good purposes. Nuclear energy and its potential uses are an excellent analogy.

With cloning the dangers are both similar and different. Intellectual and artistic genius does depend to a great degree on genetic makeup, and it would seem a solution to some of the world's problems simply to guarantee a constant and predictable supply of genius in whatever areas for which a need could be demonstrated. However, we do not understand what makes genius flower. Davis foresees complacency in a society in which genius is assured. There might then be no reason to rise above the rest, to strive to achieve excellence, or to exert the effort that Albert Einstein described as genius: "10% inspiration and 90% perspiration." If the flowering of genius depends on the sociocultural climate, complacency would kill it even before it had a chance to bud. In addition, one of the joys of creative genius is its unexpectedness and originality. Part of the beauty of a Beethoven symphony, an I. M. Pei building, or Plato's philosophy is the marvel that it arose from a single and unique individual who created the work at a precise moment in time and in a certain set of circumstances that will never again exist. If there were a thousand Beethovens who could have written the same music, it would lose its uniqueness and creativity and thus its value. Originality might cease to exist, and the human spirit would be in some way quenched.

There is also an evolutionary danger in cloning. One of the ways any species survives is through the existence of individuals that are genetically capable of adapting to a constantly changing environment. If a population were sufficiently homogenized by cloning, it could lose that capacity to adapt and an envolutionary danger would be created. By cloning only those humans who are most suitable to the present environment we would assure either the eventual destruction of the species or its marked alteration with such loss of its own characteristics that it would no longer be the same species. This is true of all species. If sufficient other species became extinct or were drastically changed, the environment and our relationship to it would be permanently affected.

Davis views the uses to which scientific technology is put as a social problem and sees potential danger as that problem becomes larger. He points out, however, "Recognition of a problem is the first step toward its solution, and now that we have taken this step it would seem reasonable to assume, until proved otherwise, that further scientific advance can contribute to the solution faster than it will expand the problem."[2,p.1283]

USES FOR GENETIC MANIPULATION

Research in genetics concerns the nature of individual cells, how they function, and equally important, how they malfunction. Cancer cells are a perfect example of cell malfunction. Marie DiBernadino of the Medical College of Pennsylvania has found that some cancer cells can undergo a degree of reversibility.[1] Transplanting the nuclei of cancer cells into frog eggs and thereby manipulating the cell environment produced cancer-free tadpoles. All the tadpoles had genetic abnormalities and all died, but none had cancer. Behavior of the cancer cells was reversed. This research into the nature of why and how cells normally divide could lead to information about why and how cells abnormally divide. The ability to produce a cancer-free tadpole indicates that cell division can be manipulated and suggests exciting future possibilities.

If a gene can be isolated or synthesized in vitro, specificity can be built into the synthesis. If a person is born without a certain body chemical, for example, an enzyme, he is now dependent on either receiving the enzyme artificially or adapting to life without it. If the gene that stimulates production of that particular enzyme could be injected into the genetic makeup of a clone, the enzyme would be produced naturally and the organism would not be dependent on receiving it from the outside.

Scientists have already found that it is possible to isolate a human gene that causes the creation of a certain substance, transplant it into the reproductive system of bacteria, and clone those bacteria, which will then produce, in copious amounts, that gene's particular product. This work has already been accomplished with the hormone somatostatin (which controls growth), and work is now in progress to do the same thing with insulin, hemoglobin and interferon (an important anti-viral agent produced by the body).*

---

*Abrams, Maxine: Frogs, asparagus and you—the real meaning of cloning, The Philadelphia Inquirer, Today magazine, p. 18, October 29, 1978.

If these experiments in cloned substances prove successful, the problem of rejection by the human body would be eliminated because the cloned substance would be genetically identical to the human body for which it is intended. Robert Weinmann of the Wistar Institute projects this process a step further. An insulin gene could be introduced into a harmless virus with which a diabetic person could then be infected. The gene attached to the virus would find its way into the body's cells, and the person would be able to produce his own insulin.[1]

Another interesting theoretical possibility for cloning is regeneration. DiBernadino postulates that every body cell has the ability to regenerate and heal itself.[1] Somehow during the aging process that ability is lost and cells begin to deteriorate and heal less rapidly when injured. The ability to clone or to reverse cell function may provide clues in enabling cells to regain the lost power of regeneration and rejuvenation. This would not necessarily ensure immortality, but it would further research about the aging process, degenerative diseases, and cell deterioration. The death of an individual cell occurs when it has lost its ability to regenerate. Reversing this process could have tremendous implications for cardiovascular, neuromuscular, and other types of diseases that result from the inability of cells to rejuvenate or regenerate.

Genetic manipulation could open doors to what has thus far been only in the realm of science fiction. Creation of a chimera is one such possibility. A chimera is a mythologic creature whose body is composed of parts of several different species, for example, the sphinx. The introduction of nonhuman genetic material into a human gene would not necessarily create a recognizable chimera, but it could alter the structure and appearance of the being and would surely affect its function. The possibilities are fascinating. The introduction of genetic material from a human being into a subhuman primate such as a chimpanzee might produce a superchimp with the strength and agility of a chimpanzee, some human intellectual capacity, and the total identity of neither. Its identity would be somewhere between the two species, and its function could be whatever its creators wished: sewer cleaner, iron worker, subject of biomedical research, or baby-sitter. The combinations and permutations are endless, awe-inspiring, and frightening. If this were to come about we would have to redefine personhood or perhaps learn to define it precisely so that an absolute line between human and nonhuman could be drawn.

The "genetic" combination of human and machine may also some day be possible. Hal, the computer in Stanley Kubrick's classic film, *2001: A Space Odyssey,* has a definite personality that elicits feeling and sympathy from the audience. How will we relate to the computer/person who lives with us and does our housework if we are not entirely certain whether it is a computer or a person?

Kass[3] divides biochemical technologies, in which is included genetic manipulation in all its forms, into three categories: (1) control of life and death by the medical arts of prolonging life and controlling reproduction, (2) control of human potentialities by genetic engineering, and (3) control of human achievement by neurologic and psychologic manipulation. It is the second category that we are concerned with here. Kass believes that genetic engineering will not only be able to make essential differences that can be transferred to succeeding generations but will also establish norms of health and illness. He therefore sees both a therapeutic and eugenic use for such technology. Injecting a normal gene into a genetically defective embryo (or even into a fully developed person) to correct a deficiency is an example of a therapeutic use. Manipulating the gene pool to create greater or fewer numbers of certain kinds of people is an example of a eugenic use.

Genetic surgery on embryos is another method of genetic manipulation. Suppose, for example, one could isolate a specific gene or area on a strand of DNA that was certain to cause a genetic defect. The embryo could be removed from its mother's body, the offending part surgically removed, and the embryo then replaced to develop on its own. Or better yet, the embryo could be grown in vitro until a thorough genetic survey is made. If a defect is discovered, the embryo could be either destroyed or surgically corrected, depending on parental preference. Instead of snipping out an observed defect, the "bad" gene could be replaced with a "good" one that had been previously cloned from one parent (either mother or father depending on circumstances) for just such an eventuality. Perhaps the embryo in utero or in vitro could be infused or injected with a virus to which has been attached a normal gene that had been previously prepared.

The first step in cloning a human being would likely require the participation of a human female in the same way that in vitro fertilization requires participation of a woman to carry the pregnancy to term. A cloned cell would be implanted in a woman's body when it reached the blastocyst stage, at least until the technology was available for a pregnancy to be carried to term in vitro. Asexual reproduction would have come of age, and men and women would be free to have children without making love, if they preferred. The gender of the resulting child could be predetermined (see Chapter 5 for a discussion of predetermination of gender), although there will be no reason why a man and woman could not carry out entirely natural reproduction if they choose. Until totally in vitro pregnancy is possible, men would still be dependent on women if they wished to father a cloned child.

Contraception will not be affected by cloning or any other form of genetic manipulation; it will be just as easy or difficult to become pregnant naturally, no matter what other alternatives to reproduction exist. The advancement of technology to the point where individual cells, entire organisms, or even whole people can be reproduced without sexual intercourse does not necessarily mean that contraceptive technology will have advanced beyond its present point. Allocation of funds for scientific or technologic research is a political decision that depends on the mood and values of the scientific community at any given time. In many ways genetic research is *less* emotionally charged than contraceptive research because of its futuristic flavor. It makes an interesting topic for television talk shows, but so do flying saucers, the Bermuda triangle, and manned space flights to Jupiter. These subjects remain in the realm of science fiction and do not affect people's everyday lives. The opposite is true of contraception, which may directly affect the life of every heterosexually active person.

Cloned cells, probably bacteria or viruses, could be used as factories or farms to produce a variety of chemicals. All biologic substances are more appropriately produced biologically than synthetically, for example, insulin and a variety of hormones. Not only would production of these substances be chemically or biologically more sound, but it would be vastly less expensive. We envision a day when all biologic and many pharmaceutic substances are produced by mass cloning of bacteria. There is no reason why cloned bacteria should have to remain in the laboratory. For example, "Appropriate design might permit appreciable modifications of the normal bacterial flora of the human mouth with a significant impact upon the incidence of dental caries."[4] This principle could be applied to other parts of the body that are subject to infection or decay, notably the respiratory system. A cloned cell might be designed to produce its own antihistamines when it comes into contact with a cold virus, and another cell could be programmed to absorb and destroy various atmospheric pollutants.

However, once cloned cells are let loose in an environment where they cannot be controlled by external forces, the risk of running amuck is almost as great as that of noncloned cells that presently have that ability. For this reason the United States National Academy in 1974 proposed a moratorium on the use of *Escherichia coli*.[4] Scientists were about to create new, self-propagating forms of *E. coli*, which is known to be a natural inhabitant of the human intestine. This new form would then have a completely unknown potential; it could become oncogenic (cancer-producing) or could mutate in thousands of ways that could not be controlled. One of the advantages of working with *E. coli* is that it is so common and reproduces rapidly; those advantages could, however, turn into disastrous disadvantages if a dangerously mutant *E. coli* strain spread rapidly throughout the country. The controversy in the scientific community was heated, but consensus was reached that potentially dangerous experiments should be halted until a means of "biological containment" could be developed. "By biological containment is meant the crippling of all vehicles—cells or viruses—intended to carry the recombinant genomes through the insertion of a variety of genetic defects so as to reduce very greatly the likelihood that the organisms could survive outside of a protective, carefully supplemented laboratory culture."[4] In other words, the cells were to be designed to self-destruct if they got away from the researchers.

REGULATION AND PUBLIC POLICY

In the conference just described (sponsored by the Recombinant DNA Molecule Program Advisory Committee of the National Institutes of Health) in which a voluntary moratorium was called on certain types of potentially dangerous research, the public was not much in evidence. Debate occurred mostly within the scientific community even though lawyers and the press were invited to attend. Some mention was made in the public press, but it died quickly. When the NIH Advisory Committee developed guidelines in 1975 for recombinant DNA research, no member of the public was on the committee.[5] In early 1976 the Committee met again, and this time the meeting was attended by several public interest groups that questioned the safety and advisability of recombinant DNA research. Callahan[5] believes that the crucial question concerns who must accept the burden of proof of the advisability of research—the scientists who wish to continue the research or their opponents. He believes that the proof of danger must be shown by the opponents.

We live in a country which still has a great faith in scientific progress, and an equally great dependence on such innovations for our economic, medical, and social well-being. In that general cultural milieu it seems pointless to blame individual scientists for wanting always to move forward. It is the culture itself which must be questioned.*

The 1976 meeting marked the beginning of active public debate about recombinat DNA research. Several states held public hearings, and in the most dramatic public outcry citizens in Cambridge wanted to block the building of a recombinant DNA laboratory at Harvard. The building went ahead only after a citizens' commission approved construction plans. Several environmental groups have also become involved in the issue. Now that the public is firmly and irrevocably involved in the issue of genetic manipulation, Callahan[5] believes they should concentrate on the following three key questions.

1. Why did it take the public so long to get involved in the issues? Scientists did not deliberately keep the public out; in fact, the press was invited to conferences from the beginning. There is always a lag between a major scientific discovery and public interest in it, but the issue of recombinant DNA research took longer than usual to pique public interest. Callahan notes that the public did not take a real interest until some noted scientists spoke out on the side of the opponents. It seems that people needed these scientists to lead them into the fray. Although Callahan does not speculate about this, it almost seems that the public at least in this instance was waiting for a group of scientists to tell them how to think. The implications of the public's apathy about genetic manipulation are frightening.

2. Now that the public is involved, what options are open and how can issues be evaluated? The first option is to turn NIH guidelines into law; this would apply only to federal grantees, not to private industry that does not receive public funds. Another option is to ignore the present guidelines and begin debate all over again. A third is to call a full moratorium on all recombinant DNA research until public policy guidelines can be developed using the democratic process. Yet another choice is to appoint a presidential or congressional commission to study ethical and socal issues. Callahan favors turning the present NIH guidelines into law and at the same time establishing a commission to further study the issues.

3. What ethical and social criteria should the public use in judging and deciding the future of recombinant DNA research? Callahan points out that there has yet to be a public discussion of the issues that addressed both content and criteria. The public needs to think about scientific progress in general and about the ethical issues of genetic manipulation in particular.

No one denies that scientists doing research on genetic manipulation have a responsibility to the public. The problem is how to discharge that responsibility without thwarting scientific goals. Dismukes[6] believes that three things must be

---

*Callahan, Daniel: Recombinant DNA: Science and the public, Hastings Center Report 7(2):20, April 1970. Reprinted with permission of the Hastings Center: © Institute of Society, Ethics and the Life Sciences, 360 Broadway, Hastings-on-Hudson, N.Y. 10706.

accomplished in devising public policy: (1) clarification of attitudes about taking risks and assessing benefits, (2) recognition of scientists' discomfort with outside regulation, and (3) examination of past practices of regulatory agencies to determine which policies will work and which will not.

Scientists are in sharp disagreement about the relative risks and benefits of recombinant DNA research. The fact that not enough is known about the process itself makes it extremely difficult to assess risks and to establish effective safety precautions. Statements of the probability of disaster will be guesswork at best and will provide little comfort for a nervous public.

The calculation of risk and benefit is further complicated by considerable divergence in what people consider beneficial and what their attitudes are toward risk-taking. Some people are gamblers; some are highly conservative. The scientific community considers the pursuit of knowledge worth a considerable amount of risk, but may differ in this from public attitudes.*

Recombinant DNA research involves taking segments of DNA from one species and inserting it into that of another. Usually this is done with bacteria because of their simple molecular composition. When the cell divides, it then has characteristics of both species. Ergo a new species is created. Danger lies not only in inadvertantly creating a species that proves to be pathogenic or dangerous in some other way but also in the unpredictability of the research and of what might happen if some of these cells escape the laboratory. The whole area is highly speculative, and the public has reason for concern.

One public policy problem involves maintaining a balance between a healthy concern for danger and the advancement of scientific knowledge and progress, all the while keeping hysteria out of the arguments. Scientists can become as hysterical as the public when their autonomy is infringed on and even when they perceive a possibility of infringement. Scientists generally fear and distrust any kind of regulation and think that all areas of endeavor are fair game for research. Regulation must be imposed, however, for scientists cannot be free to study whatever they want in whatever way they choose. Regulation applies not to the thought process but to actions derived from that thought. Thinking, however, is not funded—research proposals are. Therefore scientists feel thwarted in carrying out research when they are required to adhere to certain restrictions if the consequences may affect human beings in dubious or unknown ways. Most worthwhile and interesting research will ultimately affect people, and recombinant DNA research falls into that category. Even the most zealous scientist, if he can be described as a humane person (and most can), will realize that the risk to public safety cannot go beyond a certain point. The problem lies in determining that point.

Based on arguments about the conflict between the advancement of science and the protection of public safety, Dismukes[6] proposes that the United States Public

---

*Dismukes, Key: Recombinant DNA: a proposal for regulation, Hastings Center Report 7(2):26, April 1977. Reprinted with permission of the Hastings Center: © Institute of Society, Ethics and the Life Sciences, 360 Broadway, Hastings-on-Hudson, N.Y. 10706.

Health Service (USPHS) consider recombinant DNA research to be among the activities it regulates. The USPHS is not officially a regulatory agency (such as the Federal Aviation Agency or the Securities and Exchange Commission), but it has similar functions and could adapt to the role without major reorganization. Both the Center for Disease Control and National Institutes of Health are subordinate agencies of the USPHS and could provide technical assistance and advice. The agency should first evaluate existing guidelines and do its own research, if necessary, to ascertain significant hazards. Once data are obtained, new guidelines could be established and administered.

ETHICAL USES

Probably no other area of scientific research, including astronomy and space exploration, will have as large and as permanent an impact on human beings as genetic manipulation, or genetic engineering as it is sometimes called. There has been public debate and many people are morally opposed to the research, but on the whole there seems to be a consensus in the scientific community to get on with it. There has not been sufficient public pressure to offer more than token resistance. Almost no research projects have been halted (a few have been slowed temporarily) because of ethical issues. No one has cried "Foul!" loud enough to stop research.

Moreover, when there has been a scientific breakthrough, the general reaction has been one of wondrous excitement, in the scientific no less than the public media. Whatever ethical reservations or objections may have been voiced prior to the breakthrough have been swept away with astonishing rapidity once the actual events have taken place.*

In other area of research has this phenomenon been so evident. This is not meant to imply that research should be halted, but racing along on a research course without pausing to examine ethical issues may lead to a destination we may wish we had not reached. Ethical issues must be elucidated and discussed.

Utilitarians would probably take a position of examining the risk/benefit ratio when debating moral issues. Will continued genetic research ultimately benefit or harm humankind, and what specific areas of research will create the greatest benefit? Scientific pragmatism would be the watchword. A deontologist would look beyond research consequences to determine what if any characteristics of the research itself have elements of right and wrong. The deontologist might ask questions about the *idea* and the action of creating a new species or of cloning a human rather than being concerned only with the consequences of the act. Deontologists would ask if cloning is essentially good or bad.

A central issue has to do with power, specifically the power that present generations have over the future. Historically, every generation of young people has accused its elders of misusing power, of exercising its will over nature, or in some

---

*Callahan, Daniel: The moral career of genetic engineering, Hastings Center Report 9(2):9, April 1979. Reprinted with permission of the Hastings Center: ©Institute of Society, Ethics and the Life Sciences, 360 Broadway, Hastings-on-Hudson, N.Y. 10706.

instances of making the world worse than it was when they found it. By the same token, advancing age brings greater conservatism, and yesterday's protestors at the steps of the halls of ivy are tommorow's genetic researchers. Children become parents and must endure the indignities from their children that they heaped on their own parents. The point is that attitudes toward the power to affect the future shift with life circumstances. A childless person is more likely to be concerned about the present intellectual pleasures of the pursuit of knowledge than a person who is concerned about his progeny. An older person is more likely to want to fulfill his own goals (and worry less about the future) than a younger person.

At the crux of the issue is the power that human beings have over their own nature and that outside their immediate selves. Each generation succeeds in controlling nature a bit more than the preceding one, but in each generation exists only a tiny fraction of all the people who are yet to be. Should a few hundred existing persons and a few hundred still to be born be given power to control the nature of billions? Each measure of power that human beings win or exert over nature is also power over others because human beings and nature are inextricably bound to each other. Therefore how much power do we want to give ourselves over our present and future selves? How much liberty and autonomy are we willing to sacrifice for future generations? Should we let future generations worry about themselves, or should we take steps now to protect them? Shall we research, experiment, and satisfy our own intellectual curiosity because tomorrow we will not have to live in the disaster we may create today? Or should we take the attitude that today's research will lead to advances in solving problems that will surely be with us tomorrow and forever, for example, genetic malformation and hereditary disease, pain and aging, viral infections that decimate large segments of the population, and starvation? All these problems of human existence have some chance of being solved or at least partially alleviated by genetic manipulation.

Kass[3] addresses the issue of the dehumanizing effects of scientific progress in general and of genetic manipulation in particular. He points to the technology that has depersonalized death to a large degree and foresees a time when conception will occur in a cool laboratory rather than in a warm bed. Yes, the "product" will likely be more perfect if the process is more rigidly controlled, but "It should not be forgotten that human procreation not only issues new human beings, but is itself a human activity."[3,p.784] We could indeed have perfect nutrition if we consumed only prescribed nutrition pellets, but do we want to give up the human pleasure of a candlelight dinner and the taste, smell, and texture of delicious food?

Kass believes that genetic manipulation by laboratory production of human beings would result in drastic moral and social changes. He asks if human parenthood could and would be kept human and theorizes that the institutions of marriage and the family would erode when bearing children is no longer a strong justification for marriage. Family ties link us to both past and future; without them, Kass believes, alienation, loneliness, and depersonalization will increase. He urges caution and restraint in the matter of genetic manipulation because we lack the wisdom to know where we are headed and to what uses new technology will be put. If we acknowledge social and ethical costs, we will be likely to adopt a less permissive and more critical attitude toward scientific development. No one, scientists least of all, enjoys censorship, which by and large is a negative social stance, but to throw all caution to the wind in the area of genetic experimentation seems foolhardy. Efforts *now* to determine and weigh social costs might prevent future regulation and control.

The relationship of science and scientists to the rest of society is such that a minority controls technologic aspects of the lives of the majority. The more sophisticated and abundant the technology, the wider the gap between the minority and the majority and the greater amount of power the minority exerts over the majority. Science is the foundation on which technology is built, although technology to some extent can dictate its needs to science. "The way science is used is determined by the interests and orientation of the dominant social sectors, and there is no reason to expect this to be any less true for gene manipulation than other research."[7,p.73] The key word here is *dominant*, which does not necessarily indicate dominance of numbers. We are fast becoming a society dominated by technology, and those who provide that technology are becoming society's elite and powerful. Thus technologists can use scientific discoveries about genetic manipulation in whatever way they choose unless specific controls are placed on them.

Signer defines technology as "an institutionalized system for highly centralized and intensive control over large groups of men, machines, and events by small groups of technically skilled men operating through organizational hierarchies. Technological organization defines the roles and values of its members, not vice versa."[7,p.74] Again we see the concept of a minority exerting power over the majority. The values of scientists and technologists could easily usurp the values of the rest of society in regard to genetic manipulation. This may not necessarily be bad if society is aware of what is happening and incorporates its own values, that is, the values of the majority, into genetic technology instead of sitting back and being passive recipients of technologic happenings.

Technology, can even to some degree control the direction of basic scientific research in three ways: (1) industry, which controls technology, funds much basic research; university research funded by tax money and other public funds accounts for only about 10% of all scientific experimentation; (2) as individual scientists rise in the establishment hierarchy, their personal influence commands both research grants and the power to dictate their own areas of research; and (3) any research will be done if it is feasible to do so, that is, if it is physically possible and someone has an interest in it.[7] Given this situation, it can be seen that the scientific community will do what it wants as long as technology makes research possible. Thus the interdependent relationship of science and technology becomes evident.

Because genetic research follows a similar pattern, Signer[7] proposes the following steps to safeguard society:

1. Scientists should begin to investigate the value of their work rather than depending on a technologic definition of its value. Scientists, particularly those working with genetic manipulation, should be forced to confront the likely applications of their work. Scientists' intellectual fulfillment will have to give way, at least in part, to the establishment of societal responsibility.

2. Scientists must be aware that their research can be put to conflicting uses with different social consequences. Scientists should begin directing the uses to which their research and discoveries will be put instead of leaving them solely to technologists.
3. Science should be demystified by scientists who must take responsibility for educating the public openly and honestly about all possibilities involved with genetic manipulation. Scientists should initiate dialogues with the public in an attempt to solve problems about research results and uses.

There are reasons to both approve and oppose a scientist's right to uncontrolled experimentation with genetic manipulation. Those who support uncontrolled research state that any new knowledge is valuable in and of itself and is worth obtaining no matter what means are used, although more responsible people agree to set certain limits and guidelines about research methods. These same people see the right to know as a basic human right and any attempt to place restraints on that right as an infringement on the scientist's freedom. It is human to be intellectually curious, and to obstruct the right to act on that curiosity is to thwart human capacities. There is much room for discovery of new knowledge, and discovery will lead to important and useful social consequences. Anything that humans have the capacity to do will eventually be done and to attempt to thwart scientists from acting on that ability would be futile.

Those who oppose unrestricted scientific inquiry, especially in genetic manipulation, cite several reasons. Natural life processes are sacred, and therefore scientists have no right to intervene. This position is frequently used in an uneven and nonintellectual way; for example, these critics allow scientists to interfere with the natural process of disease without approbation. But scientists have no right to alter distinctly human characteristcs, for to do so would be to change the essential nature of humanity.

A qualitative difference in the meaning of human life would occur if the effects of research were to radically alter life as we now know and value it. The risk is too great to give up the degree of certitude we have about life's meaning and values for the uncertainty of qualities and meanings that might emerge.*

Discoveries about qualities of human life might lead to the power to control that life. Those opposed to genetic research believe that the risk of this power falling into the wrong hands is too great. A few people who have knowledge and power should not be in a position to contol the destiny of all of humanity. The familiar argument that human beings should not play God, which appears in many bioethical issues, is particularly in evidence concerning genetic manipulation. Some fear affront to God and to no small degree fear the consequences of God's wrath, and some fear damage to established religious values.

Points can be made in support of both views. The reason for all scientific inves-

---

*Gustafson, James M.: Gentic engineering and the normative view of the human. In Williams, Preston N.: Ethical issues in biology and medicine: proceedings of a symposium on the identity and dignity of man, Cambridge, 1972, Schenkman Publishing Co., p. 48.

tigation and experimentation is to increase knowledge about nature and to control it. There is nothing intrinsically wrong with *knowing,* but dilemmas arise with the use to which knowledge is put. Implicit in all scientific research is the desire to increase the human capacity for self-determination. The possible irony in genetic research is that we might determine ourselves right out of business; that is, in manipulating and changing essential human nature, we might loose those characteristics that prompted us to investigate nature in the first place. Self-improvement and self-fulfillment are generally seen as moral and desirable qualities. However, in the course of improving ourselves we must be alert not to change ourselves irreversibly unless societal values indicate that this is an appropriate path to take. It is conceivable that this could happen because some human characteristics are valued and some are not. There is reason to believe that characteristics that are almost universally considered negative (such as violent aggression) will be "bred out" by scientists with the approval of society in the not-too-distant future. We are moving toward a goal of homogenization of values and behavior, and it seems to follow that we will also move toward a goal of homogenization of genetic makeup.

Changes will be gradual; we will not wake up one morning to hear a news announcement of a new model human being. Whatever changes occur will probably not to any great extent affect the lives of those people already existing. But today's infants will see definite patterns of future change by the time they reach the end of their lives. Those human characteristics that are most valued by most people will be altered last: for example, physical existence in the form of a human body, a sense of well-being or happiness (the ancient Greeks called it *eudemonia*), a sense of bodily and spiritual integrity or wholeness in that humans can form communities and can achieve satisfaction as individuals and in concert with the community, and some kind of religious or spiritual life in which a sense of continuity with the past and with moral and religious values exists. Other characteristics that are not so commonly valued might be changed first if genetic experimentation is permitted to continue unchecked.

Everything in scientific life must be morally weighed. Every decision has costs and benefits. "The essence of tragedy is the conflict of one good with another. The conflict of good and evil is only melodrama. We often have to calculate the relative desirability of things. We pay for what we get, always."[8,p.17] A decision between two benefits is always more difficult to make than a decision between a benefit and a nonbenefit. This is true in the abortion debate that centers on prevailing rights to life, and it is true in genetic manipulation, where the ethical debate is between restricted and unrestricted control of experimentation. No one seriously believes that genetic research will be totally and permanently halted. The issue is *how* to do the research, not whether to do it at all. Should controls exist, and if so, should they be imposed voluntarily by scientists themselves or from the outside by those not actively engaged in research? History has shown that scientists have been ineffective in regulating their own endeavors; they have required outside controls. If commissions have been established to protect the subjects of biomedical and behavioral research, they will surely be needed to protect genes that are being manipulated. This may seem a contradiction: why would a gene need to be protected in the same way as a person? If the U.S. Constitution does not ensure the safety and rights of a fetus, why should a regulatory agency protect a single cell or a gene? Regulations or other controls would not be directed toward particular individual cells or even cells in the aggregate as they are toward the protection of individual human beings; rather controls would be aimed at the *results* of experimenting with individual cells. The purpose of genetic manipulation is to change or improve the species, and therefore human beings who result from experimentation with genes and cells need to be protected like any other human beings who are subjects of research.

Eugenics

Eugenics, or "good breeding," is designed to improve the condition and capacity of a species. Stock breeding of animals is an example of eugenics. Dogs are bred to ensure more perfect physical composition and to achieve species perfection. Cattle are bred to perfect the ratio of edible flesh to fat and bone, and an effort is made to improve the quality of the flesh itself, to make it tastier and more tender. Horses are bred to run faster, and cows are bred to give more milk of higher quality. Although there are ethical dilemmas involved in animal eugenics (for example, is it justified to increase the possibility of negative or hurtful genetic characteristics in animals simply to improve the positive ones?), we tend to ignore them because a social utility is served by perfecting species; we want plumper chickens and more milk in relation to feed consumed.

Human eugenics, however, is a different story. A perfect example is the Boston XYY case.[9] In the mid-1960s studies of individuals in mental and penal institutions revealed that approximately 2% had an XYY chromosome type, whereas this configuration was seen in only 0.11% of the general population. Generalizations were made, based on insufficient empirical evidence, that persons with the XYY chromosome makeup were more likely to demonstrate violently aggressive behavior than those who did not have the characteristic. The information received wide publicity, and a study was begun at Harvard in 1973 to screen male children to detect the XYY chromosome type. The study was eventually halted by Dr. Stanley Walzer, a Harvard psychiatrist, because of heated controversy about the study methods, its legitimacy, and uses to which results were to be put. About 97% of all people born with the XYY type end up leading quite normal lives. The other 3% who engage in antisocial behavior might do so for reasons totally unrelated to their particular chromosome type. No cause-and-effect relationship had been established between XYY and violently aggressive behavior, yet male children who were found to have this chromosomal configuration were stereotyped as future criminals and their parents were caused unwarranted anguish.

Another study conducted by Walzer and Dr. Park Gerald, a geneticist, involved both genetic screening and a detailed psychologic and behavioral study of children with the XYY genotype.[9] Newborn infants were subjected to chromosomal study and distinguished as one of three types: those with an extra X chomosome (Klinefelter's syndrome), those with an extra Y, and those with balanced chromosomes (one X and one Y). A 20-year follow-up study was planned that involved interviews with the parents of children with abnormal chromosomal configuration by a scientist who knew that the children were affected *and* behavioral observations and testing by a scientist who did not know which children were affected and which not. School and home behavior were observed. "An unusual component of this program has been its willingness to intervene therapeutically in the event that some specific treatable disabilities are detected."[9,p.6] Therein lies the ethical dilemma. If statistics predict that only 3% of the XYY children will engage in aggressive antisocial behavior, two problems immediately become evident: which are the 3%, and should the remaining 97% also be treated? There are other issues as well. The study assumes that future antisocial behavior can be predicted and that causes of the behavior will be genetic, but no proof exists for either assumption. *If* proof existed, what treatment modality would be used, and would benefits of any treatment chosen be worth the risks? What kind of information should be given to parents? Considering the sketchiness of information available to scientists, why would parents consent to participation in such research?

It seems that the only benefits of this study, if any can be found, are purely observational, and even this aspect is fraught with danger. If parents know why their child is being so assiduously observed (in order to give informed consent, they would have to be aware of the scientists' hypotheses), would not their behavior toward their child be affected? If they knew the hypothesized correlation between the XYY chromosomal type and antisocial behavior, would their mode of raising the child affect this behavior and thus negate the study results? Would the parents misinterpret every childhood aggressive act and punish it severely, possibly increasing future aggression by significantly altering the parent-child relationship? They could, on the other hand, adopt a dangerously laissez-faire attitude and remove all discipline and controls from the child's upbringing, thinking that whatever they did would have no effect because the child's behavior was genetically determined. Early diagnosis and screening might prove to be of some benefit *if* there were a definite treatment or a known way to prevent the antisocial behavior that *might* occur in 3% of XYY children. Giving parents the information necessary for informed consent would automatically skew results of the study, but not telling parents why their children are being observed would violate a number of ethical principles. It seems that in this instance the possible benefits are not worth the risk; in fact, it is almost impossible to isolate and identify any benefits at all.

Davis[10] describes three basic patterns that can be used in human eugenics:

1. *Selection against monogenic defects*. This approach has in the past depended almost entirely on estimates of probability; for example, statistics can predict that a certain percentage of children born to carriers of a genetic disease will be born with the disease. It is now possible to detect the presence of certain genetic diseases in utero while a decision for abortion can still be made. This eugenic method, although significant to the individuals involved, has an almost miniscule effect on the general population. Even if every fetus known to have a genetic defect were aborted, the eugenic effect would still not be statistically significant on a worldwide basis. "The reason is that most hereditary diseases are genetically recessive and therefore appear only when both parents have the same rare defective gene; and

for each such mating there will be a huge reservoir of carriers of the gene who will not be detected because they did not mate with a similar carrier."[10]

2. *Selection of especially desirable germ cells.* This approach involves the establishment of sperm banks (in the future when the entire course of pregnancy may take place in vitro, egg banks may also be established) to choose whatever human characteristics are deemed ideal or desirable by society. One might assume that parental pride would increase as superchildren became superachievers, but Davis thinks the voluntary aspect of this type of eugenic program would soon disappear and all couples would be subjected to eugenic selection.

3. *Differential reproduction of large groups.* This is a rather euphemistic designation for the encouragement of certain groups of people to reproduce and the discouragement of certain other groups. Those people who have demonstrated superior achievements would be encouraged to bear more children than those who are considered less socially desirable. This eugenic method has strong racist overtones and would not be acceptable to a society that sees itself as egalitarian. It also would not result in a statistically significant change unless the eugenic program were made nonvoluntary and coercive. Davis proposes that a compromise solution,

another eugenic approach, essentially ignored in the past, may be more likely to prove acceptable: one with the humanitarian goal of increasing human satisfaction, and decreasing misery, by minimizing the production of individuals whose genetic endowment would seriously limit their capacity to find a sense of usefulness and fulfillment in a complex world. In this approach an improved endowment would not be an alternative to an improved environment, but the two would be complementary approaches to the solution of persistent social problems*

This is an extremely value-laden view that essentially advocates preventing the birth of all individuals who cannot accomodate the present social and physical environment. It would be practical *if* one could positively identify and define all those factors that increase satisfaction and decrease misery. It also depends on knowing what capacities lead to a sense of "usefulness and fulfillment in a complex world." If this theory were to be put into practice, we would require total agreement on all subjective components of life *and* the means to achieve these desired goals. If everyone were to agree on what promotes happiness and decreases misery, individual differences would disappear and we would be a truly homogenized society. At that point it might not seem terribly outrageous to make cloning a routine part of life.

Davis finds several trends and advantages in the development of a eugenic program:

1. Since population needs to be controlled anyway, it may make sense to restrict the growth of certain population segments by various licensing or incentive procedures. The gene pool would surely be unalterably affected.

---

*Davis, Benard D.: Threat and promise in genetic engineering. I Williams, Preston N.: Ethical issues in biology and medicine: proceedings of a symposium on the identity and dignity of man, Cambridge, 1972, Schenkman Pbulishing Co., p. 27.

2. Knowledge about genetics would increase and would become more important in the study of psychology, sociology, education, and even economics. A firm genetic base might be used to measure and predict all sorts of human endeavors.

3. Those sections of the country where biology is taught without mention of evolutionary principles would be forced to acknowledge the enormous role of genetics in human development.

4. Increased knowledge could be expected to equalize the sharing of societal goods and opportunities. If it can be definitely proved that people of certain genetic makeup have more difficulty coping with the world or succeeding in it, would it not be kinder to prevent them from being born at all? This could apply to people with mental as well as physical defects. Indeed, society could define *defect* in any way it chose and could impose a genetic program that conformed to the definition and shifted with changing societal values.

Whatever eugenic or genetic technology is developed will surely be put to some use. We are too pragmatic a society to ignore or prohibit a new technologic tool without first investigating its use.

These observations about what could be done with a eugenic program are at the same time fascinating and terrifying. The potential for both good and evil is limitless. Racial prejudice could be either eliminated totally by eventually having only one race or drastically increased by restricting or encouraging the population growth of certain races. We could make human beings supremely adaptable to changing environments, or we could breed out our present remarkable ability to adapt. In creating breeds of superpeople of pure genetic makeup, however, we might wish we had not eliminated the mongrelization that adds to our hardiness and adaptability. Presumably a eugenic program would encourage breeding of intelligent people with the hope that the species would grow smarter. Society, which now depends on people with average or low intelligence to carry out some of the routine tasks of keeping the wheels in motion, would perhaps be unable to maintain itself. Automation can take us only so far. If no one wanted to be assembly line workers, keypunch operators, telephone operators, and bus drivers, the fabric of life would change. Consider what happens now during a general strike in England or Italy, where they occur with depressing regularity; life is changed for the duration of the strike because essential services are halted. Multiply that times forever if the entire world were composed of geniuses.

Evolution would be unalterably affected by eugenics, and it is impossible to know whether it would be for good or ill. Eugenics is as fascinating as it is frightening, and the desire to experiment with human genes just to see what happens is incredibly strong. To tell a scientist that intellectual curiosity must be stifled because the future of humanity rests on his and his colleagues' shoulders is to place an unreasonable burden on the scientific community. Society supports the *idea* of creative science, and to prohibit some of it would be to deny the intellectual curiosity that is an integral part of human nature.

Lederberg[11] coined the term *euphenics*, which is alleviation of genotypic maladjustment by treating affected individuals early in their development with genetic surgery and cloning. Genetic surgery could correct a defect in a particular individual, but the trait would still be passed on to offspring and would therefore have no permanent eugenic effect. Cloning will, however be available in the foreseeable future and will have the eugenic advantage of providing exact copies of specific genotypes and the additional bonus of providing all the spare parts that will ever be needed. A euphenic treatment program would, of course, hold all the dangers and disadvantages of almost any mass genetic program because one does not know and cannot predict the eventual societal effect.

The idea of a eugenic program is probably unacceptable to most people today. The racist overtones are strong, and the program would meet opposition by many groups in the United States, especially minorities. In the rest of the world where racial or subracial caste systems are more firmly entrenched in the fabric of society, suggestions of a eugenic program would likely be met with rioting and bloodshed. Imagine the effect of such an announcement in South Africa or Zimbabwe. Consider the effect on the class struggle in India. An American politician who wanted to appropriate funds for an experimental eugenic program would soon be voted out of office. The time is not yet ripe for a eugenic program, but the interesting questions are when it will be and what social, political, and economic conditions will exist before it will be acceptable to a majority of the population of any country.

GENETIC SCREENING AND COUNSELING

Gregor Mendel discovered most of the laws of heredity in the 19th century, and by the mid-1970s approximately 2300 genetically related disorders had been discovered.[12] Genetic testing of various kinds can detect a few of these disorders although these are only a handful in comparison with the total. Some tests are done after an infant is born, some are done in utero, and some can detect and predict possible defects even before conception takes place. For example, genetic testing of individual adults can reveal about 50 recessive conditions. A recessive condition is a disorder in persons who have one normal gene and one variant gene in the same location on paired chromosomes. They usually do not suffer from the disease and are known as carriers. However, if two carriers of the same recessive trait reproduce, chances are one in four that each offspring will be affected with the disease.[13] An example is Tay-Sachs disease.

Prenatal diagnosis is another way of detecting genetic disease. Various procedures make this possible; the most accurate is amniocentesis, with which samples of fetal cells and blood can be examined. Sickle cell disease and Down's syndrome can be positively diagnosed in this manner. The fetoscope is now being used experimentally to visually examine the fetus to detect some anatomic abnormalities. Fetal diagnosis allows the choice of aborting the deformed or diseased fetus or permitting it to be born. The reader is referred to Chapter 7 on abortion for a discussion of ethical issues.

Genetic screening is the application of testing techniques to large numbers of people and involves no medical procedures. It can be voluntary or involuntary. The former is already in existence, but the latter would involve coercive techniques and societal decisions regarding what to do about the results of screening. An involuntary screening program would make little sense without an involuntary eugenics program. However, there are isolated examples of mandatory testing for the presence of certain genetic diseases. Almost all states require newborn infants to be tested for phenylketonuria (PKU), which causes mental retardation. No state, however, makes treatment *mandatory* after PKU is detected. Voluntary screening can detect both individuals who are already afflicted with a genetic disease and individuals who are carriers.

Genetic counseling is done after screening has taken place. A counselor tells the parents or prospective parents what traits or defects have been found, what the statistical chances are for the birth of a defective infant, and what options are available for circumventing the birth or for dealing with a child afflicted with a genetic disease. Genetic counselors have traditionally been physicians, but more nurses, social workers, and physiologists are now filling the role.

Amniocentesis, a highly effective form of genetic screening, carries a certain physical risk although with the use of ultrasonography for fetal and placental localization that risk is decreasing. Developmental damage to the fetus could occur through the introduction of organisms or by somehow disturbing the intrauterine environment by removing amniotic fluid. Long-term studies of the intellectual and behavioral development of children who were subjected to amniocentesis during fetal life are now being conducted by the National Institute of Child Health and Human Development, but no definitive results have yet been shown.[13] For the present, amniocentesis is considered a low-risk, effective procedure.

Several factors indicate a need for genetic screening by amniocentesis. One is advanced maternal age (first pregnancy over the age of 30 or succeeding pregnancies over the age of 35), which results in increased risk of Down's syndrome and other forms of mental retardation. Another indication is a couple who have previously given birth to a genetically defective child. This is called retrospective detection, but in certain diseases, especially ones linked to dominant genes (for example, Huntington's chorea), the risk to the fetus is 50%. *Theoretically* all cases except those caused by new mutations could be detected, and selective abortion could eliminate the disease. Screening methods are not completely accurate, however, and to eliminate a disease screening and treatment would have to be made mandatory.

A utilitarian view based on cost/benefit analysis would likely be in favor of mandatory genetic screening at least for certain diseases that can be easily and positively identified, such as Tay-Sachs disease or Down's syndrome. Not only would families be spared the emotional agony and financial disaster of a defective child, but society, which bears much of the financial burden, would be relieved of one aspect of health care cost. The cost of a defective child can be reasonably calculated in terms of money and resources. Emotional costs can be acknowledged but not calculated. What of the benefit side of cost/benefit analysis? Are there personal or societal benefits to be gained by the birth of deformed children? The matter, of course, is entirely subjective and completely unanswerable. One sometimes hears of parental pleasure from the frequently sunny disposition of children with Down's syndrome, and coping with the crisis of a defective child can release strengths people did not know they had. But are these benefits? Other children have equally loving personalities, and there are more than enough family crises to test anyone's strength. Would a person honestly prefer to have a defective child than a normal one? If the answer is no, then finding a benefit becomes even more difficult. However, even if *no* benefits exist and personal and societal costs become astronomic, it does not necessarily follow that genetic screening should be mandatory.

A deontologist would look at the right or wrong nature of the act itself and seek ethical rules in any situation regardless of consequences. The obvious moral rule in genetic screening is the liberty of individuals to reproduce as they please, or autonomy. Paternalistic arguments might center on the purity or determination of the genetic pool, societal cost, and even the unnecessary grief families might experience. All these arguments have merit and all are pragmatic, but they all eventually crash headlong into the fundamental concept of personal freedom and liberty. There is no way to get around this barrier unless one is willing to change many of the principles by which we live.

There are physical reasons as well to oppose genetic screening. Motulsky of the University of Washington and Neel of the University of Michigan have found that large-scale prenatal abortion could affect the diversity and quality of the gene pool.[13] Such programs could result in an inadvertent increase in genes for certain genetic diseases. For example, detection of affected males with an X-linked disease such as hemophilia cannot yet be accomplished in utero, although carrier mothers can be detected and the gender of a fetus known. If all male fetuses of carrier mothers were aborted, the gene frequency would increase by 50% *with each generation*. There are, of course, diseases that could be eliminated by selective abortion, but the ultimate long-term effects cannot be determined. It is possible that by eliminating one disease by genetic manipulation or selective abortion, a new and far worse mutation could occur with an even greater incidence. Perhaps some diseases hold others at bay.

Why do we want to rid ourselves of genetic disease? What do we instinctively dislike or fear about people who are born different? Is it that they are sometimes misshapen and ugly? Not all are. Is it that they will die soon and cause us grief? Some live normal life spans. Is it that we are forced to do something to help them? We *could* simply throw them into pits the way lepers and other outcasts were in Biblical times. Is it that they remind us of our own mortality and lack of perfection? Not everyone is forced to think about persons with genetic disease. Do they represent an intellectual challenge to cleanse or purify the human race? We are obviously not satisfied with ourselves as we are.

Most of the fear of these different people and the drive to eliminate genetic disease is linked to a horror of what we are capable of producing and the guilt or shame that a "freak" or defective person could have sprung from a perfect and normal body. The ancients cast them out of society so that they would not have to acknowledge or deal with them (Aristotle recommended that they simply be eliminated). Moderns retreat to their laboratories to devise ways to prevent them from coming into existence.

What actually is wrong with being different or retarded or deformed? Why are we so anxious that everyone be similar, smart and physically perfect? There is, of course, nothing intrinsically wrong with being born with below-average intelligence, but society values intelligence. There is nothing immoral about ugliness or imperfection, but society values beauty and physical wholeness. Differences can be unique and interesting, but society values similarity and homogenization. These statements seem to imply that society is at fault for wanting to decrease or eliminate genetic disease. Disease or defect, if it causes suffering to the individual and to those who love him, should be fought and eliminated. Differences that are not intrinsically painful or dangerous to the individual are another matter. Being unable to cope with individual physical or psychologic differences is a grave *societal* problem, and it is then society, not fate or chance, that inflicts pain on the different person.

One must wonder why society values sameness so much, why intelligence is prized, and why we all strive to be as beautiful as possible. Parents often are blamed for bringing defective children into the world, especially if the defect could have been predicted by genetic screening or even by the couple's decision not to bear children together. Do we "then share with our ancestors the view that a defective child is a curse but then unlike them, provide no comfort whatever, other than the ascetic reward of praise or blame for socially acceptable behavior in the face of the curse"[14]? With the advent of the use of cost/benefit ratios in health care, society can find even greater justification for blaming parents and for encouraging people to do everything in their power to prevent the birth of a defective child. Even the language we use indicates societal values. *Defective, abnormal, diseased,* and so on are all negative words when used in this context, and striving for physical perfection rivals religious zeal in some quarters. This is not meant to imply that diseases or defects in and of themselves are good and are to be encouraged; what is implied, however, is that society needs to reexamine its values about those people who are born different from the average. Can we continue to discriminate against *or* reward people on the basis of physical or mental characteristics over which they have no control?

The Research Group on Ethical, Social and Legal Issues in Genetic Counseling and Genetic Engineering[15] (hereinafter referred to as the Research Group) of the Institute of Society, Ethics, and the Life Sciences described some principles it believes to be essential to the operation of genetic screening programs. The following is a summary:

1. The screening program should be based on one or more clearly defined goals that should be identified before screening begins. The Research Group believes that the most important goals are those that contribute to improving the health of persons who suffer from genetic disorders, allow carriers of a variant gene to make informed choices about reproduction, or move toward the alleviation of anxiety of families faced with the prospect of serious genetic disease.
2. The screening program should be able to demonstrate benefits to persons or couples who receive services such as providing genetic counseling, de-

tecting asymptomatic persons at birth, and detecting carriers of variant genes.

3. The screening program should also contribute to knowledge about genetic disease by determining the frequency of rare diseases and the incidence and prevalence of all genetic diseases.

4. The operation of a screening program should not begin until pilot projects have demonstrated that its goals are attainable and are flexible enough to update procedures and objectives as new knowledge becomes available.

5. Committees should be involved in planning and operating the screening program, and mechanisms must be established to assure equal availability to all members of the community.

6. Testing should be accurate. The screening program must ensure the reliability of laboratory services, whether its own or an ouside contractor's.

7. Compulsion of any kind must not exist in either the screening policies or the childbearing practices of affected couples. Voluntarism must be assured. Screening must be done only with informed consent.

8. The Research Group believed that even though there is minimal physical risk in genetic screening, psychologic or social injury could be great because the programs are relatively new. Therefore genetic screening ought to be considered a form of human experimentation and subjects protected according to DHEW guidelines.

9. All policies and procedures for screening should be disclosed to individuals being tested and to the community in which the program is located. Results of all diagnostic tests should be made available to the individual or couple.

10. Well-trained genetic counselors should be available for interpreting diagnostic tests and for explaining options available as a result of the tests. Counseling should be nondirective, that is, the counselor should inform clients but not make choices for them. There is an urgent need to define and establish appropriate qualifications for genetic counselors, but the quality and effectiveness of work done by the screening program remains the responsibility of the program director.

11. Information about available therapy and its cost, the facilities for maintaining afflicted offspring, and the risks and benefits involved should be given to all clients. Decisions about whether to participate in the program are not possible without this information. Clients' privacy must be protected at all times.

The Research Group concluded that "Even if the above guidelines are followed, some risk will remain that the information derived from genetic screening will be misused. Such misuse or misinterpretation must be seen as one of the principal potentially deleterious consequences of screening programs."[15] The most serious kind of misinterpretation involves labeling and stigmatizing people. For example, people who have sickle-cell trait are erroneously believed to be handicapped and unable to function. This can result in job discrimination and social isolation. Physical activities of school children with the trait have been restricted, and adult carriers have been denied life insurance coverage. None of these opinions is medically warranted; all are the result of public misinterpretation of fact. The Research Group believes that screening programs have a definite educational function to prevent or minimize such occurrences.

Several moral or ethical problems arise in genetic screening and counseling. The first involves telling the truth. Is an individual obligated to tell a spouse or an intended marriage partner of a known problem, or can the person say nothing and hope for the best? Is the genetic counselor obligated to tell the whole truth? Some counselors feel that even though one person is the distinct carrier of a variant gene and thus the "cause" of a defective child, it is kinder to the couple to say either that the information is not avialable or that both marriage partners are equally "responsible."

Another dilemma concerns what to do with the information generated by the testing. Should a defective fetus be aborted, should the couple resort to artifical insemination with donor sperm, or should they not reproduce at all? Should an engaged couple refrain from marrying if it is found that one carries a variant gene? If they do marry, can one partner demand of the other that they have no children together?

A group of moral problems revolves around the defective child. Should the defect be treated, and if so, how much time, energy, and money are to be invested? If the defects are very serious (the degree of severity can be viewed both objectively and subjectively), should infanticide be considered? If the child is only mildly or moderately affected, is the home or an institution the best place for him?

Various factors complicate the resolution of ethical conflicts: misinformation or misinterpretation of correct information; conflict of values between marriage partners; other family members, especially parents, imposing their views and increasing conflict; religious beliefs that may not agree with personal desire; guilt, shame, or remorse; and disagreements with physicians or genetic counselors.

Moral dilemmas and the factors that tend to complicate them can be viewed in two basic ways. The first involves a responsibility to the human community and includes such issues as cost/benefit analysis, societal responsibility to a defective child, and the like. In this view are actualized the feelings of loyalty to the self, to close others, and to the human community in general. There are also conflicts about responsibilities, that is, about which moral rules take precedence over others.

Fletcher[16] reports that most people who sought genetic screening and counseling did so because of a felt responsibility to the health of their children and the security of their family. One mother in a group of 25 couples interviewed expressed resistance to abortion for economic or psychologic reasons but spoke of the unfairness of deliberately bringing a defective child into the world. Many of the parents seemed concerned with the concept of fairness in justifying decisions. "The important note in their reasoning was that of a willing acceptance of parental and genetic responsibility. None of these parents could be described as proactive eugenecists, and only a tiny fraction reasoned solely on the basis of individual convenience."[16]

Fletcher also found that the couples were concerned about population problems, genetic responsibility, and parental values as well as their own social ethics.

None of the couples was unalterably opposed to aborting a defective fetus, particularly those who were already parents of a deformed or retarded child. Two of the couples were Catholic, four were Jewish, five had mixed religious marriages, three expressed no religious affiliation, and the rest were Protestant. The high proportion of Jewish couples probably reflects the vast publicity about Tay-Sachs disease, which affects Ashkenazic Jews almost exclusively. The low proportion of Catholics may reflect that church's deterministic attitude about reproduction. Fletcher found that the most important expressed value in genetic decision making was parental protection of a child or fetus. Protection extended to ending the life of a fetus to "protect" it from the problems of being deformed in a normal world.

Guilt is a strong complicating factor in making ethical decisions, especially on the part of women. The failure to produce a perfect baby is seen by some as not only a personal tragedy but also as a failure of "duty" to the husband. The inability to "give" him a healthy child is frequently viewed as a failure of the wifely function. Even worse, those women who internalize the expectations of society about the role of women and have no other outlet for their creative energies tend to experience more guilt than those who do not.

Two other interesting observations that Fletcher made as a result of continuing interviews with the 25 couples are that (1) the wishes of the genetic counselor are always directly or indirectly conveyed to the couple and (2) couples felt morally competent to make decisions based on the results of genetic screening without seeking nonmedical advice. From this one might infer that the role of genetic counselor should be limited to provider of facts and information about options and nothing else. Since the counselor should never make a decision for individuals or couples, perhaps genetic counselors should remove themselves from the area of psychologic therapy.

Ramsey[17] sees intrauterine screening as potentially dangerous (presumably he would, if asked, extend the concept of screening to karyotyping of individuals prior to their decision to have a child). He believes it will erode society's willingness to accept and care for abnormal children and will enlarge the category of unacceptable abnormality while at the same time narrowing the category of normality. He believes that the argument that intrauterine screening promotes a greater number of normal babies is fallacious; he maintains that the definition of *normal* simply changes and that the argument is one of semantics, not genetics or morality. Ramsey states that it would seem more human and forthright "to advocate that an individual shall not be certified to be among us—counting equally—until two days after birth, or when he can have his first check-up to determine whether he can qualify for the 'quality of life' we mean to enhance."[17] Similar suggestions have been made by James Watson, Glanville Williams, and others; the idea is literally as old as the Bible. When Ramsey makes this suggestion he seems to have his tongue firmly planted in his cheek: "this has in view the destruction and not the treatment of the needy patient."[17] He does not believe that aborting defective fetuses is an appropriate response to the problem of genetic defects.

Veatch[18] presents a case that involves several ethical dilemmas. Mr. and Mrs. Edwall heard about the Tay-Sachs screening program at their synagogue. They decided to be tested because they were both Ashkenazic Jews and were planning to start a family soon. Mr. Edwall was found to be a carrier. The genetic counselor assured the couple that they would never have a Tay-Sachs baby, but she questioned Mr. Edwall about the rest of his family. He had two younger brothers who were both married and who presumably planned to have children. The counselor suggested that Mr. Edwall contact his brothers so that they too could be tested. He thought about it and came to believe that he was "not quite a man" since he carried this sickness in his cells. He felt ashamed and refused to inform his brothers. The counselor tried in every way she could to convince Mr. Edwall to notify his brothers, but he was adamant. If both brothers and their wives were carriers, the chances were 1 in 60 of their producing a baby with Tay-Sachs disease. (The rate in the non-Jewish population is about 1 in 600, which is very high considering the tragic course and end result of the disease.) The counselor argued and pleaded with Mr. Edwall, but he still refused. Finally she wrote a discreet letter to both brothers.

Several conflicts appear in this case. Does the counselor owe absolute confidentiality to Mr. Edwall, or are his brothers in sufficient jeopardy to warrant breaking the confidence? Does the fact that the counselor never asked for Mr. Edwall's permission to contact his brothers (she only requested that *he* do it) place the breach of confidentiality in a different ethical perspective, or would that be using a technicality to get around the spirit of the principle involved? How will the policies and ongoing practices of the genetic screening program be affected by the two letters? If the public found out what the counselor did, its confidence could decrease; is this risk worthwhile compared to the necessity of giving the brothers information? To whom does Mr. Edwall owe primary responsibility—to himself in keeping private information private or to his brothers who might avoid major tragedy were it not for Mr. Edwall's personal shame based on unrealistic perceptions? How much responsibility do Mr. Edwall and the counselor have toward the brothers? They are aware of their ethnic background and presumably would be tested if they so chose. Does the counselor have a further obligation to suggest that Mr. Edwall receive some kind of psychologic help in dealing with his feelings?

POLITICAL IMPLICATIONS

Genetics and politics have always been closely linked. History and literature are filled with discussions of superpeople and superraces; the quest to improve the human species is probably as old as the species itself. Both democratic and totalitarian forms of government contribute to the likelihood that genetic manipulation will occur and research will be supported. A democracy supports the idea of genetic research for the same reason it supports all other research: principles of individual liberty and autonomy permit and encourage discovery and public disclosure of new knowledge. Unless research can definitely be shown to have harmful potential, it is generally not thwarted, although societal values determine to a large degree what kinds of research will be supported by public and private funds. Totalitarian governments can, if they are interested, support and encourage genetic manipulation by dictating avenues of inquiry to scientists and by creating whatever kinds of genetic policies are desired by those in power. They need not be bothered by public pressure, ethical considerations, or moral principles.

The best example of this in recent history was the Nazi policy of eugenics and their desire to create an all-Aryan race. Germany did not suddenly discover eugenic theories with the rise of Hitler; the idea of the superiority of Aryans had been part of the German consciousness for many years. Alfred Ploetz (1860-1940) was a central figure in the German eugenics movement of the 1920s.[19] He criticized both capitalism and socialism and thought that a eugenic society would put the good of the future above comforts of the present. He believed that the humanitarian and idealistic goals of socialism could be combined with the eugenic goal of a constantly improving biologic base to form a perfect society. His knowledge of genetics was sketchy (so was everyone else's at the time), but he was one of the first to point out that the "value consequences of applying the science of human heredity depend more on *when* and *how* it is applied than on the question of what values are inherent in the science itself.[19,p.31] This is the essential connection between genetics and politics. The term *eugenics* in Germany in the period between the world wars went through a series of permutations. One of the characteristics of eugenics was the 1929 description by Fritz Lenz in *Archive for Race and Social Biology* in which he states that the human race will genetically deteriorate unless it is prevented from doing so by giving the strong and fit advantages in propagation. From there it was only a small step to giving a disadvantage to the weak and unfit. Lenz was one of Hitler's earliest supporters and presumably had strong influence on the Fuhrer's eugenic policies.

One might have thought that Russia during the early period after the revolution would be uninterested in eugenics. But apparently not everyone was enthralled with the principles of socialism, because in 1921 both the Russian Eugenics Society and Bureau of Gentics of the Academy of Sciences were established. The journals published by both societies were mainly concerned with the geneologies of famous Russian families. The flavor, however was distinctly antirevolutionary and did not gain much respect in the scientific community. Soviet eugenic debates were important, however, because of the way eugenics was perceived outside the community of eugenicists. "What was the relation of doctrines of eugenics to the idea of Russian socialism and communism?"[19,p.33] This debate continues today and centers on the conflicts between biologic determinants of human behavior (a purely genetic-determinist view) and socioeconomic determinants (the basis of socialism). The Marxist view that social conditions determine and are the foundation of the class struggle would be in jeopardy if proof could be firmly established that eugenics can be used to create a more equal or just society.

What would be the result for the proletariat, for the lower social classes in general, and for the cause of social revolution if acquired characteristics were inherited? Most people seem to believe . . . that such a theory points to rapid social reform, whereas classical genetics, with its stable genotype, is usually considered as inherently conservative in its social implications.*

---

*Graham, Loren R.: Political ideology and genetic theory: Russia and Germany in the 1920s, Hastings Center Report 7(5):34, October 1977. Reprinted with the permission of The Hastings Center: © Institute of Society, Ethics and the Life Sciences, 360 Broadway, Hastings-on-Hudson, N.Y. 10706.

The science of genetics is applicable to human beings *if* human beings choose to apply it to themselves. However, its development is so new that greater disaster than benefit would probably result from using genetic principles to attempt to improve the human race. Many believe that science remains the best hope to correct the political and social mess we have made of the world, but to blame science or to pin hopes on it for future remedies is naive. Human beings apply scientific principles and technologic possibilities to achieve their own ends and the application of genetic principles is not likley to cure social ills that have resulted from human greed and misplaced values. Rival genetic theories have been used by rival political theorists to advocate various social and political systems. In Chapter 9 on human experimentation it will be shown how the popular scientific beliefs of the day "proved" Negroes to be not only an inferior race of people but also "natural" breeders and carriers of syphilis. These infamous beliefs led to the reprehensible Tuskegee Syphilis Study. Various social systems have thought they had proved specific groups of people (almost always minorities, it should be noted) were genetically inferior to other groups and then set out to eliminate those inferior groups, with varying degrees of success. The whole idea of racial superiority is probably scientific nonsense, but even if it is not and if one race, or a segment of a race *could* be proved superior or better in some way, then what? Action taken on this information would depend on the political and class system that dominated the society that discovered it. The *knowledge* itself would mean nothing, as does parents' knowledge that one of their children is smarter than the other. What is done about the knowledge means everything. Graham points out that a

value-free interpretation of these [genetic] theories of human heredity is persuasive only if the links of science and society are severed, and if science is viewed in abstract isolation from its setting. In fact, every scientific theory and every technological innovation *always* exists in a social and political setting, and the value impacts of these combinations can be massive.*

Thus we have the untouchables in India, centuries of slaughter of Jews, apartheid in South Africa, racism in the United States and elsewhere, Sino-Japanese wars, and every other atrocity that uses genetics as its justification, no matter how thinly veiled.

Veatch[18] presents a case in which an American accused the state of genocide. Wilbur Johnson and Mae Sanford, both black, decided to marry and have a family. When they appeared for the premarital venereal disease blood test, they learned that their state also required black applicants for a marriage license to be tested for sickle-cell disease. Sickle-cell disease is autosomal recessive; that is, both parents must be carriers before there is a risk of producing a child with the disease. When both parents are carriers, each child has a risk of 25% of having the disease. Mr. Johnson had a younger brother who died of the disease; therefore both his parents

---

*Graham, Loren R.: Political ideology and genetic theory: Russia and Germany in the 1920s, Hastings Center Report 7(5):34, October 1977. Reprinted with the permission of The Hastings Center: © Institute of Society, Ethics and the Life Sciences, 360 Broadway, Hastings-on-Hudson, N.Y. 10706.

were carriers, and the chances were 50% that he was also. About one black in 12 is a carrier of the trait. Two prospective parents who are both carriers have only three options: (1) they risk a 25% chance for each child to have sickle-cell disease, (2) they can resort to artificial insemination with sperm of a noncarrier donor, or (3) they can refrain from childbearing altogether. Mr. Johnson found all these choices unacceptable and argued that mandatory testing for sickle-cell disease in blacks is an attempt by a white-dominated society to control the reproductive capacity of blacks and thus is tantamount to genocide. The government's beneficence in providing free information to blacks is merely a guise for frightening them and discouraging them from bearing children. He refused to be tested, as did his fiancee.

Mr. Johnson's point is well taken although his rationale may not be entirely accurate. Since there is no treatment for sickle-cell disease except for a degree of palliation, there is no point in making screening mandatory. Even if there were treatment, mandatory screening for one particular minority group does raise one's suspicions about racism. Tay-Sachs disease is also automosal recessive, but Ashkenazic Jews are not required by law to be tested prior to marriage. PKU testing is mandatory for newborn infants, but there is a treatment if this metabolic disease is detected (although the treatment is by no means totally effective) and the mandatory testing is therefore based on a specific rationale. It is also likely that if a parent refused to have a newborn infant tested for PKU, that refusal would be upheld in court. Syphilis screening prior to marriage and during pregnancy is required by law in most states but syphilis is a contagious disease that affects public health and safety. Sickle-cell testing should surely be encouraged among blacks and educational programs about the disease and its effects should be increased, but one must question the state's right to interfere with an individual's right to bodily privacy and autonomy by making sickle-cell testing mandatory. "The responsibility to make informed parental decisions does not necessarily justify a compulsory information supplying program."[18,p.205]

OUTCOMES AND POSSIBILITIES

Genetic manipulation provides so much food for futuristic thought that the mind boggles. The possibilities are endless, and each day brings us closer to those possibilities. Some disasters are inevitable, but the existence of diaster does not necessarily mean that research should be halted. Erwin Chargoff, professor emeritus of biochemistry at Columbia University, said, "Anyone affirming immediate disaster is a charlatan, but anyone denying the possibility of its occurring is an even greater one."[20]

The commercial possibilities of recombinant DNA research seem most applicable in the pharmaceutical industry where genetic replacement of substances missing from the body may lead to cure or control of many genetic diseases. Manufacturing antibiotics and biologicals may be faster and cheaper using cloned bacteria than by present synthetic methods. Now that the Supreme Court has ruled that it is legally permissible to patent newly discovered life forms, genetic research can be expected to proceed at an increased rate. When all cell reproduction becomes more clearly understood, there is likelihood that the causes of cancer will also become known, and this will ultimately lead to cures. The aging process might be slowed or perhaps synchronized so that different parts of the body wear out at approximately the same time.

Possibilities in correctly genetic disease are almost limitless, as are the possibilities of using knowledge about genetic manipulation for the most socially horrendous means. The choice is ours to make.

SUMMARY

Genetic manipulation almost automatically implies cloning, although other processes are also involved in general genetic manipulation. Cloning is the exact duplication of any nonsex cell by stimulation of that cell to begin mitosis and from there to grow into a complete organism that is an exact genetic duplicate of its parent. The description sounds simple and in theory the process is, but cloning has been in experimentation for decades and so far only bacteria, viruses, plants, and amphibians have been successfully cloned. Human beings have not and probably will not be cloned for several more decades.

Other forms of genetic manipulation include somatic cell alteration, germ cell alteration, reversal of differentiation of somatic cells, and recombinant DNA.

The uses to which genetic manipulation could be put are almost endless and the potential for both good and evil is also limitless. The nature of humanity could be unalterably changed, but there is no way to predict exactly what changes will occur; therein lie both excitement and danger. If we find a cure for cancer, we might at the same time tip the evolutionary balance to create a scourge far worse than cancer. Whether the risk of all genetic research should be taken depends on society's values and what it sees as acceptable directions for genetic research.

Regulation of research is a hotly debated issue. Scientists are suspicious of any attempts to control or stop inquiry; they maintain that new knowledge is useful, not only for its own sake but also for the benefits it can provide to human beings. Some religious leaders and lay people believe that experimenting with life processes is too dangerous for human beings and that whatever good might result is not worth the risks taken. Several attempts at federal regulation have been made, but they are all fairly impotent. It took the public a relatively long time to become interested in genetic research, and it still does not command the vociferous attention of other bioethical issues perhaps because the public does not see genetic manipulation as a direct concern to their own lives. Only a minority are actively concerned about the future.

Ethical issues in genetic manipulation revolve around what will be done with the knowledge gained from research and what the social and political costs will be. Will we permit ourselves to be dominated by technology at the expense of humanitarian ideals, or can the two coexist? Should scientists be permitted to experiment with the nature of life (and presumably to alter it as they see fit), or should they be restricted from doing so? If restraints are imposed, what boundaries will be established?

Eugenics, or "good breeding," is used to improve the condition and capacity of a species. Animal breeders have been using eugenics for centuries, but the principles applied to human beings raise complex issues. Should natural selection be interfered with? If so, what genetic qualities should be bred into humans of the future and what qualities eliminated? Three basic patterns can be used in human genetics: (1) selection against monogenic defects, (2) selection of especially desirable germ cells, and (3) differential reproduction of large groups. Each has advantages and disadvantages, and each has serious racist overtones. Genocide or certainly a significant alteration of specific groups of people is a distinct possibility in eugenics. The decision to adopt a particular eugenic program would be so dangerous and value-laden that it would seem a foolhardy course of action. It also is unlikely that the majority of people are now ready to put such an idea into practice.

Genetic screening is the process by which some genetic traits or defects are detected in carriers, fetuses, or people who already have a genetic disease. Genetic counseling is the providing of information to people about the results of the screening. It usually involves a discussion of statistical chances for bearing a child with a specific genetic disease or trait and treatment or prevention options available to parents or prospective parents. Genetic disease or the trait is detected by chromosomal karyotyping of any human cell or fetal cells by amniocentesis. Genetic screening is a valuable detection tool, particularly for groups of people especially prone to certain genetic diseases, but making it mandatory is another matter and involves principles of liberty and autonomy. There are probably diseases that could be eliminated by prohibition of reproduction or selective abortion, but the long-term effects of such drastic action cannot possibly be predicted.

Truth telling, confidentiality, personal privacy, paternalism, and autonomy are all issues in genetic screening and counseling. It seems likely that the debate about these will increase in intensity as science and technology create more possibilities in the realm of genetic manipulation.

REFERENCES

1. Abrams, Maxine: Frogs, asparagus and you—the real meaning of cloning, The Philadelphia Inquirer, Today magazine, p. 15, October 29, 1978.
2. Davis, Bernard D.: Prospects for genetic intervention in man, Science **170**:1279-1283.
3. Kass, Leon R.: The new biology: what price relieving man's estate? Science **174**:779-788, November 19, 1971.
4. Sinsheimer, Robert: Troubled dawn for genetic engineering, New Scientist: The Weekly Review of Science and Technology (London) **68**, October 16, 1975.
5. Callahan, Daniel: Recombinant DNA: science and the public, Hastings Center Report **7**(2):20, April 1977.
6. Dismukes, Key: Recombinant DNA: a proposal for regulation, Hastings Center Report **7**(2):25, April 1977.
7. Signer, Ethan: Gene manipulation and the role of science. In Wertz, Richard W., editor: Readings on ethical and social issues in biomedicine, Englewood Cliffs, N. J., 1973, Prentice-Hall, Inc.
8. Fletcher, Joseph: The ethics of genetic control, New York, 1974, Doubleday & Co., Inc.
9. Roblin, Richard: The Boston XYY case, Hastings Center Report **5**(4):5-8, August 1975.
10. Davis, Bernard D.: Threat and promise in genetic engineering. In Williams, Preston N.: Ethical issues in biology and medicine: proceedings of a symposium on the identity and dignity of man, Cambridge, Mass., 1972, Schenkman Publishing Co.
11. Lederberg, Joshua: Experimental genetics and human evolution, Bulletin of Atomic Scientists **22**:5-6, October 1966.
12. Beauchamp, Tom L., and Walters, LeRoy: Comtemporary issues in bioethics, Belmont, Calif., 1978, Wadsworth Publishing Co.

13. Friedmann, Theodore: Prenatal diagnosis of genetic disease, Scientific American **225**(5):34-42, November 1971.

14. Callahan, Daniel: The meaning and significance of genetic disease: philosophical perspectives. In Hilton, Bruce, et al., editors: Ethical issues in human genetics: genetic counseling and the use of genetic knowledge, New York, 1973, Plenum Publishing Corp.

15. The Research Group on Ethical, Social, and Legal Issues in Genetic Counseling and Genetic Engineering of the Institute of Society, Ethics, and the Life Sciences: Ethical and social issues in screening for genetic disease, New England Journal of Medicine **286**:1129-1132, 1972.

16. Fletcher, John: Moral problems in genetic counseling, Pastoral Psychology **23**:47-60, April 1972.

17. Ramsey, Paul: Screening: an ethicist's view. In Hilton, Bruce, et al., editors: Ethical issues in human genetics: genetic counseling and the use of genetic knowledge, New York, 1973, Plenum Publishing Corp.

18. Veatch, Robert M.: Case studies in medical ethics, Cambridge, 1977, Harvard University Press.

19. Graham, Loren R.: Political ideology and genetic theory: Russia and Germany in the 1920s, Hastings Center Report **7**(5):30-39, October 1977.

20. Powledge, Tabitha: Recombinant DNA: the argument shifts, Hastings Center Report **7**(2):19, April 1977.

BIBLIOGRAPHY

Abrams, Maxine: Frogs, asparagus and you—the real meaning of cloning, The Philadelphia Inquirer, Today magazine, p. 14, October 29, 1978.

Beauchamp, Tom L., and Walters, LeRoy: Contemporary issues in bioethics, Belmont, Calif., 1978, Wadsworth Publishing Co.

Callahan, Daniel: Recombinant DNA: science and the public, Hastings Center Report **7**(2):20-24, April 1977.

Callahan, Daniel: The meaning and significance of genetic disease: philosophical perspectives. In Hilton, Bruce, et al. editors: Ethical issues in human genetics: genetic counseling and the use of genetic knowledge, New York, 1973, Plenum Publishing Corp.

Callahan, Daniel: The moral career of genetic engineering, Hastings Center Report **9**(2):9, April 1979.

Davis, Bernard D.: Prospects for genetic intervention in man, Science **170**:1279-1283, December 18, 1970.

Davis, Bernard D.: Threat and promise in genetic engineering. In Williams, Preston N., editor: Ethical issues in biology and medicine: proceedings of a symposium on the identity and dignity of man, Cambridge, Mass., 1973, Schenkman Publishing Co.

Dedek, John F.: Contemporary medical ethics, New York, 1975, Sheed & Ward, Inc.

Dismukes, Key: Recombinant DNA: a proposal for regulation, Hastings Center Report **7**(2):25-30, April 1977.

Fletcher, John: Moral problems in genetic counseling, Pastoral Psychology **23**:47-60, April 1972.

Fletcher, Joseph: The ethics of genetic control, New York, 1974, Doubleday & Co., Inc.

Friedmann, Theodore: Prenatal diagnosis of genetic disease, Scientific American **255**(5):34-42, November 1971.

Golding, Martin P.: Ethical issues in biological engineering, UCLA Law Review **15**:443-479, 1968.

Graham, Loren R.: Political ideology and genetic theory: Russia and Germany in the 1920s, Hastings Center Report **7**(5):30-39, October 1977.

Gustafson, James M.: Genetic engineering and the normative view of the human. In Williams, Preston N.: Ethical issues in biology and medicine: proceedings of a symposium on the identity and dignity of man, Cambridge, Mass., 1972, Schenkman Publishing Co.

Kass, Leon R.: The new biology: what price relieving man's estate? Science **174**:779-788, November 19, 1971.

Leach, Gerald: The biocrats, New York, 1970, McGraw-Hill Book Co.

Lederberg, Joshua: Experimental genetics and human evolution, Bulletin of Atomic Scientists **22**:5-6, October 1966.

Nelson, James B.: Human medicine: ethical perspectives on new medical issues, Minneapolis, 1973, Augsburg Publishing House.

Powledge, Tabitha M.: Recombinant DNA: backing off on legislation, Hastings Center Report **7**(6):8-10, December 1977.

Powledge, Tabitha M.: Recombinant DNA: the argument shifts, Hastings Center Report **7**(2):18-19, April 1977.

Ramsey, Paul: Screening: an ethicist's view. In Hilton, Bruce, et al., editors: Ethical issues in human genetics: genetic counseling and the use of genetic knowledge, New York, 1973, Plenum Publishing Corp.

The Research Group on Ethical, Social, and Legal Issues in Genetic Counseling and Genetic Engineering of the Institute of Society, Ethics, and the Life Sciences: Ethical and social issues in screening for genetic disease, New England Journal of Medicine **286**:1129-1132, 1972.

Roblin, Richard: The Boston XYY case, Hastings Center Report **5**(4):5-8, August 1975.

Signer, Ethan: Gene manipulation and the role of science. In Wertz, Richard W.: Readings on ethical and social issues in biomedicine, Englewood Cliffs, N.J., 1973, Prentice-Hall, Inc.

Sinsheimer, Robert: Troubled dawn for genetic engineering, New Scientist: The Weekly Review of Science and Technology (London) **68**, October 16, 1975.

Vaux, Kenneth: Biomedical ethics, New York, 1974, Harper & Row, Publishers, Inc.

Veatch, Robert M.: Case studies in medical ethics, Cambridge, Mass., 1977, Harvard University Press.

Watson, James D.: The future of asexual reproduction, Intellectual Digest **2**(2):115-125, 1971.

Williams, Preston N.: Ethical issues in biology and medicine: proceedings of a symposium on the identity and dignity of man, Cambridge, Mass., 1972, Schendman Publishing Co.

Wojcik, Jan: Muted consent: a casebook in modern medical ethics, West Lafayette, Ind., 1978, Purdue Research Foundation.

4

Overpopulation

PROBLEM OF OVERPOPULATION

Too many people live on earth. In many places we are physically too close together, much too close for comfort, and in total there are too many of us for available natural resources. The phrase "population explosion" is accurate. In 1850 approximately a billion people lived on earth; in only 80 years that number doubled, and in only 40 more years the original billion had tripled. If the present growth rate continues, the world population will reach 8 billion by the year 2000.

Not only are the sheer numbers frightening, but growth rates in different areas of the world cause varying problems. Those areas that can least afford a population growth—Latin America, Africa, the Middle East (except Israel), and Asia—are experiencing the highest growth rates. The countries of North America and Europe that could easily absorb an increased population have the lowest growth rates.[1] About a third of the world's population is in adolescence, although in poorer countries where the population is expanding at a more rapid rate, the proportion of people in their childbearing years is even greater. Thus the population explosion is only beginning, and if present trends continue it can and will worsen.

Perhaps we should look further at this staggering number. For example, all of the more than three billion people alive on earth today could be packed—one per square yard—within the confines of metropolitan Chicago, and almost 1.5 billion could be put into Detroit and its suburbs. But bear in mind that at our present rate of growth this would be the situation, not in a few Chicagos and Detroits, but over the whole face of the earth, including deserts, mountains, polar icecaps, and oceans. And this is not in some dim, incalculable millenium, but in a few hundred years—hardly longer than from Columbus' first glimpse of America to the present day.*

One person per square yard. The image that invokes is horrifying: hordes of people as far as the eye can see, standing upright with their arms at their sides because if they swing their arms or hold them akimbo they would encroach on the next person's square yard. Given the likely social and emotional climate, a fight to the death would ensue. This chapter will explore some of the implications and

---

*Augenstein, Leroy: Come, let us play God, p. 55. Copyright © 1969 by Harper and Row, New York.

ethical considerations of drastic population growth and the effect it would have on human beings as they function as individuals and in groups.

We are already experiencing the effects of runaway population. In Calcutta every morning municipal "street cleaners" make early rounds to collect the bodies of those who starved to death overnight and were placed on the street to be picked up for mass burial; no morning goes by without a considerable collection of bodies. In New York City during rush hour in the subway the trains are so tightly packed with people that a woman whom I saw faint did not fall to the ground because the press of people held her up; it was only when the mass of people shifted for a station stop that she swayed, fell, and was nearly trampled. Two thirds of the nations of the world are sinking into poverty so rapidly that no amount of foreign aid from more developed countries will be able to stem the tide of starvation *unless* the number of people to be fed is substantially reduced.

Some people in highly developed technologic countries think that an expanding population is good for business and thus good for the economy. Industry needs mass markets to consume the goods and services it produces, and increased number of people are needed to manufacture the products, a situation that leads to a rise in employment and consumer spending. There is, however, a point at which this argument becomes self-defeating. When increased technology leads to increased automation, unemployment will become a problem and leisure time will increase to the point at which wear and tear on the already endangered environment will become unmanageable. The environment will no longer provide resources necessary for production of the goods and services we covet. This kind of economic speculation is an exercise in futility because population trends are hard to predict, except in terms of gross figures on a worldwide basis.

Demographers have more cause to blush than amateur weather forecasters. They not only missed the post-war baby booms, for instance, but also the falling birth-rates that followed them in the 1960s. Population forecasting is fiendishly difficult. The future size and structure of a population depends on a long list of factors—from death-rates at each age group to the age of marriage, the proportion of women marrying, average family size and how far babies are spaced out—factors which are continuously changing, are independent of each other and may have opposite effects.*

Causes

The causes of the population explosion are so complex that leading sociologists and demographers do not understand them. Some contributing factors, however, seem clear. Perhaps the greatest single factor is not so much an *increased* birth rate, but the *decreased* death rate, specifically in two areas: increased life expectancy and a decline in infant mortality. At the beginning of the Christian era life expectancy was about 30 years; today in Western countries the average is about 72 years.[1] With more infants surviving to reach sexual maturity (this is a truer description of developed countries than undeveloped ones, though infant mortality has been steadily declining all over the world), the number of births naturally in-

---

*Leach, Gerald: The biocrats, New York, 1970, McGraw Hill Inc. pp. 50-51.

creases. Both the increase in life expectancy and the decrease in infant mortality result from technology and scientific progress; the greatest single event probably was the development of the germ theory of disease. Once we got rid of the idea that spirits and hobgoblins were killing people and began decimating germs, we began the spiral to out-of-control population growth. It could safely be said that no one regrets the development of the germ theory or wants to return to the witch doctor phase of health care, but we *did* open a Pandora's box of population growth when we started washing our hands, sterilizing our surgical instruments, and injecting ourselves with antibiotics.

As technology increased in Europe and North America, large families were no longer necessary or fashionable. People moved off farms and into cities to take advantage of what technology and industrialization had to offer. Birth control techniques were improved to the point where a couple could control the number of children they had. As the cost of living rose, children became an economic burden and family size decreased. This situation did not develop in the rest of the world, which remained largely agrarian and technologically underdeveloped (with a few notable exceptions such as Japan and South Africa). Birth rates in underdeveloped countries are still high, but death rates are beginning to decline because the developed Western countries are exporting medical, industrial, and agricultural technology.

For a variety of reasons the export of birth control knowledge and use has not been as successful as the export of automotive technology and new ways of planting fields and harvesting crops. Little research has been done to determine why people in poor countries continue to bear more and more children, even when they are surrounded by mass starvation—even when they themselves have stomachs that constantly rumble with hunger. A woman whose body has been ravaged by the birth of too many children, who has watched her infants starve to death, and who is pregnant yet again is an enigma to us. We cannot imagine what her thoughts, feelings, and needs are. The United Nations has declared overpopulation to be the most pressing world problem of this century and the next and has mounted vigorous birth control campaigns, especially in India, the Orient, Latin America, and Africa. Yet birth rates continue to rise despite increased dissemination of birth control information. Industrialized countries have complacently assumed that as soon as birth control information and technology become readily available to the masses of people who appear to need it most, they will begin to use it and the birth rate will drop. This has not occurred. People resist artificially controlling their procreative powers for a variety of reasons: tradition, superstition, what is seen as an economic need, culture, sexual taboos, fear of change, and suspicion of technology. Until we discover what motivates people to keep bearing children even in the face of certain starvation and death, the population explosion will continue.

Another issue overrides even the discovery of cause: does one nation or a group of nations have the right to try to control the population of another nation or group? Or at its basic level, does one human being have the right to force, coerce, or even convince another human being not to have a child? Do the needs of society in general preclude the unrestricted personal rights of people to use their bodies as they choose? These questions are the crux of ethical issues involved in population control and the basis of the exploration of various problem areas throughout this chapter.

Consequences

The problem is not so much the number of people but the number of people *in relation to* the amount of resources available: air, water, food, space to grow food, and room to move about without bumping into someone at every turn. The alternative to controlling world population is death by starvation or by personal or international violence. If I am hungry and my children are too weak from hunger to move, I may use my last shred of strength to kill you for the piece of bread you hold in your hand. It is not likely that I will feel guilt, for the morals and customs that accompany mass starvation will have made that kind of guilt a quaint anachronism. Not only would I kill you for a piece of bread, but you might face death if you stepped into my allotted personal territory, drank a drop of my water ration, or came near my air purifier. You would kill me too if you perceived that I was threatening you in any of these ways. Violence and death are the major consequences of overpopulation. There are others.

Even in areas of the world where people might not be literally starving (the United States, Canada, and some of the wealthier European countries), food would be scarce and expensive, especially foods that require much land to produce such as meat (with the exception of poultry) and produce. Most of our diet would likely consist of synthetic food substitutes. Living space would also be a problem, for there would be no place to get away from it all, and group living would be the norm. (Even now we have an inkling of what is to come: to camp in any of the several national parks in the Western United States in summer, it is necessary to make a reservation months in advance.) As a single person I would never be permitted to live alone in the spacious two-bedroom townhouse I now occupy; a small room in a vast complex for unmarried people would probably be my allocation. Problems that plague any overcrowded urban area today—dirt, rats and other vermin, crime and violence, poor sanitation, lack of privacy, and noise—will multiply by a thousand. The hideous picture comes into focus:

For multitudes, adequate clothing is rare. Education is a novelty. Rotting teeth and festering sores are daily companions. Brains and bodies are permanently damaged by lack of proper food. Sapped by disease, gnawed by hunger, devoid of hope, with pain as a daily companion, life itself is torment. Often they resemble walking skeletons. They are the living dead of the earth.*

Suicide would increase. The ethical problems of euthanasia and prolongation of life discussed in Chapter 12 would no longer be moral dilemmas, for society might not be able to afford to keep those people alive who showed the slightest sign of weakening. Pollution would be so widespread and pervasive that we would no more venture outdoors without our gas masks than we would now without our clothes.

---

*Frazier, Claude A. Is it moral to modify man? p. 52, 1973. Courtesy of Charles C Thomas, Publisher, Springfield, Illinois.

While population is increasing technology will be advancing, but will scientific discoveries be enough and in time to overtake the population explosion? For example, building the Aswan Dam in Egypt was one of the greatest engineering feats of all time. The waters of the Nile backed up behind the dam are used to irrigate new land and increase food production by an estimated 20%. But during the building of the dam the population of Egypt increased 30%; the net result is that Egypt is now 10% further *behind* in feeding its population than before the dam was started. Being 10% behind is better than 30%, but that is a small consolation. Technology was not sufficient to solve the problem. Will medicine and science be able to keep up with the epidemics that are certain to arise as a result of overpopulation? Will social scientists be able to cope with the violence and aggression that will breed when we are all living on top of one another?

One of the direst consequences of overpopulation would be changes in the way we live. Look at a photograph of Jones Beach in New York City on a hot summer Sunday; it is difficult to see the sand for the people. The entire United States shoreline from Maine to Florida, from Washington to Southern California, would look like that every day, every summer. National parks would have been decimated for their trees and the land area used for living space. Private transportation would be a thing of the past; world oil supplies would be depleted, and nuclear-powered transport would be operated by government and big business.

What would we do for recreation and pleasure? What about sex, which is generally considered recreational and pleasurable? Augenstein[2] reported an experiment with rats that was conducted by the National Institutes of Health. The experimenters built four large pens with runways connecting the enclosures; in each pen were comfortable resting and sleeping areas. Equal numbers of males and females were put into the enclosure, and an overpopulated situation was created. Very soon the two biggest and most aggressive male rats established harems by sleeping at the foot of the runways leading to the enclosures. When the animals came down the runway, females were allowed to pass but males were chased away. In the two center pens where there was a predominance of males, problems began to develop. Experimenters observed growing neurotic behaviors, notable among them abnormal sex practices. When females came into heat, the males copulated with them relentlessly until the females dropped from exhaustion. During pregnancy the females did not establish nests as is usual among rats, and when the pups were born their mothers simply dropped them and walked away, left them to be cannibalized by the others. The males indulged in homosexual behavior and tried to copulate with females even when they were not in heat, which is very unusual for rats. This experiment conjures up a vision of what our "sex lives" could be like if we reached this stage of overpopulation.

Since the physical oppression of women is an aggressive behavior sometimes engaged in by men who feel threatened, we could expect an increase in rape and other forms of sexual assault as a result of overcrowding. In many cultures women are seen as property on a par with land, cattle, and other forms of material wealth, and thus slavery for women or the establishment of harems might be the norm as men fought for and bartered whatever they owned to gain a bit of land or food. If

KANSAS SCHOOL OF RELIGION
UNIVERSITY OF KANSAS
1300 OREAD AVENUE
LAWRENCE, KANSAS 66044

women were organized into harems or sold into slavery, both male and female homosexuality would increase. Those men who had little or no access to available women would turn to each other, as would women who might seek comfort, solace, and sexual gratification from each other. It is unlikely that except for a lucky few sex would continue to be seen as recreational and pleasurable.

What about the way we work? Since there would not be sufficient jobs for everyone who would get them and what would everyone else *do* all day? They could not move around much, as recreation would be severely limited and no one would have much money. The only commodity in ample supply and equally available to everyone would be time: time to think about the miserable state of affairs, to develop neuroses and psychoses, to hatch plans for getting a bit more of everything, to grow bored, short-tempered, and murderous.

Possible remedies

In India and Japan the government has mounted a widespread birth control campaign with advertising, free materials, door-to-door and village-to-village information teams, and even financial incentives for sterilization. The Indian birth rate *increased* 1.2% during the first 16 years of the campaign, but the rate in Japan declined rapidly during the same period.[3] The change in the latter probably resulted from two factors: Japan is an island where overcrowding tends to be more noticeable, and the industrialization and Westernization of the country increased rapidly after World War II.

If population cannot be controlled, then food and space must be increased. We must decide whether to use land for growing food or housing people. Vast land areas *are* now unpopulated, but for a reason: they are deserts, dense forests, polar ice caps, mountain ranges, and places like the Steppes of Asia and river jungles of South America. The cost of making this land either arable or hospitable for living is probably too enormous for any government or group of governments to undertake. There are also possibilities of growing food in the sea, culturing microbes for protein, using algae as nutrition, and breeding whales and dolphins for food if the increasing number and magnitude of oil spills does not make ocean farming impractical. All these ideas are possible, and research is going on in these and other areas, but practical application of the research is still far in the future and will require billions of dollars in capital expenditure. Will it then be too little and too late—another Aswan Dam? Exporting people to other planets is another idea but is more fantasy than workable. Interstellar or even interplanetary transport is so far in the future that by the time the first load of emigrants was ready to take off for Alpha Centauri, we would have all starved to death or killed each other in another way. By that time, at our present rate of population growth, the earth would be so solidly packed that humanity could not survive. The universe beyond the earth offers no escape, for though the future may hold an answer, we may not survive long enough to make use of it.

When the population reaches a certain point, large numbers of people will die by war, disease, and starvation. That is one way to control population, however undesirable. We see it beginning now. The crude death rate, infant mortality, and the death rate from a variety of diseases are higher in inner city ghettos populated by poor people than in areas where living conditions are not so harsh. Health and social welfare professionals work to stem this tide of high death rates, but their work will be for naught in the event of overpopulation. Controlling population size by condoning or possibly encouraging mass suffering is not the answer to the problem.

There remains only one workable solution to avert disaster: birth control. We simply must decrease and somehow continue to regulate the number of people who are born. Whether it is done voluntarily or by government mandate, it must be done. This position is taken by many economists, demographers, social planners, and politicians, but it is not universally popular. The effects of birth control on various aspects of our lives may not all be popular, but it seems the only viable alternative to mass misery and death. The following approaches could be taken to lower the birth rate; ramifications of all will be discussed throughout the chapter.

1. Voluntary cooperation of all families (it is a common myth in North America and Europe that poor, nonwhite families have more children than do middle- and upper-class whites) to have no more than two children. This method is called zero population growth: the two children replace their parents, but total population does not increase. The concept is gaining popularity very slowly, and a massive extensive public education program would have to be mounted. Voluntary limiting of family size is least likely to work in those countries where the birth rate is most out of control.

2. Mass worldwide distribution of free birth control devices with accompanying education about use. This is beginning through the United Nations, but the process is long and slow and attitudes about interference with sexual functioning are extremely difficult to modify.

3. Voluntary sterilization of one of the couple (the surgery involved is faster and less complex for a man than a woman) after they have had two children.

4. Compulsory birth control programs ranging from very stringent (compulsory sterilization) to relatively relaxed (for example, higher tax rates for a family with more than two children). The methods suggested include requiring a license to conceive, with heavy fines for noncompliance; adding contraceptive drugs to the water supply during certain months to limit the number of conceptions per year; mandatory abortion after the two-child limit has been reached; and compelling those couples who have not yet had two children to adopt the "surplus" children of other couples.

All these suggestions for compulsory birth control are highly controversial. Some are probably quite immoral in and of themselves though perhaps not so immoral when viewed in comparison to the alternatives. All would require long and vociferous public debate, and all involve incredibly complex ethical issues. We cannot, however, continue to reproduce at the rate we are now. We must stop ourselves.

CROWDING, AGGRESSION, AND VIOLENCE

Violence has become a way of life in all parts of the world; as population increases, so does violence. In Bombay or Calcutta a man might put a knife through your heart on a crowded street in broad daylight for the apple you hold in your hand. In parts of Africa CARE workers who distribute food drop the sacks from helicopters because when food was distributed by hand the workers were killed or badly injured in the human stampede. Even with the helicopter drops it is not uncommon for the hungry to trample each other to death in their rush for the food. In the United States we are not yet killing each other for apples or sacks of grain, but murders are committed because some can no longer tolerate the crush of people or pace of life. Americans are more and more dealing with their feelings of anger, hostility, frustration, and hopelessness by physically lashing out at each other. Half of all murder victims know their assailant, and domestic violence is increasing. Police in large cities, particularly in crowded areas, know that when people are cooped up together because of bad weather, when they are trapped in large crowds, or when their tempers are frazzled by heat, humidity, and closeness, the murder rate increases. Some think that human beings enjoy violence and are not likely to change.

For 600 years the citizens of ancient Rome watched with pleasure circuses in which men killed each other or were killed by wild animals. Hundreds of thousands of gladiators thus perished in municipal arenas to the delight of the public. Today we get vicarious thrills out of seeing actors die violent deaths nightly on television in our living rooms.*

Hoagland[4] reports that in 1 week the violence displayed on television included 114 murders, 143 attempted murders, 52 justified killings, 14 cases of drugging, 13 kidnappings, 7 cases of torture, 1 massacre scene in which hundreds were killed, plus assorted muggings jailbreaks, robberies, thefts, and burglaries. Football, a much more violent sport than baseball, has surpassed the latter in national spectatorship, and hockey, more violent even than football, is rapidly gaining popularity. Passers-by always slow down to see as much as possible of a traffic accident and seem vaguely disappointed if there is not much blood. Movies that portray violence, particularly sexual violence, seem to do a large box office business and are much in demand by the public.

The relationship between crowding and physical violence is close. Animal studies have shown that crowding beyond certain limits, either in nature or in captivity, leads to a breakdown in social order, fighting to the death, cannabalism of the young, and severe alteration of certain reproductive processes. In this way the population of species of lower animals is controlled when it exceeds a certain density or passes a critical point in the survival of the species. Some "primitive" societies also experience war, famine, and disease on a cyclic basis for much the same reason.[4] Reduction in population may also be a by-product of overcrowding. The cause-effect relationship may work in several ways.

These cyclic fluctuations of populations with crowding have been demonstrated with rats, mice, hares, monkeys, lemmings, deer, and many other species, including a host of insect species. Among mammals, the dying off with crowding is characterized by overactivity

---

*Hoagland, Hudson: Biological consideration of agression, violence and crowding. In Williams, Preston, editor: Ethical issues in biology and medicine: proceedings of a symposium on the identity and dignity of man, Cambridge, 1973, Schenkman Publishing Co., pp. 66, 68.

of the adrenal cortex called upon via the hypothalamic pituitary axis to meet competitive stresses. The stress response mechanism ultimately breaks down if the stresses of crowding are sufficiently prolonged and severe. The overstressed adrenocortical system may produce atherosclerosis, hypertension, and enhanced susceptibility to infectious agents and a variety of other endocrine and metabolic disorders resulting ultimately in increased death rates, thus reducing the animal population.*

Concentration camp victims were known to have had overactivity of the adrenals, and hypertension tends to be more common in crowded ghettos than it does in more spacious areas. It could therefore be predicted that overpopulation will cause disease and death from stress reaction in addition to increasing aggression and violence. Another view is that the long history of tension and stress resulting from overcrowded ghetto conditions, particularly in black urban America, causes a generational and unrelenting rage associated with hypertension.

Hoagland reports some fascinating experiments to enhance or reduce aggressive behavior in certain animals. The physiologic basis for these experiments is instinctual behavior, some of which exists in quite elaborate patterns, for example, imprinting of newborns to their mother, web spinning of spiders, squirrels burying nuts for the future (they exhibited the same burying behavior even when confined to a room with a concrete floor), mating rituals, and migration over great distances. Instinctual behavior can be changed by chemically or electrically interfering with certain neurologic tracts once they have been isolated. For example, normally docile cats that would not attack rats will do so efficiently and violently when certain areas of the lateral hypothalamus are stimulated. They exhibit all the stalking and killing behaviors of their species even though they had never been taught to stalk or provoked into doing so. Conversely, aggressive behavior can be controlled. A Norway rat is a particularly savage and completely untamable animal that bites and slashes at the slightest provocation. Following bilateral amygdalectomy (the amygdala is part of the brain's limbic system, which is one of the loci of emotions) the rats could be handled as pets, stroked, and put on one's shoulder.

Electrodes can be implanted in the limbic brain of any number of animals and their behavior controlled by telemetry. In Delgado's dramatic example a ferocious Spanish bull charges a man in an arena who is armed only with a telemetric stimulating box. When the bull rushes forward, head lowered in full charge, the man pushes a button and the bull halts. He pushes another button and the bull turns and trots away like a huge docile pet. Films of this experiment are breathtaking. The implications for humans are even more fantastic; they will be discussed in detail in Chapter 8 on behavior control. Suffice it here to say that experiments on humans have produced similar effects and could be honed to a fine sophistication in the future. If overcrowding breeds violence, and all indicators are that it does, and if we continue to increase our population, the time may come when no one will dare venture out without his telemetry box to ward off attackers.

---

*Hoagland, Hudson: Biological consideration of agression, violence and crowding. In Williams, Preston, editor: Ethical issues in biology and medicine: proceedings of a symposium on the identity and dignity of man, Cambridge, 1973, Schenkman Publishing Co., pp. 66, 68.

TERRITORIALITY

Territoriality is a characteristic of most animals that live in groups, particularly those that are competitive within their own species and that compete with other species for food. The more complex the social hierarchy of a species, the greater its instinct for defense of territory and the more it will use aggression and violence. Humans, the most complex animal, have the most complex territory to defend: home, possessions, family, community, country, religious and political beliefs, status, job, and everything else they hold dear. Humans are kept constantly busy figuring out new ways to acquire more territory and increasingly violent ways to defend it. Humans use aggression to obtain and hold everything they have, from a spouse (competing with other members of the same sex) to a job to personal property. The nature of the aggression is more or less violent as the situation warrants or is perceived. As territory becomes scarcer as numbers of people increase, the amount of violence used in territoriality will increase.

Human beings attack each other violently for two major reasons: (1) when they perceive themselves (including family, possessions, and beliefs) to be threatened and (2) when there is an interference with the cerebral mechanism that controls violent aggression, that veneer that protects us all from being at each other's throats whenever we *feel* angry and aggressive. Severe overcrowding will affect these two cause-effect relationships. If one's personal territory becomes increasingly smaller and more aggression had to be used to obtain it in the first place, it will be seen as more precious; thus any real or imagined threat will be met with faster and stronger violent counterattacks. What is valued most is protected most strongly, and when personal territory becomes one of the most highly valued commodites, people may fight to the death for it.

As we begin to live squashed more and more closely together, our veneer of self-control will grow thinner. Aggravations that today we accept with minimal irritation may tomorrow send us into tirades of violent rage. When we are caught in a traffic jam that takes an hour to unsnarl, we may sit in our cars and curse and fume for a while, then settle down to wait. If we are *really* frustrated we might blow the horn or pace up and down by the side of the road. But if we live in a world where the traffic piles up like this every day and if we are on our way home to the same kind of crowded conditions and have not been alone for weeks, frustration could easily reach the point of violence.

Many social scientists believe that humans are instinctually territorial, having an innate compulsion to acquire, preserve, and defend territory, and in this respect are no different from, albeit more sophisticated than, mockingbirds, eagles, and lions. If this characteristic is indeed genetic and thus ineradicable, the drive to violently defend territory and to acquire new territory will increase as the number of people on earth increases. Ardrey[5] believes the territorial imperative is stronger in humans than the sexual drive; he makes this point by asking us to compare the number of men who died for their country with the number who died for women. The number of the former would surely be impressive, even after one subtracts those men who went to war because they were forced to by their government and not out of a sense of patriotism or even a conscious sense of territorial defense.

Territoriality may indeed be instinctual in humans, but we can temper that instinct through neocortical functioning. We do the same in other areas. Sex is one of the strongest drives we have and is certainly genetic and instinctual, yet we control our impulses by the exercise of socially and culturally learned behaviors. When two people meet and find they are sexually attracted to each other, they do not immediately act on their sexual urges. Instead they channel them in a socially approved direction, such as conversing or flirting. So too can we channel our urges for acquisition of territory.

Certain stressors override inhibition of our territorial or sexual urges. War is one of those stressors, as are civil strife, famine, revolution, and other forms of social upheaval or disaster. The incidence of rape increases drastically during war, as does the taking of booty. One might say that women are seen as part of general booty, or the spoils of war. Looting, encroaching on other people's personal territory, increases immediately after any natural or man-made disaster. Not long ago I lived in an apartment complex that experienced a serious fire. It was the lead story on the 11 o'clock news that night, and before midnight I began to see strangers poking around in the burned apartments looking for things to loot. During the Watts riots of 1965 violent looting caused more destruction and personal damage than the riots themselves. These are examples of territoriality gone awry when stress becomes so overwhelming or need so great that societal, cultural, and personal inhibitions break down temporarily. But if the stress of overpopulation, crowded living conditions, and shortages of all basic commodities were *not* temporary, then the inhibitions would be permanently discarded. The process has already begun. On the evening news of a local Philadelphia television station the reporter told about the "newest fad in street crime": young toughs running up to people on crowded streets in daylight, ripping gold chains off their necks, and then racing off into the crowd. Incursions like this into other people's personal territory will become a way of life rather than a newsworthy novelty if the current population trend continues.

Awareness that the stress of overcrowding leads to breakdown of aggressive inhibitions—that if some societal conditions are not alleviated, violent aggression will increase more rapidly—should warrant political concern and action. However, solutions initiated with less than complete understanding of the problem will be less than adequate. In addition, overcrowding may cause a loss of individuality, a sense of alienation, and perhaps anonymity, a breeding ground for anger and resentment that can flare up into aggression if kindled in the right way.

Montagu disagrees with Ardrey's theory that territoriality in humans is genetic and unalterable.

In humans, on the contrary, the rules governing property are culturally determined and are learned; there is no pattern of signals common to the whole species. Hence, the diversity in different societies of such rules, and the variety of conditions encountered in which aggression in defense of property is permitted. Furthermore, territoriality, in those species that display it, seems to insure some sort of regulation of density. In humans it does not.*

---

*Montagu, Ashley: *The Nature of Human Aggression*, New York, 1976, Oxford University Press, p. 243.

Montagu goes on to say that territorial behavior depends largely on environmental conditions; for example, hamadrayas baboons in crowded zoos become extremely territorial, a behavior they do not exhibit under natural conditions. The United States Department of Fisheries in a study conducted by Langlois found that bass, if they were placed in shallow ponds with much vegetation, tended to be territorial and cannibalistic.[6] When the vegetation was cleared and the ponds deepened, the bass had more room to move around and could see the food thrown to them; they then stopped eating each other and began to live together quite amicably. Vervet monkeys show the same kind of behavior: when crowded together they become territorial and aggressive, but when they live in open country and have sufficient room to roam about, they live peaceably with each other. Hundreds of examples could be given, but it seems obvious that certain species' demonstrations of territoriality depend on environmental conditions. *Homo sapiens* is one of those species: the more crowded we are, the more nervous, short-tempered, aggressive, and violent we become.

Discussing territoriality in humans is difficult and complex. We do not simply spray urine on rocks and bushes and then snarl warningly at others who cross our self-proclaimed boundary. Defense of our property or territory depends on a wide variety of variables: how much we value the property and how hard we worked to get it, what we feel about it, in what way we perceive the encroachment on our territory, what other life experiences are going on at the same time, and what environmental or sociocultural conditions exist. The more we value the property or territory, the harder we will defend it, and the more dangerous the threat is perceived to be, the harder we fight for what we have. The more personal the property is, the greater our defense of it; that is, we will fight hardest for whatever means the most to our personal happiness.

We can also discuss territoriality in terms of closeness or remoteness to our personal selves: people who are close (family), things that are close (home, pets, personal possessions), people who are physically remote but emotionally close (members of a religious or professional group), abstract concepts or ideologies, and physical territory that is remote (nation). Physical territory is intertwined with emotional closeness; for example, we may feel remote from the vastness of the United States, but we feel a sense of territoriality about a homeland or motherland. This phenomenon is clearly seen in American Jews' attitude toward Israel, a country they may perceive as an emotional or spiritual homeland even though they choose to make the United States their actual home. They support Israel with money, and many volunteer to help physically defend it each time it is attacked. An attack on Israel is perceived as a personal attack on every Jew. In the United States this attitude is interesting and unique and is sometimes viewed by non-Jews as anti-American, leading to increased anti-Semitism. American Catholics have a sense of loyalty to Vatican City, but this is loyalty more to the Pope or to the symbolic seat of the Church than to the physical territory. There is one commonality, however: an attack on the Pope or the Vatican would be seen as a personal attack by American Catholics. The territory is remote, but the ideology is close.

When human beings are crowded into particularly small spaces, their territoriality becomes strong. Lorenz and Leyhausen[7] described this characteristic in prisoners of war. When the prisoners were moved to a new camp, the first thing each man did was to "stake out his territory" by choosing a bed in the barracks and dividing it from the rest of the room as best he could with pieces of clothing or string or by hanging a blanket in a strategic way. This distribution of living space was performed by all prisoners shortly after their arrival, and the process was acknowledged and respected by everyone. This behavior can be extended to other situations. Lorenz and Leyhausen[7] make the observation that increasing population density increases the tendency of an individual or family to mark off his or their own boundaries with even greater precision, to bolt doors, and to greet intrusions by strangers ("unauthorized persons") with distrust or open antagonism.

People can accommodate changes in living conditions and drastically reduced space, as the prisoners of war did, but only for short periods of time and if external conditions are perceived as making accommodation necessary. But if the crowded conditions continue for too long (the length of time people can tolerate crowding depends on a number of internal and external variables), tensions rise, quarreling and aggressive behavior increase, and violence breaks out.

Whether humans are genetically and instinctually territorial or this characteristic is a learned cultural and societal behavior does not seem to matter. What *does* matter, and what will have a profound effect on our future, is that we do not *like* to live too close together. Over and over we have seen from animal behavior studies, from observation of life in crowded cities, and from personal experience that when we are forced to live in close proximity to other human beings for long periods of time, when we do not have sufficient personal space, and when there is no opportunity to get away from it all, we grow snappish with each other, develop new neuroses and increase our old ones, are suspicious and paranoid, and lash out physically at the slightest provocation of threat. We begin to kill each other. There is little doubt that continued overpopulation will increase these behaviors and lead to a life that will be intolerable for most people.

Personal and international consequences

Overpopulation is an international problem caused by the most personal of human behavior: sexuality, or more specifically, unprotected sexual intercourse. The relationship between the act of intercourse, generally viewed as positive and pleasurable, and death by starvation, generally viewed as negative and pain-filled, is direct but remote. The relationship does exist; it is not an abstract concept. The hard fact is that the more acts of unprotected intercourse that take place, the more people will starve. The relationship is at the same time simple and complex, as are solutions to the problem. Theoretically one could solve the problem of overpopulation simply by reducing the number of acts of unprotected intercourse. But when the theory is applied to human beings, both individually and as members of national groups, the problem increases in complexity so much that it appears unsolvable.

The scope of the problem is best demonstrated by an example in a case study by Warwick, Merrick, and Caplan.[8] In a Latin American country both private and government organizations dispense contraceptives to all people who request them regardless of age or marital status. No one inquires whether the individual is married, and no consent is required. Considerable debate and criticism have been generated. Some leaders feel that the distribution of contraceptives to young unmarried women has led to an increase in "moral looseness" and a breakdown in traditional controls on sexual behavior. They also think that giving contraceptives to married women without the consent of their husbands has led to increased adultery. Spokesmen for the agencies distributing the contraceptives say that their only aim is to prevent unwanted births and that they are not "moral policemen." They also maintain that individuals have the right to determine the number and spacing of their own children. The moral dilemma presented is this: "To what extent is freedom of contraceptive choice and availability a higher priority value than local social or religious traditions and beliefs with respect to sexual behavior?"[8,p.17]

In his commentary on the issue Merrick[8] maintains that freedom of contraceptive choice need not threaten morals but that the manner in which information is given and contraceptives distributed could offend local sensitivities. In this case it does not appear to be social sensitivities that are at issue but a more basic question of whether access to contraception causes a moral breakdown. This hypothesis would be impossible to prove, and local leaders are not likely to put it to the test because of the strongly held belief that an unwanted pregnancy (or the risk of one) is a lesser evil than religious abrogation or the disturbance of male domination in society. Merrick thinks, as many do, that local authorities should be educated or convinced of the fact that pregnancy need not be a sanction for sexual activity, but he does acknowledge the risk of advancing one's own beliefs over local custom. The best interest of the people involved may not always be clear. The strong conviction that family planning is in the best interest of local populations may be counterproductive. "If there is a lesson in this case for American population assistance policy in the Third World, it is that attempts to understand how family planning and reproductive behavior relate to individual welfare are justified even if their main objective is not to increase acceptance of family planning."[8,p.17]

Caplan[8] thinks that the question asked at the end of the case is part of a larger moral issue: is it ever morally justified for one group of individuals to replace the moral values of another group with its own values? A desire to respect cultural diversity can lead, Caplan says, to "moral paralysis" among individuals concerned with population issues. Some believe that Western medical organizations by virtue of their size and power would inevitably alter the social and sexual mores of cultures if they intervened in attitudes and practices related to family planning. This belief maintains that since one value is as good as another, values should not be imposed; consequently Western medical organizations should not intervene in the contraceptive practices of other cultures. The imposition of medical technology on underdeveloped countries has not been an unqualified success and could be seen as coercive and unworkable. Caplan believes that because people express individual opinions and hold certain beliefs, all values should not be given equal moral weight. In the case of the Latin American nation in question he sees no place for "blind adherence to crude ethical relativism" (the belief that all values are equal).

"Any intervention into a sensitive area such as sexual behavior will prove disruptive to some degree; surely the agency has a duty to help the recipients anticipate and cope with such changes. However, disruption to prevailing values in itself is not a sound ethical reason against intervention."[8,p.17] This position implies that cultural values should be changed when they are based on misinformation, superstition, fear, or compulsion, particularly when the rights of individuals are clearly denied because of reliance on erroneous values.

The dilemma illustrated by this case is what faces population experts and family planners. There is also another issue: when a right of an individual (in this instance, to bear as many children as one wants) comes in conflict with the needs of the larger society (for adequate space, food, and air), what is to be done? In general it depends on what rights have to be given up to meet the larger needs. In population control the right at issue is one's *unrestricted* reproduction, and the need of society is adequate living space and resources for the rest of the population. In the Socratic method of solving moral problems one moral principle must take precedence over another. Prevention of starvation is more important than an individual's right to reproduce indiscriminately. Avoidance of the mass aggression and violence that would result from overcrowding is a higher priority than the right to bear children. Individual and cultural values related to reproduction are less important than feeding the world's population. In other words, the eventual fate of the world should take priority over the right of an individual couple to have an unrestricted number of children. Preservation of the *humanity* of the species supersedes all individual, cultural, and societal values, beliefs, and needs. Some feel that a solution does not have to choose one side over the other, that the species can be protected while permitting unrestrained individual reproduction. This is reminiscent of Charles Reich's theory in *The Greening of America* that individuals need not be concerned with changing the world because individual personal change will ultimately and collectively change the world. Some think this theory was developed to disguise the failure of some of the liberal movements of the 1960s and has succeeded only in producing a greater degree of self-absorption.

Another issue is that the socioeconomic development of some countries, particularly those of the Third World, influences the value of the individual, which is then reflected in increasing birth rates. In some countries people are seen as labor or political strength, and the philosophic concern of Americans and other Westerners with individual rights loses importance in countries that are striving for socioeconomic power.

War as a result

War is undoubtedly an efficient way of at least partially controlling population size, and if the next war is nuclear, even in a modified form, we will not have to worry about overpopulation. But governments claim to be working hard toward avoiding war, although individuals are not always completely opposed to it. We must, however, face the fact that as population size and overcrowding increase, so does the likelihood that violent aggression will lead to war.

Montagu[6] describes modern war as a fairly unemotional, nonhostile state of affairs. In his view it is started by statesmen with calm deliberation, directed by generals who never go near a battlefield, and fought by soldiers who have little personal contact with or feeling about their enemy. This seems an oversimplification, especially with respect to the role of individual soldiers. During the United States' last major war troops engaged in a great deal of hand-to-hand combat with the Vietnamese, and as it was mainly a guerrilla war, individual battlefields were small, often the size of a village consisting of a few huts. Soldiers *did* become personally involved with their enemy. The Arab-Israeli war, one of the most prolonged in modern times, is highly personal. But for the most part wars are started for economic and political reasons, not because of an inability to inhibit feelings of rage and aggression. The average soldier is a servant of his government and has no particular anger or feelings of aggression toward the enemy except as he perceives the enemy to be an individual who is trying to kill him.

The nature of future wars may change because of the continued erosion of inhibitions against violence resulting from overcrowding. Wars may not occur between nations; wars of overpopulation will more likely resemble the gang fights that have become so much a part of big city life. The fights in the 1950s that were romanticized and set to music by Leonard Bernstein in *West Side Story* had become a deadly game by the 1970s and could be a routine way of life by the turn of the century. In certain parts of Philadelphia (and presumably in other cities), Neighborhood Protective Associations organize volunteers to patrol the streets looking for suspicious people and unusual occurrences. They are unarmed and work in cooperation with the police, who do not have enough manpower to adequately protect high-crime neighborhoods.

So it has begun. When we cannot now rest quietly in our beds at night but must take turns pacing the streets to protect ourselves from hoodlums, we can easily project what life might be like in another 20 or 30 years. The concept of the mercenary, a soldier who fights for any country that will pay him without needing to feel a loyalty to that country, may become more popular; we may see armies of "protection" who for a price will guarantee the safety of one's territory. Or perhaps a band of thugs will turn on their employer and take his own territory from him. Gang warfare may develop to a frightening degree of sophistication. Aggressive violence may become the norm rather than the exception, and fights to the death over small plots of land may be common.

RELIGIOUS VIEWS

Thomas Malthus, a minister in the Church of England, was the first person to begin writing seriously and objectively about the population problem. In his 1798 essay "On Population," Malthus postulated that "misery and vice" in the form of war, famine, disease, malnutrition, and other factors over which humans have no control determine birth and death rates. At the time he wrote this, the population of earth had not yet reached 1 billion. Although misery and vice may or may not be the *cause* of fluctuations in the birth and death rates, there is a strong correlation between the two. Malthus almost 200 years ago urged people to exercise voluntary restraints on birth. Since no modern form of contraception existed (women were then using homemade devices in an effort not to become pregnant, the most common of which was a sponge dipped into a variety of herbs and other substances and inserted into the vagina to soak up semen), one must assume that Malthus's idea of voluntary restraint was to refrain from intercourse. No wonder the population continued to increase! Malthus proposed three hypothetical propositions that are generally still held to be true by today's demographers[9]:

1. That large numbers of people feel a need to control the number of children they produce and will do so under the right conditions (the felt-need hypothesis).
2. That motivation to exercise fertility control can be increased (moral restraint hypothesis).
3. That conditions favorable to the exercise of fertility control can be improved.

These three hypotheses form the basis for worldwide population control.

Except for Roman Catholicism and Orthodox Judaism, most of the world's great religions do not have much to say about population control as a *religious* issue; they seem to view it more as a secular and practical concern. Official Catholic doctrine, however, reinforced by encyclicals from every modern Pope, forbids use of artificial birth control, but what the Church preaches and what individual Catholics practice are not the same. Many parish priests are advising their parishioners that although the Church forbids birth control, individuals are free to attend to their own consciences and needs in the matter of family planning. No longer are priests whispering this in the privacy of the confessional; they are preaching it from the pulpit on Sundays. And the number of Catholics disobeying the Church's edict is increasing.

In a national sample interviewed before and after Pope Paul's visit (October, 1966) to the United Nations, 58% of the Catholics, compared with 55% of the non-Catholics, felt, before the Pope's visit, that the Catholic Church should ease its disapproval of contraceptive methods; directly after the Pope's visit, 55% of the Catholics and 52% of the non-Catholics still felt the same way. Catholic opinion was, however, influenced somewhat more than non-Catholic opinion by Pope Paul's statement at the United Nations calling upon the United Nations to ensure "enough bread on the tables of mankind and not to encourage artificial birth control."*

This contradictory statement by Pope Paul, repeated in essence by Pope John Paul II shortly after he assumed the papacy, may be seen to ignore the needs of individual Catholics and the world population as a whole.

One might expect the birth rate in countries that are predominantly Catholic (more than 80% of their total population) to be very high. On the contrary, the birth rate in Argentina is 21.8 per 1000; Belgium, 16.4; France, 17.7; Ireland, 22.2; Luxembourg, 15.6; Austria, 17.9, and Italy, 19.2. In comparison the United States has a birth rate of 19.4, and Bulgaria (the lowest of all countries for which data was available), 15.4.[9] These figures are from the world population data sheet compiled by the Population Reference Bureau in Washington, D.C. The Church's condem-

---

*Dyck, Arthur J.: Religious factors in the population problem. In Cutter, Donald R., editor: Updating life and death: essays in ethics and medicine, Boston, 1969, Beacon Press, p. 143.

nation of contraception, although important because it represents the official policy of a religion with several hundred million adherents, is decreasing in importance for individual Catholics. It must not, however, be discounted, because the Church is a powerful influence in international politics and can by the imposition of its moral theology impede the dissemination of birth control information and devices to those who need it.

Orthodox Judaism is as adamant about artificial birth control as Catholicism although for different reasons, and the influence of this branch of Judaism on sexual practices is barely felt in terms of world population because the proportion of Orthodox Jews to the rest of the population is less than a fraction of 1%, a number that is statistically insignificant. Orthodox Judaism has specific rules about when a husband and wife are permitted to have sexual intercourse and when they are prohibited from doing so. The prohibitions are geared to the woman's menstrual cycle, and the times she and her husband are permitted to have intercourse coincide with her most fertile period. Combined with the prohibition against artificial birth control, these rules almost ensure that the Orthodox Jewish couple will "be fruitful and multiply." The number of Jews who adhere to these rigid proscriptions is small (although increasing among younger people in the United States), and Jews generally practice artificial birth control.

In the United States and Canada the birth rate of Jews is below that for zero population growth and in Europe is quickly approaching it. In Israel, however, which has fewer Jews than New York, government officials encourage large families, and although birth control is practiced and is not illegal, it is not regarded favorably by government. This, however, is more for political and practical than religious reasons: to prevent Arabs from outnumbering Jews as citizens of Israel.

Hinduism, Buddhism, and Islam have no official sanctions against birth control, but great masses of people with these religions personally believe abstinence the only acceptable method of contraception. This is an ironic reversal of the situation seen in Catholicism, in which official policy and individual practice differ in the opposite way. We can perhaps infer from this phenomenon that people will make up their own minds about how they use their bodies regardless of official religious doctrine.

In 1937 the Mufti of Egypt issued a *fatwa* (proclamation) stating that husband and wife by mutual consent could take measures to prevent semen from entering the uterus. In 1961 in Turkey and in 1964 in Jordan similar *fatwas* were issued. Islam is, however, a very male-dominated religion, and most Moslem women who live in the Middle East are illiterate and then had no way of knowing about the existence of the *fatwas*. In an effort not to lose any of their social dominance, their husbands neglected to tell their wives that they could control the number of children they conceived. Many of the men also are illiterate and could not read the *fatwa*, but men of Islam have greater access to more informal modes of communication and dissemination of information. Because they are not forced to stay home or to remain silent in public as women are, it can be assumed that they had a greater chance of knowing about the existence of the *fatwa*.

Once women began finding out that they could control their reproductive functions, however, they began using contraception with increasing frequency. Women's obtaining this knowledge resulted from two major factors: (1) government and private organizations, as part of a worldwide population control effort, began disseminating information with teams of workers going into villages to establish clinics and informal classes, and (2) Jihan Sadat, wife of Egyptian President Anwar Sadat, urged her husband to take steps to improve the life of Egyptian women through education, health care, home economics, and birth control. As a result, some Egyptian women lead lives that although primitive and circumscribed by American standards are far more liberated than many of their Arab neighbors. The Shah of Iran, before he was deposed and exiled in 1979, also took steps to accomplish the same sort of advances for the women of his country, again largely because of his wife's urging. When the Ayatullah Khomeini took over and established an Islamic Republic in Iran, he negated all the rights the Shah had allowed women to exercise.

In most countries a woman's place in society is linked closely to her role as childbearer *and* to the social interpretation of that role. The less a woman is linked to the role of *involuntary* childbearer, the more her social status increases. In addition, the more education and knowledge a woman has, the less likely she is to bear unwanted children; this will eventually have a strong effect on world population. Thus in the interest of both the population problem in general and women's place in society in particular, women should be encouraged to seek and use birth control.

India, whose population is 85% Hindu, has a birth rate of 40 to 43, and Pakistan at 49 to 53 per 1000 has the highest birth rate in Asia, exceeded in the world by only a few African countries. Official religious doctrine seems to have no correlation with birth rates. Dyck points out that

if we limit the study of the influence of religion upon fertility control to the influence exerted through promulgated doctrines and if among these doctrines we focus only upon those specifying acceptance or rejection of contraceptives, religion will not be interpreted as extremely important in understanding or solving the population problem.*

Desired family size seems to have more to do with actual family size than does the influence of official religious doctrines on individual lives.

Personal religious beliefs, however, do affect the practice of fertility control. A distinction must be made between spacing of children and total number of children born. No religion prohibits the reasonable spacing of children (even the Catholic Church has no sanctions against this as long as the method used is natural, such as breast-feeding, rhythm, or abstinence, none of them by any means foolproof), because the health of the mother is protected so that she can bear more children. Therefore the wider spacing of children may lead to a decrease in the birth rate. Many Moslem, Hindu, and Buddhist girls marry as soon as they reach puberty or even before, and even if they were to have a child only every other year it is

---

*Dyck, Arthur J.: Religious factors in the population problem. In Cutter, Donald R., editor: Updating life and death: essays in ethics and medicine, Boston, 1969, Beacon Press, p. 145.

theoretically possible to give birth to 20 children before fertility ends or their bodies become completely exhausted.

Religious beliefs can influence a person's response and reaction to his environment (1) in the form of circumstances that perpetuate one's religion (the continued existence of the world as it is viewed) in reward for piety and (2) because the believer is provided with an environmental orientation shaped by God and to a lesser extent by humans. Each of these factors has a bearing on the motivation to control family size. The following are some examples:

1. Hinduism demands that a father be buried by one of his sons. As long as there is a relatively high infant mortality in countries that are primarily Hindu, such as India, women will keep bearing children to ensure that a son survives to bury his father. Moslems also need sons for burial duties.
2. All major religions except Buddhism have doctrinal injunctions to marry and bear children; this encouragement is deeply ingrained in the societal and cultural practices that arise out of religious beliefs.
3. Moslems and Hindus see children as a blessing from God; therefore, the more children one has, the more one is considered to be blessed. This is not only a source of personal satisfaction but a matter of public pride as well. When a man walks down the street followed by many children, he is regarded with respect by his peers.
4. The concept of *kismet* (fate) is very strong in Islamic belief. Since Allah (God) controls sexuality and everything else in nature, it is Allah who controls fertility and barrenness. Therefore it is thought useless to attempt anything to thwart the will of Allah. A true belief in the tenets of Islam rests on a belief in the beneficence of divine providence; therefore to take measures to control fertility would make one appear to be less than pious.
5. The Hindu belief in *karma* is a reliance on a natural reaping and sowing in human cyclical functions. There is also a doctrine of *ahimsa* (noninjury). Any effort to prevent conception can be seen as injury to life and as interference with the natural life cycle.
6. Gauchos of South America consider it unmanly and cowardly to engage in too much rational forethought, which is seen as a failure to accept what fate has to offer. This is another view of the proscription against thwarting God's will.

This theme of fear of God is seen over and over in every religion and in all its many forms is probably the single most potent force that causes people to refuse to use artificial birth control. It is a belief so deeply ingrained in the consciousness of many millions of people, particularly those who lack an education and who live away from major centers of culture, that it seems unshakable. Teams of educators, health professionals, sociologists, and anthropologists can forever go from village to village and even from person to person in an effort to teach people about birth control, but unless they can somehow integrate the information into the actual religious beliefs of the people they are trying to help, all the financial and tangible incentives in the world will be useless. A transistor radio or television set pales in comparison to the wrath of God.

Marxist communism, although not a religion, is the dominant political philosophy of the two largest countries on earth, the Soviet Union and the People's Republic of China. The Chinese maintain that they adhere completely to Marx's theory, which states that overpopulation cannot exist in a socialist state because any inequity between resources and demand for those resources is a function of the capitalist mode of production. The belief implies that science will progress faster than population size and consequently whatever problems arise from the disparity between population and resources will be solved by technology. The theory has not worked in practice, and with their population approaching one billion the Chinese communists have begun to demonstrate some flexibility in regard to the sanctions against birth control. The health and prosperity of the nation were clearly in jeopardy, and thus premiums were placed on education, health, protection of women and children, equality between the sexes, and industrial development of the state. All these priorities were in conflict with the unrestricted bearing of children; therefore two actions were instituted that had a tremendous effect on lowering the birth rate: (1) mandatory late marriage (men must be 30 and women 25) and (2) severe sanctions against having more than two children per couple. With the current Chinese desire to move into the modern industrial world it can be assumed that these sanctions will be even more rigidly applied. The Russians, although rejecting Malthusian principles of overpopulation, have clearly demonstrated that industrial development of the state has assumed a higher priority than unrestricted bearing of children.

RACIAL AND IDEOLOGIC CONSIDERATIONS

In most international discussions of population and economic development, an ideological argument frequently skews the considerations. The advocacy of population control is taken to be the ideology of affluent whites, and it may be rejected by spokesmen of Asia, Latin America, and Africa. Likewise within the United States there is increasing resentment in the black ghettos toward organizations, usually white dominated, that advocate family planning. The economically deprived, who are often also the dark-skinned, resent the exhortations (as they hear them) of affluent whites advising them to limit their population. They may respond by rhetorical resistance to ethnic suicide or genocide.*

They may have a point. Perhaps the wealthy of the world are evading their responsibility to the poor, whom they have been exploiting for centuries, by saying that the poor are creating the problems of the world by overpopulating it. This is, of course, an oversimplification of the problem, but it is a fact of history that light-skinned wealthier people have tended to exploit and subjugate dark-skinned poorer people.

A dilemma is involved in solving or at least alleviating some of the Third World's problems. On the one hand, massive birth control programs cannot be imposed on any nation by any other nation (notably white, wealthier, industrialized

---

*Shinn, Roger L.: Population and the dignity of man. In Williams, Preston, editor: Ethical issues in biology and medicine: proceedings of a symposium on the identity and dignity of man, Cambridge, 1973, Schenkman Publishing Co., p. 83.

ones) without some anger and perhaps violent consequences. Even if people of a particular nation could be compelled to accept birth control, the nation's problems would not be solved simply by instituting the program. On the other hand, no economic or industrial aid program will do much to solve the problems of Third World countries unless they voluntarily take measures to stop their trend toward over-population. In addition, those countries giving aid must begin a population control program of their own if they are not to be seen as condescending or racist by the countries receiving their aid. Large industrialized nations need to control their population as much as underdeveloped ones, although for different reasons. The United States and West Germany, for instance, are not on the verge of mass starvation, but they are beginning to choke on their own waste products, run out of natural resources, and permanently upset the ecologic balance.

A number of Christian theologians including Kenneth Boulding, Lynn White, William Pollard, and others think that the use of technology will not solve problems created by technology in the first place. They believe that a reformation of religious spirit is needed to increase reverence for nature and decrease the kind of destructive arrogance for the impermanence of resources that science and technology have demonstrated. In terms of overpopulation, they feel that developing new forms of contraceptive technology and convincing the masses to use it will be less effective than voluntarily changing attitudes about humans' relationship to nature and responsibility for it. This view has philosophic merit; no one could argue that it is wrong or immoral. It is simply not likely to happen in our lifetime. There are now and will continue to be many individuals and influential groups of people who espouse this view and put it into practice in their own lives, but it seems unlikely that the government and corporate structure of the Western industrialized countries will suddenly reverse their trend toward even higher technology and seek new, closer relationships with nature.

It may make sense to say that we cannot use a method to solve a problem created by that method in the first place, that technology cannot solve problems created by technology. But can we place the blame of overpopulation solely on technology? The move toward industrialization and away from agrarian life did require large numbers of people to serve industry, but that is not the answer for most of the Third World countries, which for the most part are not industrialized. Only religion, culture, and values can redirect reproductive priorities. During the past 40 years or so we have seen in the West a gradual shift in ethical values toward existentialism, individualism, and an emphasis on the rights and freedoms of the individual. Freedom to "do one's own thing" became the hallmark of a successful life, and we began to turn into a society of disconnected individuals; the *idea* of community lost ground. As we began to disconnect from each other we also pulled away from a responsibility toward the species, and even the back-to-nature movement of the past generation seems to·be more an individual search for freedom and fulfillment than a manifestation of responsibility toward the future of humankind. This is not to say that individualism is bad; on the contrary, most of the great thinking and accomplishments of history can be attributed to individuals. But when the quest for personal freedom supersedes the needs of the community, we begin to dig our own graves.* Regard for others and a sense of individual freedom depend to some extent on the population density of an area in question. When density is low, the freedom to move about, reproduce, and lead a highly individualized life-style is relatively high. As population density increases, people begin to feel re-straints on the way they live and how they think about prohibiting the growth of population both from within by increasing birth rates and from without by immi-gration. Consequently the more freedom and individuality a society wishes to have, the more controls it must place on itself in regard to population density. This may seem contradictory, but we have seen that overcrowding increases aggression, vi-olence, and territoriality, which are *not* conditions that foster a feeling of personal liberty and a life-style that includes individual rights.

Freedom and coercion in reproduction

To what extent may a society limit the freedom of an individual to reproduce? The question is probably one of the most basic in the problem of overpopulation and is the essential moral dilemma. The right to reproduce, to use one's body as one chooses, is considered by most societies to be a basic personal option right. Yet when that right is exercised without restraint, society suffers and its existence is threatened. A threat to the existence of any society automatically implies a threat to continuation of personal rights. At the 1967 World Conference on Church and Society held in Geneva, members came to conflicting conclusions about this issue. In Section IV on Man and Community in Changing Societies, Paragraph 60 states, "Responsible parenthood is not just a matter of individual family concern: it must be accepted as an integral part of the social ethic of the day." Paragraph 105 states, "Every couple has a right to make its own responsible decisions on the planning of its own family in accord with its moral and religious convictions."[10,p.88] The United Nations is involved in the same kind of conflict: their stated goal of ensuring indi-vidual liberty can be seen as running counter to another of their goals, controlling population.

Many population experts agree that zero population growth is desirable; they also agree that this cannot be achieved on a purely voluntary basis, no matter how much education and technology is made available. But disagreement begins about *how* to accomplish zero population growth. Some wonder why societies that force people to risk their lives for their country by going to war balk at forcing people to control their reproductive processes. Highly industrialized societies feel little con-straint about spewing known carcinogens into the air and packaging them into pro-cessed food, but they will not consider some form of mass conception-control pro-gram via the public water supply or other similar method. It is an interesting dichotomy of values. If a society assumes a philosophy that dignity of the individual is important, then it must allow a life-style in which it is possible for a person to live with dignity. Overpopulation leads to the kind of life-style in which human

---

*There are, however, instances when the desire for personal freedom *should* supersede the needs of the community, for example, when various groups such as blacks, homosexuals, and women demonstrate for civil rights. Although violence can never be morally sanctioned in these instances, it has on occasion proved to be an effective demonstration of rage and frustration.

dignity cannot exist for the vast majority of people; thus dignity demands some limitation of population size. But forced limitation can be equated with the destruction of freedom and liberty. The only ethical solution, therefore, is voluntary limitation of population size, and we have seen that this does not work, at least not in the past. What, then, is the solution?

In almost all societies some personal rights are curtailed during crises, for example, gas rationing during periods of shortage or war, curfews in communities that have experienced a natural disaster, searching all vehicles on certain highways after a prison break, a ban on nonessential personal travel during a severe blizzard, the draft, and so on. Many think that the population problem has become enough of a crisis to warrant curtailment of the personal right to bear more than two children. They reason that the past failure of voluntary restraint is sufficient reason to curtail some personal freedom. Others feel that the solution lies somewhere between total freedom and rigid coercion. More subtle forms of persuasion and pressure can induce people to limit the size of their families, such as higher social and cultural esteem and prestige given to small families and childless couples, heavy taxation on families with more than two children, housing restrictions for large families, educational priorities given to children from small families, and very heavy propaganda.

Is this form of coercion—and it *is* coercion—more or less morally correct than restricting family size by law and enforcing it by mandatory sterilization and mandatory abortion for those who manage to evade sterilization? This kind of coercion could be seen as morally more correct, that is, less evil than more restrictive measures, because it does not totally restrict personal liberty and choice. On the other hand, it could be seen as morally less correct, or more evil, because it is more insidious and hypocritical than overt law and could provide a false sense of freedom when in reality many of the good things in society will be denied to people who continue to have large families. The moral dilemma and practical problem is similar to that involved in desegregation of public schools. Society has in essence said to blacks, "We are desegregating the school system; you are free to send your children to school with whites. If you want to, you can spend large sums of money transporting them to the better suburban schools. Or we can institute busing, but of course we would not want white children to go to school in inner cities, so those schools will remain mostly black anyway. Or if you live in the inner city, as most of you do, you can escape the generally poor educational system by sending your children to prohibitively expensive private schools, as whites are doing. Or you can move to the suburbs, but we know you can't afford that, so you are stuck with *de facto* segregation."

Which is more moral for a society to do, give blacks the illusion of desegregated public schools while at the same time blocking their every effort to achieve an education equal in every way to that which whites have come to expect, or simply to tell them straight out that they are not wanted in white schools? Any civil libertarian will argue strongly for the former on the premise that even though the actual fact of opportunity for equal education will not be guaranteed with desegregation, the *chance* that it could occur is significantly increased when schools are desegregated. Consequently the number of black children whose education will improve increases. The analogy is not exact, but one could assume that a partly coercive restriction on fertility with which people could maintain the illusion of freedom if they wished would be more palatable to society than the absolute curtailment of that freedom. If both individual dignity and social order are to survive, a compromise must be reached between unrestrained personal freedom and absolute coercion.

It seems obvious that some form of coercion will have to be instituted eventually, and therefore it might be more productive for population experts to begin comparing forms and degrees of coercion rather than continuing to debate whether coercion will be necessary. The two extremes appear to be mandatory sterilization and abortion at government expense at one end of the continuum and continuation of what we are doing now in most parts of the world at the other end: making birth control information available to people, asking them politely to use it, but ultimately leaving the choice up to the individual. Every society decides how restrictive it wishes to be in controlling forms of human behavior, and it seems inconsistent not to control reproductive behavior as well. We are limited in how fast we can drive our automobiles; why not limit the speed with which we increase population? One law is instituted to prevent highway deaths; the other law could be seen as a prevention of societal death.

Garrett Hardin has proposed a six-stage schedule to solve the population problem[11]:

1. Abolition of "compulsory pregnancy." Hardin phrases the idea this way instead of referring to abortion on demand or universal abortion. He believes that any woman who stays pregnant when she does not wish to be is being compelled by society to be pregnant. This should considerably lower the birth rate.
2. Altering our basic idea of the world from a "cowboy economy" to a "spaceship economy"; that is, we must accept the confines of this world and realize that resources are limited and the wide open range of unlimited personal freedom is a thing of the past.
3. A persuasive stage of population control in which people must be voluntarily led to see where unrestricted fertility will lead. Hardin admits that this is not a permanent solution but must be a precursor for more restrictive measures.
4. Limited amounts of social engineering to further nudge people into a realization of the seriousness of the problem. Changes could be small at first, such as eliminating tax deductions after the first two children or some other symbolic act such as lowering the social esteem of larger families.
5. Definite coercion based on the conviction of the vast majority of people that some form of coercion is desirable.

In other words, to be quite blunt, what one has to say at some point is that in a world in which we must control population, we cannot be infinitely tolerant of acts. We may be infinitely tolerant of beliefs, but not of acts. The act of having a child is an act of warfare against society if it is one child too many. So we have to be quite blunt about this.*

6. Children belonging to the community rather than to individual parents. The concept of personal ownership of children will not exist. Hardin does not say exactly how this would contribute to a decrease in the birth rate, but presumably he thinks that people would be less likely to have children if they could not exercise complete control over them.

Steps one through three have already been accomplished, but the jump to step four involves crossing the barrier between voluntary and involuntary controls. The population of the earth is at the hurdle at this very moment; a decision must be made soon while there is still sufficient structure left in society to be able to make that kind of decision.

Hardin and Callahan[12] have engaged in a debate over the concept of the "lifeboat ethic." Hardin postulates the metaphor of the nations of the world as a group of lifeboats. A rich nation is compared to a large lifeboat filled with rich people and poor nations to smaller, much more crowded lifeboats. The poor continually fall out of their boats and swim around in the water for a while, hoping to be admitted to one of the larger, richer lifeboats or in some other way to benefit from its advantages. The primary way to be admitted to the lifeboat is through immigration; the way to procure the benefits is through food and agriculture assistance programs and other forms of economic aid. The ethical question posed by Hardin concerns what the passengers on the rich lifeboat should do. In what way are they obligated to the passengers swimming in the water?

Hardin argues that if the United States or any other rich lifeboat were to take on all the passengers who wanted to climb aboard, it would sink and all would drown. Even if the lifeboat could take on a few additional passengers without placing it in serious jeopardy, ethical questions would arise about which passengers to admit and which to let drown. He also argues against sharing the benefits of the rich lifeboat with the overcrowded poor, basing his argument on comparative population growth. At their present rates the United States population doubles approximately every 87 years and the Third World about every 35 years. To run a kind of communal lifeboat to which all the nations would contribute according to their ability and from which all would withdraw according to need would be a mistake. The right of each nation to use the common lifeboat would not be matched by an equal responsibility to maintain it. Countries that are seen as irresponsible in terms of birth rate and food production might become more so because they would always have someone to bail them out, and if they continued to be provided with food, they might continue to reproduce at their present rate. In the long run the population of the entire world would be in jeopardy. Hardin believes that the humanitarian "sharing ethic" would eventually destroy the rich lifeboats.

Callahan finds Hardin's proposals troubling even though he agrees that it makes

---

*Williams, Preston: Ethical issues in biology and medicine: proceedings of a symposium on the identity and dignity of man, Cambridge, 1973, Schenkman Publishing Co., p. 163.

a certain amount of sense in terms of future possibilities. He thinks it amounts to a deliberate decision to allow people to starve to death when we have the power to save them. One might even see it as a kind of mass act of passive euthanasia.

> Of course most of us will not personally have to observe the emaciated bodies, or help to dig the mass graves necessary to cover the millions of corpses—and that is surely a small consolation. An even greater blessing is that we can continue about our own business, unburdened of sentimental humanitarian impulses. . . *

Callahan also points out a pragmatic error in Hardin's argument: the rich lifeboats are not completely self-sustaining but need to import natural resources (oil is the prime example) and cheaply manufactured goods from the poorer ones to maintain their economic system (we could, of course, lower our standard of living, but then we would not be such a rich lifeboat). In addition an assumption is made that the poorer lifeboats are not as smart or as competent as the richer ones and that somehow they got themselves into this situation on their own; Callahan finds this assumption untrue and condescending. He does not agree that "perfect justice" is the only solution (an example of perfect justice is the government of the United States giving the entire country back to the Indians because it was stolen from them in the first place). Instead he urges the cessation of exploitation and repression and the provision of some compensation for past injustices. In other words, we do not need to give away all our goods and food to the poor lifeboats, but we must not exploit them in order to keep our own lifeboat luxuriously afloat and should do what we can to help without inflicting our self-righteous attitudes on them. He believes that the United States has nowhere reached its limit in the ability to give food aid to underdeveloped countries and that to continue to refuse the kind of help we are capable of providing will be to ensure their continued enmity. Furthermore, no poor lifeboats are in immediate danger of sinking; even some minor action could help keep them afloat. Aside from these pragmatic considerations, the most telling point Callahan makes is the following:

> There is always something attractive about proposed hard and hard-nosed decisions. They appeal to our sense of no-nonsense realism, and to our desire to once and for all be rid of nagging problems which we never seem to solve in any happy way. They are all the more attractive when their ultimate appeal is to our own self-interest. And they are positively irresistible when they promise the possibility of both doing well and doing good. We would all like to live in a moral universe guided by a magic hand which guaranteed that any act in our own best interest was also an act in the interest of all. Ours is not that kind of universe—or only very rarely. But there is no reason to go to the other extreme, really the obverse side of the same coin, and assert that own best interests will be served by deliberately allowing people to starve. There are also moral interests to be served, of which survival is only one. If we are to worry about our duty to posterity, it would not hurt to ask what kind of moral legacy we should bequeath. One in which we won our own survival at the cost of outright cruelty and callousness would be tawdry and vile. We may fail in our efforts to

---

*Callahan, Daniel: Doing well by doing good: Garret Hardin's "lifeboat ethic," Hastings Center Reports 4(6):3, December 1974. Reprinted with permission of The Hastings Center: © Institute of Society, Ethics and the Life Sciences, 360 Broadway, Hastings-on-Hudson, N.Y. 10706.

help poor countries, and everything Dr. Hardin predicts may come true. But an adoption of his course, or that of triage, seems to me to portend a far greater evil.*

Group and societal implications. Some moral issues involved in overpopulation can be defined in terms of societal implications. The first concerns perception of the problem. Developed Western nations are very fond of telling underdeveloped ones that they have a population problem. In view of the degree of overcrowding and starvation that exists in some places, this might be a reasonable conclusion. However, some countries (notably in Africa and Latin America) do not agree and simply feel more hostile toward countries whose paternalistic attitude forces a view of the population/resource ratio through the eyes of a nation with different values. The imposition of one's own moral values on someone else is just as risky and morally questionable when nations are involved as with individuals. Poor countries cannot simply be told what their problems are by demographers who are not aware of all the social, cultural, and racial implications that led to the imbalance.

A second moral issue involves the purpose of population studies. Governments and large private foundations spend millions of dollars to send researchers to underdeveloped countries to gather population data. They often return with neatly documented causes of the problem and lists of proposed solutions. Whose problems will be solved? Are the conclusions drawn from the findings warranted; that is, does the government or foundation "prove" a need for family planning or fertility control because *it* sees a need for it, or do the people who were researched also see the need? Do the people of India really *want* the United Nations to come swooping into their villages with transistor radios as rewards for vasectomy, or do some of them accept what is being done either because they do not understand the implications or because they feel powerless to resist the paternalistic "goodness" of the United Nations workers? This is not meant to imply that all demographers or population researchers are racists intent on genocide; it is an effort to differentiate between perceived and actual needs and problems. Do researchers sometimes confuse what a country needs and what they want the country to need?

Another issue involves the moral vision that guides and controls population programs. There *will* be such programs because rich nations see a need for them and will ensure that they are developed and implemented, probably by trying them to military or other forms of economic aid ("We will sell you a certain number of fighter planes if you guarantee to sterilize a certain number of your citizens"). The issue involves the moral foundation on which the programs will be based. How will the values and aspirations of the people involved be taken into consideration? What priorities will be established? For example, in areas where mass starvation is rampant will the first action be to provide food itself and a means to continue the food supply, or will it be the establishment of a family planning program? Will countries with a population problem be threatened with a discontinuation of their foreign food aid unless they take steps to lower the birth rate? To many people it seems

---

*Callahan, Daniel: Doing well by doing good: Garret Hardin's "lifeboat ethic," Hastings Center Reports 4(6):3, December 1974. Reprinted with permission of The Hastings Center: © Institute of Society, Ethics and the Life Sciences, 360 Broadway, Hastings-on-Hudson, N.Y. 10706.

immoral to prevent a woman from ever having more children if the survival of her two or three children is so threatened by malnutrition and consequent disease that they will likely die. In those areas of the world where blessedness is measured in part by the number of one's children, can a nation in good conscience reduce people's capacity to feel blessed? How would the social order be affected? Population planners tend to have a homogenizing effect; that is, when deciding how to prevent the world from being consumed by its own fecundity, they tend to forget or dismiss the incredibly wide variety of attitudes about sexuality, fertility, parenthood, and social responsibility. The homogenizing process arises from assuming that as soon as the problem is explained to the people who are seen to be the cause, they will immediately see the error of their ways and drop their centuries-old values in the name of preventing mass starvation and death.

Veatch[13] offers an example in which food was used as an incentive for sterilization. In a very poor country in Asia where the population was doubling every 21 years, the Family Planning Council recommended drastic action because the survival of the country was in jeopardy. Every citizen who voluntarily agreed to be sterilized would be given coupons redeemable for about $20 worth of food. Any individual who voluntarily requested sterilization after having no more than two children would also receive the $20 food coupon, as would any citizen who brought to a government clinic a person who subsequently was sterilized. The council defended its action by saying that the program was entirely voluntary, that no one would be penalized for having more than two children, and that government was not forcing its views on the private values of individual citizens. The traditional religion did not look with favor at human intervention in God's fertility plan, but it was believed that only a small minority of the population found religious objections to the council's proposal.

Opinions vary about the morality of such a program. Those who see value in a food incentive for sterilization view it as a way to prevent restrictions on freedom. Granting an option for sterilization now (with a gentle nudge from the government) avoids the further limitations that unrestrained population growth would entail. Slight coercion now is morally better than severe curtailment of freedom later. Not only would a restriction on population growth *prevent* limitation of future freedom, but it might *promote* the granting of even greater freedoms: education, a variety of options in jobs and life-styles, and higher income per capita. If this were the case, even people who did not take advantage of the incentive program would ultimately benefit. Governments of most countries (this Asian one is most likely no exception) interfere in the lives of citizens by regulating their personal behavior to some degree: some sexual practices, the number of spouses allowed, certain restrictions on unfettered mobility (traffic laws), and the like. Advocates of the council's proposal ask if it is any less moral to restrict (or at least ask citizens to voluntarily restrict) the number of children when there are restrictions on the number of spouses one may have, the speed at which we drive, or the amount of untaxed income we may earn. They argue that prevention of anarchy and breakdown in the social order depend on voluntary and involuntary restrictions on human behavior. If incentives to control behavior seem artificial or coercive, the same is true of compulsory education, marriage licenses, and the payment of social security taxes to ensure freedom from poverty in old age. Planning for the national future by limiting the birth rate is seen as no more coercive than trying to prevent mass poverty of the elderly retired in a country. Planning for the future is a gamble and the ultimate stakes are survival. Those who approve the council's plan see no reason not to tip the odds in favor of humanity in this slightly coercive way rather than slant them toward destruction by doing nothing.

Opponents of the council's proposal argue that incentives or bribes would not be necessary if people were motivated to have fewer children by other means (for example, education). If they are not properly motivated, then bait becomes an unacceptable alternative. Another moral objection is that the bargain offered by the council is not fair: it offers a temporary solution (food that is consumed) to an individual's problem (starvation) while in return gaining a permanent step (sterilization) in solving a national problem. Government thus gives itself an unfair advantage although the individual is in the same socioeconomic situation when his food coupons are used up. If this plan were to have any justice, the advantage should be more equitable: a lifetime supply of food for the individual and his family in return for voluntary sterilization or continued food coupons as long as the individual uses some effective form of temporary contraception.

In countries such as the one discussed above, children are more than a source of blessing or joy; they are a sort of social security system. Parents depend on their children as a source of support in their old age, and because of the high infant mortality rate a large number of children must be born to ensure the survival of a few. To deprive a couple of support in their old age by future children is to condemn them to a future of possible starvation. This is seen as immoral and unjust by those opposed to this food incentive plan. The government claims that no one would be forced to participate in the plan or deprived because he or she chose not to participate (people would not have less food; neither would they have more). This too could be seen as immoral; forcing people to choose between two evils (foregoing the food now and depriving one's existing children of needed nutrition, or foregoing future children and depriving oneself of sufficient food in later years) is an evil in itself. Asking extremely deprived people to choose between food and sterilization is not fair. By offering extra food to those who consent to be sterilized the government is making a value judgment about which group of people is the more deserving. One must assume that food in this country is scarce and that allocating it is a matter of serious concern. Why are people who agree to be sterilized seen as more valuable than the aged, chronically ill, and children? What is this society saying about its own values; is it moral for this government to impose its own values so that some citizens will profit from meager resources at the expense, and possible death, of others? Opponents of the plan think not. The government is also saying that population growth is the single most important problem facing the country, not that it is one of a series of equally important issues. In saying that it must make other, more far-reaching decisions about the value of some people over others, what other steps will be taken to solve the problem, and the possibility that this slightly coercive incentive will lead to other measures that are blatantly coercive or that severely restrict the freedom of one or several groups of citizens. If a little incentive seems to work, will not more incentives work faster and better? It is a dangerous road on which to begin a journey; some feel the destination will be immorality and social injustice.

This example and the moral issues involved in it in many ways represent an accurate and realistic portrayal of the choices facing many of the world's countries. Proposed solutions to the problem may vary from the theme of a food incentive for sterilization, but the basic issue remains the same. If demographers and other population experts agree that population can be controlled by zero population growth, what methods can governments devise to ensure that citizens work toward that goal? Is coercion required, and if so under what circumstances and to what degree? This appears to be the basic moral issue in achieving zero population growth and thereby controlling population.

Racial and cultural implications. The contraceptive pill, the most effective form of artificial birth control now available, was developed mainly by the United States pharmaceutical companies. Major clinical trials (testing on humans required by the FDA before a drug is considered safe for sale to the general public) were performed with poor Puerto Rican women chosen mainly because it was difficult to find large numbers of women in the United States who were willing to undergo this kind of experimentation and because it was thought that if things went awry, they would be less likely to take political or legal action than more sophisticated American women. There may have been some racism on the part of the pharmaceutical companies, but a more realistic view of their choice of Puerto Rican women is that they wanted to keep any possible trouble on an island out of the mainstream of American life and the American press.

Some 20 years after mass marketing of the contraceptive pill studies are now revealing that although it is as effective as was originally thought, it is far less safe. Women in record numbers are bringing suits against pharmaceutical companies and are demanding recompense in other ways. Part of the anger revolves around the way in which the original clinical trials were run on poor uneducated women who could be expected to keep their mouths shut if anything went wrong or who might not even know if their bodies were somehow harmed during the course of the experiments. Currently in the United States there is a move toward increasing safety standards for contraceptive pills, which would require longer, more intense, and more expensive testing by companies before the drug is put on the market.

Some international population-assistance organizations have proposed a countermove: lower restrictions for testing and marketing contraceptive pills in underdeveloped countries. Health ministers in several countries have embraced the idea, as has the United States Agency for International Development (AID)[14] The major argument is that experimental caution and control over how the experiments are conducted are not warranted in poor countries because they lack the medical establishment to make the controls meaningful. Behind this official reasoning seems to lie the desire to hurry development of an even more effective means of fertility control. The World Health Organization (WHO) is concerned that contraceptive pills and devices developed for Western women might be inappropriate for women in underdeveloped countries because of their poorer nutrition and general health. The suggestion raises major questions: where should the clinical trials be carried out, what standards should be used to control the experiments, how should subjects be protected, why should differences in standards (from what is generally acceptable in the West) be permitted, how much testing should be required before the drug is released, and how much medical monitoring should occur after the drug is on the market?

Contraceptive pills could be tested in the area where they will be used. Dosages and effects that are worked out for women in the West may be totally inappropriate for women who are smaller in stature and who suffer from endemic malnutrition and anemia and from different kinds of infections and infestation of parasites. WHO has organized a network of clinical research centers in the United States, Europe, Brazil, northern and central Africa, and Asia to test both established and experimental contraceptives. Funds come from WHO and from the United Nations Fund for Population Activities (UNFPA). This arrangement would seem equitable, but it is not always. For example, Depo-Provera, the injectable contraceptive, was clinically tested in only 10 of the 20 research centers, 8 of them in underdeveloped countries. Testing was not done in Canada, England, West Germany, and Belgium; the United States did not participate because the FDA under pressure from Congress and consumer groups withdrew its conditional approval for the drug to be tested. Yet knowing this, WHO and UNFPA went ahead and permitted testing to be done in 10 countries.[14] This organizational network appears to defeat its own purpose. Tests are not distributed equally among the 20 participating countries. Decisions for participation must be based on national standards, and because more developed countries usually have higher standards for drug experimentation, underdeveloped countries are usually picked for the riskier trials and thus we have the problem of using the poor and ignorant as experimental subjects. One wonders if it is a coincidence that those countries used for the beginning stage trials are usually inhabited by dark-skinned people. One also wonders why many Third World countries become anti-imperialist and antidemocratic and why they embrace communist-socialist ideologies. Many Americans resent the political inclinations of countries the United States has been feeding for so long. But the provision of charity does not give one the right to cruelly mistreat an individual or country accepting that charity.

Obtaining informed consent in these countries is sometimes such a low priority that it is ignored. When health authorities are faced with problems of survival, mass starvation, and constant outbreaks of disease for which there is insufficient medicine, it is not surprising that the concern for obtaining informed consent takes a back seat. Another problem compounds the informed consent issue: some rudimentary knowledge of anatomy and physiology is necessary for the consent to be informed, and for the most part people in underdeveloped countries have little of this knowledge or what they have is erroneous. What to do? Educate people sufficiently so that their consent will be informed? How can one understand the concept of a 5% risk of a blood clot unless one understands what a blood clot is? Researchers are chemists and physiologists, not teachers, and it is not feasible to ask governments to provide the necessary basic information. If they were able to do so, they would have already. Should the clinical trials not be conducted because informed consents is impossible to obtain? While appearing very noble, that alternative leaves the women of the country either without effective contraception or with a drug that was tested on other and possibly quite dissimilar women. Which is worse, to risk danger during clinical trials or death and starvation from a lack of adequate fertility control? The poor and illiterate in many countries do not have the option of free choice because either they live in some form of dictatorship, no matter how benevolent, or they are so debilitated by malnutrition and hopelessness that they lack spirit to engage in the active questioning and dialogue that is so much a part of informed consent. Many researchers believe that informed consent is impossible to obtain and thus stop making the effort. Physicians in underdeveloped countries usually come from the upper privileged class, whereas research subjects are members of the lower class. The concept of command and obedience is so ingrained that an atmosphere conducive to free choice and informed consent is not likely to exist.

WHO has made an effort to surmount these barriers. All researchers are required to submit information on the risks, inconveniences, and benefits to the subjects and how this information is to be communicated to subjects. A human-subjects committee of WHO reviews the proposal before funding is approved. WHO can also exercise control by using national researchers as much as possible to carry out research in their own countries. WHO cannot dictate standards of control to individual countries about experimental procedures; it can only approve or withhold funds for research. It would be naive to assume, however, that because WHO approves funding for a particular experiment based on the researchers' stated intentions, controls and guidelines are adequately established and met. WHO is short of personnel and cannot police or even investigate every experiment it funds. Once the money is dispersed, it is for all intents and purposes the researchers' to use as they see fit. One could compare WHO's supervisory capacity to that of the International Red Cross during World War II when it inspected prisoner-of-war camps and accepted as reality only what the Germans chose to show them. There is one final disadvantage (or advantage, depending on one's point of view) to the way in which WHO approves and supervises funding: they can fall back on the basic UN principle of maintaining national sovereignty and not interfering in the internal affairs of member nations. But because of this eyes can be closed to a great deal of unethical experimental behavior.

Another ethical issue in international contraceptive use is the distribution of drugs. How much prior testing should be required, and how safe is safe? Should there be a double standard; that is, can a drug be distributed to underdeveloped countries after less testing than in more developed countries that have stronger demands for tighter safety controls? Should the severity of a country's population problem be used as a rationale for skimping on test procedures? Many argue that the risk of overpopulation and mass malnutrition and starvation is greater than a few women succumbing to pulmonary emboli or suffering the consequences of lesser side effects. This view supports the principle that a few may be sacrificed for the ultimate good of many, a concept that will be discussed more fully in Chapter 9 on human experimentation. The essential issue, of course, lies in the nature of the sacrifice and the ultimate benefit and in one's view of how the two compare.

It is relatively easy for a Western health professional to grasp the concept of individual informed consent or imagine one or even several women agreeing to a test and then experiencing side effects of drugs because they could not understand the explanation that was given. What is almost impossible for us to comprehend is the specter of mass starvation, bodies being stacked in unmarked mass graves, thousands of people being so hungry and weakened by malnutrition that they lack the strength to crawl to a source of food on the rare occasion that there is one. There is nothing in our experience to help us to comprehend the enormity of this. Thus if researchers or physicians native to countries where these conditions exist demonstrate an attitude of thinking it permissible to sacrifice a few women to eliminate this horror, how can we be certain they are acting immorally? If they are convinced that their actions are good, correct, and consistent with their standards and values, are they not indeed behaving in a way *they* think is moral?

In some countries contraceptives are distributed by nonphysicians and no continuing medical supervision is required; Pakistan and Thailand are examples of this. Is it ethical to provide people with potent drugs without medical follow-up?

The largest user of Depo-Provera in the world is the McCormick Missionary Hospital in Chiang Mai, Thailand, where thousands of women are given injections with no follow-up. Dr. Edwin McDaniel, chief of obstetrics, gynecology, and family planning, feels that Thai women are so desperately in need of effective fertility control that to deny it to a majority of them because time, money, and personnel are not available for adequate follow-up would be wrong. He also feels that many women would not avail themselves of the injection if they had to be subjected to the pelvic examination, blood tests, and history taking that many would view as embarrassing or unacceptable because of religious taboos. Given limitations of time and resources, McDaniel has made a decision about how he can be most helpful to the greatest number of women.[14]

This position is logical and realistic as well as dangerous. Is Depo-Provera, considered unsafe by the FDA, ready for such massive use without appropriate supervision? How urgent is the need to control fertility in Thailand *in comparison to* the need to gather more accurate data on the efficacy and safety of Depo-Provera? Should some of the funds available be diverted from the actual provision of contraception to improving the structure of the health care system there so that better medical supervision will become possible?

Who should take the lead in defining and attempting to solve these ethical problems? Agencies of the United Nations are restricted by their policies as already described, although WHO does have a human-subjects committee. The International Planned Parenthood Federation (IPPF) contributes heavily to private and government family planning research activities; it is particularly interested in controlling world population and thus would most likely lean toward continuing research and distribution of contraceptives even in view of ethically questionable practices. National governments can be seen as understandably biased in their efforts to find an effective means to control population. On the other hand, they could be biased against having research done on citizens of their country, citing fears of exploitation, racism, and possible attempts at genocide as reasons. Given the history of white exploitation of dark-skinned people, national leaders have a perfectly reasonable fear of research. Can research in underdeveloped countries be seen as exploitation, unwarranted experimentation, and an intrusion on individual rights? Or can it be seen as an honest and humanitarian effort to control the world's population and prevent mass death by starvation?

What is now badly needed is an impartial, international, interdisciplinary, and properly qualified private body which can analyze the questions of ethics and contraceptives in depth and make recommendations without fear of bureaucratic repercussions from donors and family planning organizations. To be effective, this group must solicit the cooperation of the national and international organizations active in this field, and benefit from their experience and opinions. To be credible, it will have to remain independent, and represent the interests of the poor and the powerless throughout the world, whether those interests should be found to require latitude or greater caution in setting and enforcing standards.*

One of the issues that this international body could tackle is the ethics of one country providing foreign aid for the specific purpose of controlling another country's population size. There is considerable debate about whether population growth speeds or retards economic and industrial growth. Some claim that high birth rates are the result of underdevelopment because of colonial economic systems, high unemployment, and consequent despair and hopelessness on the part of the populace. The opposing view is that increasing population acts as a spur for economic growth to provide more jobs and for evolving social structures (from agrarian to industrial) and that foreign aid policy depends on the view of population growth held by the country giving aid. The United States has adopted a policy that overpopulation is detrimental to a country's development, and thus more than half the funds currently available for fertility studies comes from the United States. It has justified its interference in the private lives of citizens of other countries by saying that the countries themselves have identified population growth as a major problem and have requested help. A donor country (the United States or any other) can say that it responds to a country's call for this kind of help in the same way that it responds to requests for help in educating its citizens, increasing its agricultural capacities, or defending its borders. The ethical considerations are the same: *laissez faire* is no longer a workable or desirable foreign policy. This attitude is opposed only by people who are strongly opposed to artificial conception control.

However, ethical problems still arise in providing this kind of foreign aid. Do recipient countries feel a pressure to establish or increase existing population control programs to achieve economic aid in other areas? Some countries do not care and go about their population business as they choose; for example, in 1974 the Ministry of Health in Argentina restricted the sale of contraceptive pills (the pre-

---

*Warwick, Donald: Contraceptives in the third world, Hastings Center Reports 5(4):12, August 1975. Reprinted with permission of The Hastings Center: © Institute of Society, Ethics and the Life Sciences, 360 Broadway, Hastings-on-Hudson, N. Y. 10706.

scription must be signed by *three* medical authorities) and prohibited the dissemination of birth control information.[15] Another issue concerns whether donor countries are using increased aid for population control as an excuse to decrease aid in other areas, as the former is generally much less expensive than the latter. Are education, agriculture, and defense being sacrified for a decreased birth rate? What about donor countries supporting population research in countries that have explicitly racist policies? Zimbabwe and the Republic of South Africa are two examples; both wholeheartedly support family planning for blacks while encouraging whites to have large families. This is also true of their immmigration policies; whites are encouraged to immigrate and emigration is discouraged by heavy economic sanctions. Should the donor country tacitly support apartheid by providing funds to those who perpetuate racist practices?

MASS STERILIZATION

Sterilization of large groups of people was first practiced by the Nazis in the interest of eugenics by prohibiting non-Aryans from breeding. India has the world's record number of sterilizations, approximately 12 million, all done in the name of population control. Many countries engage in sterilization of the masses, some doing it for anyone who requests it or can be coerced into it and others choosing certain groups of people, for example, blacks in Zimbabwe and South Africa, to be first when sterilization is considered as a form of population control. Some countries that do not give priority on the basis of race may do so using other criteria such as physical or mental defects, certain types of criminal records, or "socially deviant" behavior. The issue of mass sterilization involves compound ethical dilemmas. Are certain groups "worthy" of sterilization? Should all members of the group (and how many individuals constitute a group large enough to be designated a mass, as in mass sterilization?) be sterilized, and if not, what criteria should be established? Will society as a whole benefit from the sterilization of certain groups, and how can that benefit be demonstrated? How can the rights of an individual be compared with the rights of a particular group and those of society at large? Can whatever benefits accrue from mass sterilization be gained in any other way, or is sterilization the only answer? How can one be certain?

Because mass sterilization is an issue of such enormous proportions, the focus here will be narrowed to a discussion of one group of people, the mentally retarded. This is done mainly for ease of considering the problem, though this is also an ethical dilemma that is receiving widespread attention. However, all the ethical considerations involved in the issue of sterilization of the retarded can be applied to any other group of people in any country.

We must assume that sterilization of the mentally retarded is done on an involuntary basis because it is impossible to know if the consent of a retarded person is informed. If the parent or legal guardian gives consent because the person is so retarded that he cannot understand the implications of the surgery, then the sterilization must be regarded as even more involuntary even though he may present himself to the surgeon willingly and trustingly.

The arguments for sterilizing the retarded cover a wide range of philosophies. The first argument appears to be quite humane. Many mentally retarded people are capable of enjoying sexual pleasure and are not so retarded that they do not recognize the source of their pleasure; sex is a physical demonstration of love and closeness just as it is with the nonretarded. As pleasurable and positive as sex is, however, pregnancy or potential fatherhood would be physically and emotionally debilitating and traumatic, an experience that is difficult enough for people of normal intelligence and perhaps incapacitating for the retarded. The solution, according to this argument, is to sterilize the retarded so that they are free to enjoy sex without the possibility of pregnancy. This argument makes two assumptions that may or may not be true: that pregnancy would be too traumatic for the retarded person to handle and that the retarded are not capable of being adequate parents.

The second argument in favor of sterilizing the retarded concerns the children that might be born to them. Childrearing is a difficult, complex, and mentally and emotionally taxing task for the most intelligent among us. For the retarded it could be an impossible job causing both parents and children to suffer, the latter from physical and emotional deprivation or possibly even abuse.

Another argument for sterilization of the retarded concerns their apparent inability to manage impermanent forms of conception control. This is a particularly weak argument. An IUD requires almost no management, and if a retarded woman can be taught to brush her teeth (and only the most profoundly retarded cannot), she can take a pill every day. The insertion of a diaphragm or use of a condom is admittedly a bit more complex, and sterilization is indeed a guaranteed form of birth control, but it cannot be assumed that all retarded people cannot manage the alternatives.

A more abstract philosophic issue concerns whether sterilization of the retarded denies them a full place in the moral community (those who are responsible for their actions and who are held responsible by the rest of the community) by the dehumanizing act of preventing them from having full control over their bodies and by unduly invading their bodily privacy by removing a basic physiologic function. The fear of people who oppose sterilization of the retarded is that they will be treated as things rather than as people or will be used as a means to the end of releasing society from the burden of caring for children of the retarded.

To sterilize them involuntarily . . . is to do them unnecessary and dehumanizing violence. It is to regard them first of all as incapable of making a responsible decision about sterilization, thus ruling them out of membership in this respect; no defender of involuntary sterilization could deny this. It is, second, to regard their sex lives and childbearing and childrearing lives as so controlled by irresponsible impulses that the people may just as well be managed like objects in those areas of life. Third, it is quite possible and indeed likely, according to this position, that sterilization is sought for the mildly retarded in order to make their custody easier, in which case the people are treated in that respect as means only, not as ends in themselves.*

The answer to these arguments revolves mainly around characteristics of the moral community and the place of the retarded in that community. It can be ar-

---

*Neville, Robert: The philosophical arguments, Hastings Center Reports 8(3):34, June 1978. Reprinted with permission of The Hastings Center: © Institute of Society, Ethics and the Life Sciences, 360 Broadway, Hastings-on-Hudson, N.Y. 10707.

gued that membership in the moral community is directly related to the capacity for taking responsibility and that an inability to take responsibility precludes membership. Thus the retarded are not being denied full humanity because they do not have the capacity for it. The moral community is an ideal that when applied to reality needs to recognize that many people do not have full membership: children (although their potential for full membership exists), certain criminals, the aged senile, the mentally ill, and the retarded. A person who cannot be accorded the full rights of membership in the moral community is assigned a guardian (or proxy as it is sometimes called) such as a parent, prison warden, attorney, or hospital administrator. The proxy is then expected to act in the best interest of the partial member by exercising his own full moral responsibility on the other's behalf. Granted, this is an ideal (though all philosophic theories are couched in the ideal) and frequently does not work well in practice. A proxy can perhaps be seen as a crutch to aid the retarded in coming closer to achieving full membership in the moral community; that is, the retarded may need help in certain areas of life, such as sex and procreation, but may be quite capable of managing alone in other areas, such as maintaining a job. Thus deciding to sterilize the retarded can be seen as a morally correct act if viewed in this context.

One could also use this argument to say that to avoid unwanted pregnancies, unsterilized retarded people should be prevented as much as possible from having sexual intercourse and that sterilizing them permits them to enjoy the fulfilling aspects of a sexual relationship. This position can be seen as a choice between two evils rather than a choice between an action that is morally correct and one that is not. It can be said that sterilization of the retarded does them a service by permitting them to enjoy sex without the possibility of pregnancy. Viewed in this context, involuntary sterilization can be seen as a decision made out of a choice between a moral good and a moral evil rather than between the two evils.

The crux of the argument involves two opposing premises: that involuntary sterilization fosters more complete membership in the moral community by increasing the chances of morally responsible behavior, or that it denies an individual the right to control his own body and its functions and that personal liberty is abrogated by the unwarranted imposition of the values of some parts of society on others.

SUMMARY

Too many people live on earth. This simple statement has vast implications: insufficient habitable land to support the multitudes, a dwindling supply of natural resources, overcrowding to the point at which aggression and violence become a routine part of life, mass starvation on an even larger scale than we see now, and all manner of other horrors.

The causes of overpopulation are complex and so intertwined that no single one can be seen as the cause of all the others. One important factor in addition to the increasing birth rate is the decreasing death rate, a result of medical technology and most notably of the development of the germ theory of disease. Countries that have remained mostly agrarian continue to have high birth rates although their death rates are decreasing, and industrialized countries had decreasing birth rates;

thus technology can be seen as both a positive and negative force in overpopulation. Resistance to change leads people in many cultures to continue to have many children for a variety of reasons such as religious requirements, the perception that the more children one has, the more blessed by God one is, the need to give birth to large numbers of children so that some will survive to take care of their parents in old age, a fear and distrust of medical intervention in natural reproductive processes, and a sense of moral outrage at being told how to control something as personal as sexuality and reproduction.

Other consequences of overpopulation include air and water not fit for consumption, insufficient space to live, constant personal violence, a resurgence of currently conquered disease because of a lack of health care, rampant unemployment, increased suicide, a total depletion of natural resources and a dependence on chemicals for nutrition, an increased use of nuclear power, and the return of slavery perhaps—all on a global scale.

Various remedies have been suggested since overpopulation was first recognized as a problem more than 2 centuries ago. Some are more coercive than others and some are more effective, but none of the proposals has been shown to be an absolute answer. One suggestion is a person-to-person education campaign about methods of birth control. This is time-consuming, expensive, and reaches only small numbers of people. Another idea is to convert deserts, forests, and oceans to arable areas. This is also expensive, and the fruits of this labor might be too little too late. And transporting people to other planets is not practical in the foreseeable future. Lowering the birth rate seems to be the most effective and practical remedy and could be accomplished in a number of ways, such as voluntary cooperation of all families to have no more than two children, mass distribution of free birth control on a worldwide basis, voluntary sterilization of one of the partners of a couple, and various forms of compulsory birth control though these are highly controversial and some are probably quite immoral. But *not* forcing people to limit the number of children they bear can be seen as immoral if unrestricted births will mean the eventual destruction of humanity.

Violence and aggressive territoriality will increase as a result of overpopulation. People attack each other for two major reasons: when they perceive themselves to be threatened and when there is interference with the cerebral mechanism that inhibits attack. Both of these phenomena will increase in intensity when we begin to overcrowd each other. We *will* be threatened more frequently, and the psycho-emotional climate of daily life will weaken inhibition against attack. Violent incursions into other people's personal space will increase, as will the ferocity of the defense and counterattack.

In terms of the international consequences of overpopulation a variety of moral issues are raised. The basis for all these issues concerns whether it is ever morally justified for one country (usually an industrialized developed one) to impose its values on another country (an underdeveloped one) by coercing the latter in a variety of ways to decrease the size of its population. Should one country intervene in the personal practices of the citizens of another? Can a government take it upon itself (with or without aid and encouragement from outside governments) to limit the family size of its citizens?

Although overpopulation is not specifically a religious issue, the Catholic Church has become a full participant in the debate over moral issues. What the Church in an official capacity preaches (banning of any artificial form of birth control) and what individual Catholics practice are often not the same. The Church itself often seems contradictory, at the same exhorting Catholics not to use birth control and urging governments to prevent starvation. Orthodox Jews do not practice artificial birth control either, but their numbers are so small that they do not make a statistical difference in population size. Hinduism, Buddhism, and Islam have no official sanctions against artificial birth control, but again individuals vary greatly in their beliefs.

An important international issue in the ethics of overpopulation concerns whether rich nations are morally obligated to help poor nations control the size of their populations. The rich (and usually light-skinned) have been exploiting the poor (and often dark-skinned) countries for centuries; the former now tend to blame the latter for causing the world's population problems. Any effort to control the size of another nation's population may be met with anger and resentment; the more coercive the effort, the greater the anger. At the same time, no economic or social development programs can be expected to make much headway if a population is increasing out of control. The right to reproduce, to use one's body as one sees fit, is viewed as a basic right; any effort to curtail that right is seen as immoral by many and essential for the survival of the species by many others. The voluntary limitation of family size has not been successful to any appreciable degree, and complete unrestricted reproduction will lead to mass starvation and death. The ethical dilemma seems to be unsolvable.

What kind of control should a government exercise on its own citizens, and how much coercion (in the form of extra food, better housing, or products like transistor radios) to be sterilized is morally acceptable? Will a little coercion lead to more? Is any amount permissible? Should poor countries that have the most serious population problems be used in the experimental testing of new forms of birth control, and should safety standards be lowered to achieve faster results? How can truly informed consent be obtained from people who are the subjects of these experiments when they have a limited understanding of their bodies? Can birth control devices or drugs about which there is some question of safety be distributed to underdeveloped countries without adequate medical supervision in an effort simply to make birth control available to those who want it?

The ethical ramifications of mass sterilization are many and must be explored in relation to population control. As with other issues, there are reasons to favor it and to oppose it.

REFERENCES

1. Frazier, Claude A.: It is moral to modify man? Springfield, Ill., 1973, Charles C Thomas, Publisher.
2. Augenstein, Leroy: Come, let us play God, New York, 1969, Harper & Row, Publishers, Inc.
3. Erlich, Paul R.: The population bomb, New York, 1968, Ballantine Books, Inc.
4. Hoagland, Hudson: Biological considerations of aggression, violence and crowding. In Williams, Preston, editor: Ethical issues in biology and medicine: proceedings of a symposium on the

identity and dignity of man, Cambridge, Mass., 1973, Schenkman Publishing Co.

5. Ardrey, Robert: The territorial imperative, New York, 1966, Atheneum Publishers.
6. Montagu, Ashley: The nature of human aggression, New York, 1976, Oxford University Press.
7. Lorenz, Konrad, and Leyhausen, Paul: Motivation of human and animal behavior: an ethological view (B. A. Tonkin, translater), New York, 1973, Van Nostrand Reinhold Co.
8. Warwick, Donald, Merrick, Thomas W., and Caplan, Arthur: International population programs: should they challenge local values? Hastings Center Reports 7(5):17, October 1977.
9. Dyck, Arthur J.: Religious factors in the population problem. In Cutler, Donald R., editor: Updating life and death: essays in ethics and medicine, Boston, 1969, Beacon Press.
10. Shinn, Roger L.: Population and the dignity of man. In Williams, Preston, editor: Ethical issues in biology and medicine: proceedings of a symposium on the identity and dignity of man, Cambridge, Mass., 1973, Schenkman Publishing Co.
11. Williams, Preston: Ethical issues in biology and medicine: proceedings of a symposium on the identity and dignity of man, Cambridge, Mass., 1973, Schenkman Publishing Co.
12. Callahan, Daniel: Doing well by doing good: Garret Hardin's "lifeboat ethic," Hastings Center Reports 4(6):1-4, December 1974.
13. Veatch, Robert M.: Case studies in medical ethics, Cambridge, Mass., 1977, Harvard University Press.
14. Warwick, Donald: Contraceptives in the Third World, Hastings Center Reports 5(4):9, August 1975.
15. Warwick, Donald P.: Ethics and population control in developing countries, Hastings Center Reports 4(3):2, June 1974.

BIBLIOGRAPHY

Ardrey, Robert: The territorial imperative, New York, 1966, Atheneum Publishers.

Augenstein, Leroy: Come, let us play God, New York, 1969, Harper and Row, Publishers, Inc.

Bayles, Michael: The legal precedents, Hastings Center Reports 8(3):37-41, June 1978.

Callahan, Daniel: Doing well by doing good: Garret Hardin's "lifeboat ethic," Hastings Center Reports 4(6):1-4, December 1974.

Dyck, Arthur J.: Religious factors in the population problem. In Cutler, Donald R., editor: Updating life and death: essays in ethics and medicine, Boston, 1969, Beacon Press.

Ehrlich, Paul R.: The population bomb, New York, 1968, Ballantine Books, Inc. 1968.

Frazier, Claude A.: Is it moral to modify man? Springfield, Ill., 1973, Charles C Thomas, Publisher.

Gaylin, Willard: Sterilization of the retarded: in whose interest? Hastings Center Reports 8(3):28, June 1978.

Hoagland, Hudson: Biological considerations of aggression, violence and crowding. In Williams, Preston, editor: Ethical issues in biology and medicine: proceedings of a symposium on the identity and dignity of man, Cambridge, Mass., 1973, Schenkman Publishing Co.

Leach, Gerald: The Biocrats, New York, 1970, McGraw-Hill Book Co.

Lorenz, Konrad: On aggression (Marjorie Kerr Wilson, translator), New York, 1966, Harcourt, Brace and World.

Lorenz, Konrad, and Leyhausen, Paul: Motivation of human and animal behavior: an ethological view (B. A. Tonkin, translator), New York, 1973, Van Nostrand Reinhold Co.

Montagu, Ashley: The nature of human aggression, New York, 1976, Oxford University Press.

Neville, Robert: The philosophical arguments, Hastings Center Reports 8(3):33-37, June 1978.

Shinn, Roger L.: Population and the dignity of man. In Williams, Preston, editor: Ethical issues in biology and medicine: proceedings of a symposium on the identity and dignity of man, Cambridge, Mass., 1973, Schenkman Publishing Co.

Thompson, Travis: The behavioral perspective, Hastings Center Reports 8(3):29-32, June 1978.

Veatch, Robert M.: Case studies in medical ethics, Cambridge, Mass., 1977, Harvard University Press.

Warwick, Donald: Contraceptives in the Third World, Hastings Center Reports 5(4):9-12 August 1975.

Warwick, Donald: Ethics and population control in developing countries, Hastings Center Reports 4(3):1-4, June 1974.

Warwick, Donald: The moral message of Bucharest, Hastings Center Reports 4(6):8-9, December 1974.

Warwick, Donald, Merrick, Thomas W., and Caplan, Arthur: International population programs: should they challenge local values? Hastings Center Reports 7(5):17-18, October 1977.

Williams, Preston, editor: Ethical issues in biology and medicine: proceedings of a symposium on the identity and dignity of man, Cambridge, Mass., 1973, Schenkman Publishing Co.

5

Artificial insemination

HISTORY AND DEFINITIONS

In 1884 a wealthy Philadelphia businessman approached Dr. William Pancoast, a professor at Jefferson Medical College, to ask if anything could be done about his childless marriage. Pancoast was perplexed and discussed the problem with six students in his human anatomy class. The wife was examined (the examination was described as "very complete, almost as perfect as an army examination"), but the infertility seemed linked to the husband, especially after he admitted to having had gonorrhea in his youth. After a few months of medical treatment without success a student suggested using a "hired man," the best-looking student in the class, whose semen could be injected into the wife's uterus while she was under anesthesia. Dr. Pancoast approved the experiment without consulting either the husband or wife. A son was born who resembled the husband, but Dr. Pancoast began to have mixed feelings about what he had done. He eventually told the husband, who was delighted and asked only that his wife never be told how she had conceived their child. Everyone involved in the incident agreed to keep silent about what had occurred. Years later Dr. Pancoast died, and the incident would have died with him except that in 1909 Dr. Addison Davis Hard, one of the six students, published an article about it in *Medical World* and met the son, who was then 25. In his article, "Artificial Impregnation," Dr. Hard recounted what was most likely the first documented case of human artificial insemination; he also suggested some eugenic improvements in the human race.[1] The 1909 article marked the beginning of experimentation into and arguments about artificial insemination that still continue today.

Artificial insemination is a relatively simple procedure. Semen obtained through masturbation is introduced by a sterile syringe into the woman's cervix or uterus when she is ovulating. It is hoped that fertilization and implantation will take place naturally and the pregnancy proceed as usual. About 20% of artificial insemination attempts are successful.

There are two kinds of artificial insemination: homologous, or artificial insemination by the husband (AIH), and heterologous, or artificial insemination by a donor (AID). AIH is more common by far and is used if no known cause for infertility exists or if the woman's vaginal or cervical secretions are somehow inhospitable to her husband's semen. It can also be used if the husband's sperm are viable and motile but low in number. In this case several samples of his semen are collected, usually several days apart, kept frozen, and then mixed together to produce the required concentration of sperm. AID is used when the husband is found to be totally aspermatogenic or if evidence shows that he is a carrier of a genetic disease. A suitable donor is located or frozen sperm from a sperm bank is used, but in neither case are the identities of the donor and recipient made known to each other. An effort is usually made, however, to match some of the physical characteristics of the donor to the recipient mother or couple. AID is also used when a single woman wishes to become pregnant.

Artificial insemination is now considered to be a routine part of the treatment of infertility, although for the couple it usually is their last hope to have a child and is far from routine for them. Many couples see artificial insemination as the final effort to conceive before they consider adoption, which may involve a wait of 5 to 10 years.

LEGAL IMPLICATIONS

To date no legal problems have arisen from AIH when the husband is the biologic father of the child, the legal husband of the mother, and consequently the legal father of the child. The fact that his semen was introduced into the vagina of his wife by a syringe rather than his penis makes no *legal* difference. There are legal implications of AID, however, and these tend to be complex. The legal issues involved with AID will be discussed in this chapter. Individual cases that come to litigation are hampered because few legal precedents exist and only a few state statutes concern aid.

One of the major legal issues concerns the question of adultery of a specific and modified kind. Adultery is considered a criminal act in almost all states. Although adultery usually involves physical contact between the man and woman, with AID the child conceived is not biologically related to the woman's husband, and the biologic father of the child is not the husband of the wife. Can it be said that the crime of adultery has taken place? Would the woman therefore be a criminal and her husband an accessory to the crime, assuming he had consented to AID? If AID is a crime, then the resulting child would have to be considered illegitimate. Many might scoff at the use of this seemingly old-fashioned term, but the problems for the child could be enormous. Whose name would the child be legally permitted to use, would he be eligible for inheritance, and would he have to be legally adopted by his mother's husband? Is the mother's husband legally responsible for supporting the child?

If the mother is charged with the crime of adultery, could she possibly be jailed or lose custody of her child? These eventualities *could* happen but usually do not as long as the husband has consented to AID. Rarely would a judge convict a woman of adultery merely because AID had taken place. The law also generally recognizes the legitimacy of a child conceived in wedlock even if the child is not the husband's. If the husband wanted to challenge the legitimacy of the child, he would have to institute a suit against his wife and prove it was not his. Until it was proved that the child was not his, he would be considered the legal father. In AID when the husband consents to the procedure, he also consents to assume all responsibilities of fatherhood and will be considered the legal father of the child.

If AID takes place without the husband's consent, the legal problems become thornier. One can assume that in some cases the husband might be angry and want to take legal action against his wife. Can the husband name the donor as correspondent in a divorce suit? If the identity of the donor is confidential, can the physician performing AID be named instead? If adultery is defined as requiring physical contact between the wife and the biologic father of the child, would the husband have grounds for a suit? If the husband brings suit, can the identity of the donor be revealed, and if so, can he be made legally responsible for his biologic child? If the identity of the donor cannot be revealed or if records were not kept accurately, and if the physician is somehow named as correspondent or legal father, what can be done if the physician is a woman?

The technology of artificial insemination has proceeded farther and faster than the legal statutes and precedents that apply to it. This has happened in many areas of health technology and is probably a reflection of the different rates at which the wheels of technology and legality turn. For example, if a husband divorces his wife several years after successful conception with AID, is he still considered the legal father of the child? If his legal fatherhood remains intact in the state in which the AID was done, will it remain intact if he or his former wife move to another state?

In 1967 a man divorced three years earlier was charged by the District Attorney of Sonoma County, California, with willful nonsupport of his wife's 6-year-old child conceived with his consent by AID. The wife had refused such support, but the man was found guilty. Even though he may have agreed to the venture, can such a husband disown the child as illegitimate when born? If the husband is not in any sense the child's real father, according to the courts, then who is the father of the child? The anonymous donor? If so, could the donor claim the child, or at least visiting rights? Can the child claim a share in his biological father's estate? If the identity of the donor becomes known can the husband sue him for child support? One way around this problem is for the husband to legally adopt his offspring by AID.*

No federal statutes exist regarding the legitimacy of AID children, and only one state, Oklahoma in 1967, has passed a law declaring the child to be the legal responsibility of the woman's husband. In all other states problems are solved one case at a time. One dilemma concerning the legality of artificial insemination involves what happens when a physical and technical fact crosses the boundary of common sense and practicality. For example, a sample of donor semen could be used to father about 30 children. Consider the possibility of 30 irate husbands all suing one unsuspecting man for child support. This possibility exists, but the impracticality of this situation is ludicrous. Accusing a donor or even the attending physician of adultery is legally possible, but what person would *believe* it actually is adultery? By no stretch of the imagination could the public or a jury be asked to equate masturbating into a sterile receptacle with a physical act of sex—one would have to legally define AID and sexual intercourse as the same thing.

---

*Utopian motherhood: new trends in human reproduction, by Dr. Robert T. Francoeur, p. 32. Copyright © 1970 by Robert T. Francoeur. Reprinted by permission of Doubleday & Company, Inc.

Whereas AID without the consent of the husband may or may not constitute legal adultery, many think it violates the sanctity of the marriage insofar as a woman may become pregnant without her husband's knowledge and consent and then expect him to assume responsibility for the resulting child. The husband in this instance ought to have some legal recourse, perhaps the right to an uncontested divorce or the absolution of his financial responsibility to the child.

ETHICAL AND SOCIAL ASPECTS

The ethical and social ramifications of artificial insemination revolve around two major issues: (1) the nature of sexuality, breeding, and the concept of parenthood and family and (2) how far the technology involved will and should lead us. Various aspects of these two major issues will appear in the following discussion.

Single women

Single women provide an example of both the sexual and technologic issues. More single women, both lesbians and heterosexuals, can be expected to seek AID as the means for having a child without marriage or even the most casual sexual relationship with a man (which could turn out less casual than she had anticipated if the man later chooses to assert his rights as father).

Single-parent families are common in the United States. Most did not start out that way or occur by specific design, but increasing numbers of women who find themselves pregnant are deciding to rear the child alone. More single women are attempting to adopt a child, and because of the logistic and social difficulties they encounter, AID might be a logical answer for them. It is also a practical solution for a lesbian who does not wish to have intercourse with a man and because of legal or societal sanctions cannot adopt a child.

The increase in the divorce rate, changes in child custody laws, and the increase in single-parent families in general are stressful to society. Can the American social conscience accept a woman who feels she has no need of a husband or a father for her children?

Many women who become single parents prefer not to be and have not deliberately chosen the role. Lesbians, however, choose the role of single parent or raise the child in a two-parent family in which both are women. (Male homosexuals also raise children alone or in couples, but this is much less common than with female homosexuals). This practice is radical and unacceptable to many people.

There are several commonly held objections, both practical and moral, to single women having children with AID.

Given the structure of our society, it is easier and more practical to bring children into the traditional two-parent family for several reasons: the child is less likely to be subjected to denigration by his peers, there is no risk of social ostracism of mother and child because of their family structure, financial supports are often stronger, another parent is available in the event that one dies, and there are advantages to having both masculine and feminine influences on the child's development regardless of the child's sex.

In addition to the practical objections there are at least three common moral objections. The first is a belief that the traditional two-parent family is sacrosanct.

A deliberate attempt to begin a nontraditional family is seen as immoral and an affront to the institution of marriage. Judeo-Christian tradition holds that marriage is the appropriate milieu for procreation. Yet though the familiar passage in Genesis, "Be fruitful and multiply," tells us to procreate, it does not say that conception and birth must occur within the bounds of a socially sanctioned relationship. One could argue that a single woman who chooses AID is fulfilling that directive.

Another moral objection views conception by AID as adultery, a position that was discussed previously. A third is the opinion that a woman has no right to use a man simply because she needs a biologic act that only he can perform. One might compare this issue with the practice of some men choosing a wife solely for bearing children. It is traditional and legally permissible in many cultures for a man to discard a wife who has borne him no sons. From Biblical times to the present men have used women for their childbearing capabilities, and one could ask if a woman's use of a man's semen for the same purpose is any more or less moral. One might consider it to be more moral because it is far less taxing emotionally, physically, and financially for a man to masturbate, hand his semen over to a physician, and walk away than for a woman to conceive, bear, and raise a child.

Another objection to single women using AID, although not so loudly stated, is the idea that a woman may neither need nor want a man in her life. Although fatherless households are common in the United States, some people still balk at the idea of a woman deliberately choosing to eliminate the man in creating her family. His services are needed, but *he* is not. This is difficult for people to understand, especially in a male-dominated society, and is therefore considered unusual, sick, or somehow deviant. Consequently it is strongly discouraged. This strong negative reaction is understandable because the nuclear family with a mother and father has been the foundation of Western society and a fundamental social norm. In addition our society has been functioning on the premise that women are dependent on men as sources of love, satisfaction, income, and social status; as these ideas begin to fall apart and as some women learn to depend on themselves and on each other for these needs, they are finding that they can manage without men in many spheres of activity. Although the vast majority of women prefer to function as a parent in partnership with a male parent, those who are choosing AID are in most cases finding that they can be successful and lead fulfilling and satisfying lives.

Religion

The Catholic Church and some dioceses of the Episcopal Church have expressed the opinions that AID is contrary to God's will, adulterous by nature, and harmful to the sanctity of the family. Because of its impersonal nature it is thought to dehumanize sex and reduce women to the position of mere breeder.

It is interesting to note that most Catholic theologians do not appose AIH; on the contrary, they see it as moral and good, as long as the semen is not obtained from the husband through masturbation, which is prohibited by the Church in all circumstances. The Catholic proscription of masturbation, sometimes called onanism, derives from the story of Onan in Genesis. According to law, Onan was required to "lie with" his brother's wife after he died and provide offspring in his brother's name. Onan knew that his offspring would not count as his own, so every time he lay with Tamar he "spilled his seed on the ground" and refused to impregnate her. What Onan did was displeasing to God, who then took Onan's life. What is not certain in the story is whether God's displeasure concerned the wasting of the seed or Onan's refusal to obey the law. Onan may have been punished by death for his pride and disobedience rather than for wasting his seed. The story does not specify whether Onan actually masturbated or merely practiced coitus interruptus, but the Catholic Church interprets the story as a proscription against masturbation. This makes it difficult to obtain semen for AIH, for the husband must have his spermatozoa aspirated from his testes by needle puncture, an uncomfortable method often less satisfactory than obtaining semen through masturbation. Thus the Church condones AIH by sperm aspiration but condemns procreation through means other than husband-wife copulation.

AID, however, is unconditionally condemned by the Church for three major reasons: (1) it is considered laboratory breeding of human beings and is as unnatural as any other clinical manipulation of the life process, (2) it is against natural law because the husband has not copulated with his wife, and (3) an injustice would be done to the children, who would be considered illegitimate because AID is viewed as an act of adultery.

Many moral theologians have argued against the Catholic view. The first reason, concerning laboratory manipulation of a natural process, may be countered by the idea that human beings with more control over their natural lives can rise to a loftier moral plane where they are free to devote themselves to activities that will improve the quality of their lives. In other instances the Church looks with favor on interference with other life processes (for example, pharmacologic intervention in various diseases) that allows people to transcend a base concern for survival.

Should men attempt to suppress their reasoning faculty and the emancipating fruits of it because there are risks entailed? To transcend natural restrictions, to seek ends by means devised through choice rather than by physical determinism, is a human and spiritual victory. With many of us it is a matter of reasoned conviction that our march toward freedom and control is an irreversible trend. Man's moral and spiritual need is to exercise his moral faculties, including those of self-control as well as control over external circumstances. His task is not to suppress and deny his intellectual faculties.*

Many fear and consequently wish to prohibit any technologic advance. Some think that possible future techniques or knowledge could not be controlled and might be used to do evil. This argument has been around a long time; one can imagine that ethical debates raged over the first use of fire. Knowledge and the use to which it is put *can* be controlled and in some cases probably should be, but to prevent a childless couple from conceiving because of the fear of some remote scientific evil seems not in the best interest of intellectual inquiry or the health professions.

The second reason the Church prohibits AID, that it is unnatural because the

---

*Fletcher, Joseph: Morals and medicine, Princeton, N.J., 1954, Princeton University Press, p. 117.

husband has not copulated with his wife and because the donor is required to masturbate, may be countered in two ways. The couple *have* copulated—and probably more frequently and more diligently with the intent of procreating (in the Church's view, the primary reason for copulation) than those who are not thinking about fertility or hoping that a child will not result. A couple who has had and will most likely continue to have natural intercourse for the express purpose of conception would seem to come closer to fulfilling the Church's requirements than a couple who has intercourse without the desire to have children. The fact that their copulation does not result in conception is an accident of nature and punishing the couple by denying them AID would seem an injustice that is incongruent with the tenents of the Church.

Masturbation was discussed in reference to the story of Onan. In the interpretation of many non-Catholic theologians God's anger with Onan results from his deception and refusal to obey the law rather than his masturbation, the method he used for disobedience. In addition there are those who oppose masturbation for its own sake because they see it as a selfish, uncreative, and unproductive act. If masturbation is considered immoral for those reasons, however, then surely the donor who masturbates for the sole purpose of contributing to the creation of a new life should be seen not only as *not* immoral but as praiseworthy.

The Church's third reason, that AID is an act of adultery resulting in an illegitimate child, seems to be a rigidly legalistic and mechanistic view of the bonds of marriage. To argue that placing a syringe filled with the semen of a total stranger into a woman's vagina is an act of adultery seems inhumane and unjust. Adultery is usually considered to involve physical contact, that is, carnal knowledge between the spouse and the lover, and the deception of the spouse, that is, the husband or wife sneaking out of the marriage vow and engaging in clandestine trysts with a lover. In AID there is no physical contact and the husband is fully aware of the procedure and has given his consent.

Two Biblical stories suggest that conception may take place between a man or woman and someone other than the spouse. The first and most important concerns the law that caused Onan so much trouble. If a man dies leaving his wife childless, the dead man's brother is required to impregnate his sister-in-law, and the resulting child will have her dead husband's name and all the inheritance rights that would have accrued to him (Deut. 25:5-6). In Genesis 16:2 to 17:22 we find Sarah, who is childless, advising her husband, Abraham, to copulate with the maidservant so that he could have a child. The maid, Hagar, did conceive, and Sarah became so jealous that she treated Hagar so harshly that she ran away. God made Hagar return to Sarah and Abraham, and she bore a child. Presumably God was pleased by the unselfish act of Sarah and Abraham, and when Abraham was 100 years old and Sarah 90, Sarah conceived and eventually bore Isaac.

Thus Biblical precedent does exist for children to be born outside the technical bonds of marriage. The question whether a child resulting from AID is illegitimate does not exist if AID is not considered adultery. Although almost no statutes exist about the ligitimacy of an AID child, precedent has shown that the courts generally consider an AID child to be legally that of the husband and wife. As AID becomes more common, the issue of legitimacy will be raised less frequently.

Protestants are divided about AID as about many moral and ethical issues. In general, conservatives view the marriage bond in terms of what is seen as God's desire for monogomy: copulation should take place within marriage or it should not take place at all. AID might be seen in this view as adulterous. But Protestant theologians have not made definitive statements about the moral correctness or permissibility of AID, which thus has not officially been decreed adultery. However, nowhere in the Bible is there a specific injunction in favor of monogomous marriage; there is only a prohibition against adultery, which provides leeway in the interpretation of the definition of AID as adultery.

Protestants, like Reform and Conservative Jews, as a rule debate which traditional Biblical commands (both positive and negative) should be obeyed in modern life and in light of modern technology. Those who tend to relax their observance of strict injunctions maintain that moral sensitivity and human relationships are more important than certain rules and the institutions created by those rules. Many also argue that no commandment can be proved a clear expression of God's will and that therefore no conduct specifically must be performed or prohibited. Theologians are awash in a sea of ambiguities about what is good and moral in view of the difference between historical situations and new situations, current technolgic developments, and anticipated future changes. Religious liberals can point to almost any moral issue in health care and show how technology or knowledge transcends or at least circumvents traditional religious values.

Many theologians oppose AID as a solution to a childless marriage, but there are few objections to adoption for the same purpose. If a child conceived with AID is considered illegitimate even though he sprang from the wife's body, what about an adopted child related biologically to neither the husband nor the wife? The child is legally adopted by both parents, but even when an AID child is legally adopted by the woman's husband, many religious leaders still consider him illegitimate. The issue of adultery and the legitimacy of the child resulting from AID can be complicated by theologians who are perhaps more concerned with abstract concepts and religious appearances than they are with the people involved. Sometimes moral and psychologic issues become confused, especially as they relate to fertility and legitimacy.

Social policy

AID, especially as it becomes more widespread and popular may involve potential social and logistic problems. There is a possibility of incestuous conceptions and even more likely of the children of one donor marrying each other. Even though accurate records might be kept matching donor and recipient, no prohibitions exist presently about the number of times a donor may contribute his semen or the number of private physicians, clinics, or sperm banks that may collect the semen of an individual donor. Artifical insemination goes on all over the country, and it is not likely that a donor's history of donation is investigated—nor does a mechanism exist to do so. Consider the possibility that a young man who has many or all of the attributes of a desirable donor—good looks, intelligence, absence of known genetic defects, and excellent health—moves around the country contributing his sperm to as many as dozens of wives of infertile husbands, and perhaps he has a brother who is an equally desirable donor and who also chooses to help in this way. The possibility exists that when dozens or hundreds of children of these two men reach maturity some may marry each other. The only way to prevent his kind of incest is with yet another aspect of technology, the computer. A sperm donor's clearinghouse could be established to determine whether a particular donor's semen has been previously used. The passage of legislation forbidding use of a donor's semen in more than one insemination would greatly reduce the chance of inadvertent incest between AID children. Incest is one of the most deeply ingrained taboos in almost all cultures. Much of the repugnance stems from the idea of physical sexual contact between close relatives, but it is known that in societies and even extended families where incest is widely practiced, the incidence of birth defects increases. This is one of the major reasons in addition to religious proscriptions why marriage between siblings and in some instances first cousins is prohibited by law in the United States and elsewhere.

Those opposed to AID have made the arguments that the physician would have too much power and might select only donors that were pleasing to him and that somehow the ratio of male to female children (nature provides 105 males for every 100 females) could be significantly altered. A kind of Orwellian specter of people made to order has been created by alarmists who see physicians using AID to fulfill their own eugenic fantasies. These fears are unfounded. The number of children who would result from AID compared to the total number of natural conceptions is so small that it is and would continue to be statistically negligible, especially if viewed in the context of the world and not of only technologically advanced countries. The argument that physicians will become all-powerful in the selection of donors assumes that a physician makes choices based on his own personal preferences. The possibility certainly exists that a physician might use a blue-eyed donor to inseminate a woman who comes from a long line of brown-eyed people because he happens to prefer blue eyes. But the chance of this happening is small in relation to the number of physicians performing AID, and when compared to the number of natural conceptions, it is insignificant. AID in no way resembles the practice of eugenics with which a certain genetic or chromosomal makeup is favored through planned breeding. As much chance is involved with the child who results from AID as with the child who would have resulted if the husband's sperm had impregnated his wife or if in different circumstances the woman had married the man whose donated sperm impregnated her. Human breeding now occurs almost completely by random selection (except insofar as we are attracted to and marry people whose characteristics we like and admire) and AID will not change that random selection.

Opponents of AID point out that the world is already overpopulated and say that infertile couples have a moral obligation to adopt existing homeless children. This argument cannot carry much weight for two reasons. First, the number of AID procedures performed in lieu of adopting an existing child would not significantly affect the birth rate, and in addition those countries experiencing the most severe population growth are generally underdeveloped ones where AID is almost never used. The second reason involves the issue of personal choice and the freedom of an infertile couple to overcome their childlessness as they choose. Adoption is an act of such far-reaching social and psychologic consequences that to adopt a child for any reason other than a strong desire of both husband and wife to be parents would be foolhardy. To do so out of obligation to do something about over-population in the face of one's own infertility also would not be a wise decision. A couple who is infertile must make their own choice and should have the freedom to remain childless, treat the infertility by a variety of methods including artifical insemination, or adopt a child.

Predetermination of gender. Another technologic possibility inherent in artificial insemination is the predetermination of gender, a technique that has implications far beyond the treatment of infertility. It has been known for many years that the shape and size of a gynosperm (or X sperm, which results in a female offspring) and androsperm (or Y sperm, which results in a male offspring) differ and that they can be separated from each other by use of a centrifuge or electrophoresis or the application of chemicals to the sample of semen to make the different types of sperm sink to the bottom of the container at different rates. Thus it is easy simply to remove the gynosperm before artificial insemination if a male child is desired or the androsperm if a female child is desired.

In the available literature about gender predetermination and preference, no source reported that a majority of those surveyed would prefer female children. Campbell[2] reported that at Tietung Hospital of the Anshan Iron and Steel Company in China a technique was developed to determine the gender of a fetus as early as 47 days after conception by withdrawing a small amount of amniotic fluid via the cervix. The technique was developed ostensibly for family planning, and for the same purpose women were offered abortions after gender had been determined. Of the 100 women having experimental gender determination tests, 30 opted for abortion and 29 of the aborted fetuses were female.

Consider what could happen in a country in which the ratio of males to females is increased by even a small percentage. Because many men would not be able to marry, cultural values would change. Perhaps marriage and the family would decrease in importance leading to a more generalized bachelor existence with, as Etzioni puts it, a kind of frontier-town mentality causing an increase in aggression and violence. Men would have fewer women with whom to engage in sexual activity, a situation the could lead to a rise in homosexuality and prostitution. On the other hand, marriage and the family could increase in importance and desirability simply because opportunity would become rarer for men. Shopping for spouses, the payment of male dowries, and polyandry (one woman having more than one husband) could become prevalent and result in all kinds of legal and ethical questions: which husband would be father to which children, who would be responsible for supporting whom, how would sexuality be affected, and how would the traditional qualities of marital fidelity, intimacy, and loyalty be affected?

The entire character of society in general could change. Presently in our society men tend to be more aggressive and violent than women and are more often convicted of violent crimes. There would likely be an increase in physical violence, particularly rape. In those classes and cultures in which males are more highly valued than females there might be an even greater disproportion of males, resulting in interclass and interracial tension.

An imbalance in the numbers of males and females could give rise to a kind of supply-and-demand situation. As the number of women decreased, their value might increase leading to an eventual evening out of the gender ratio or to a sudden increase in the number of females conceived by artificial insemination. Some scientists and sociologists feel that a sudden increase in the number of males born would soon correct itself because society would seek to emulate the balance of nature. A correction would be quickly sought because societal problems would be evident. Westhoff and Rindfuss[3] in a 1970 National Fertility Study found that 63% of childless women wanted their first child to be a boy, and Fidell found the same was true of 85% of the female undergraduates at California State University at Northbridge. Because of the influence of the women's movement, however, it is likely that the number of women desiring firstborn males will decrease. Nonetheless, since firstborn children regardless of their gender tend to have characteristics that are considered more masculine than feminine (for example, assertiveness, aggressiveness, and independence), a preponderance of firstborn males might change the character of society in ways that are not be predictable.

If firstborn children really do reap a disproportionate share of the good things in life—or if people become convinced they do—then a campaign could arise to increase the proportion of firstborn girls. Cults dedicated to the increase of a single sex might appear, and political factions might pressure sex-control policies that seemed to complement their other aims. If an imbalance in the sex ratio became too threatening, governments would surely enforce new ratios, perhaps by means of premiums and fines on the model now imposed in India. Politicians might also decide to manipulate ratios for "positive" reasons. A nation bent on making war, for instance, could breed millions of male warriors.*

Postgate[4] proposes gender control as the only means of checking the world's too rapid population growth. As the number of men increased in relation to the number of women, the percentage of women as potential mothers would decrease (and it could be predicted that more women might refuse to bear children as they saw the ratio tipping out of their favor), and men would realize that they would have to breed more women or face severe problems. This would not only decrease the total population but would tend to balance the gender ratio, and natural sex selection could then ensue.

Postgate acknowledges that while the imbalance exists (he does not estimate how long, but presumably it would last several generations or perhaps a century) women would not be particularly happy, fulfilled, or even safe. Rape might increase, and women might be used as rewards for aggressive males, be kept out of the job market as men in the majority would compete for available jobs, and be unable to travel safely for fear of kidnap or capture. Those who favor gender selection as a way to control the total population seem to view the resulting situation only statistically and not in terms of what it would mean to the lives of the human

---

*Campbell, Colin: The manchild pill, Psychology Today, 90, August 1976. Reprinted from Psychology Today magazine, Copyright © 1976 by Ziff Davis Publishing Co.

beings involved. But whatever eventual good might accrue to society has to be weighed against the harm that would come to both women and men. A society filled with many more men than women could reduce women to slavery at worst and a sort of refined concubinage at best. Campbell comments that

Dangerous or not, sex control appears finally to be inevitable and unstoppable and in some ways this fact is the most disturbing theme of all. Too many scientists are working on it for it to go away, and no doubt the work itself is fascinating and compelling. The commercial market for sex control would be tremendous. In any case there are no real precedents in our society for not inventing something. A ban would seem totalitarian and medieval. We tend to think of technological progress as a rational force since technology itself is rational in many ways. Yet, as we have seen in the case of sex control, there are also dreams at work, and ancient aspirations.*

PSYCHOLOGIC ASPECTS

One can become so involved with the technologic and ethical aspects of artificial insemination that it is easy to forget human beings are involved. When thinking about artifical insemination one tends to visualize sperm being carefully prepared and inserted into a vagina. But the sperm and the vagina belong to people, usually a husband and wife who have come to realize that they cannot have children naturally and will have to depend on technology to aid them in this seemingly simple function.

What effects does infertility have on the emotions of wife and husband, on their images of themselves as a functioning man and woman, and on the marriage?

The women's movement has made great strides in helping women find satisfaction in areas other than motherhood and realize that procreation is not the only function of a woman. But a huge gap exists between the *choice* not to become a mother and the *inability* to do so. A woman of my acquaintance made the decision when she was very young not to marry or have children and arranged her life accordingly. She had a sporadically active sex life and used conception control haphazardly. As she grew older and never became pregnant, even after having taken many chances, she became convinced that she could not become pregnant and completely stopped using conception control. At age 37 she became pregnant and was shocked out of her complacency. She chose to have an abortion and to be sterilized at the same time because she really did not want a child. But the night before her surgery she said, "Well, this proves at least I could do it if I wanted to." Perhaps her need to prove herself a "real woman" was so great that she unconsciously planned the pregnancy, though it may actually have been an accident. But the satisfaction she expressed in being able to become pregnant was real. Imagine the plight of a woman who has tried and tried to become pregnant and cannot accomplish this act that seems almost totally out of her control. She walks along the street, sees pregnant women or mothers with children, and wonders why the rest of the world (or so she sees it) can have children and she cannot. Her self-concept will surely be diminished, with negative feelings spilling over into other

---

*Campbell, Colin: The manchild pill, Psychology Today, 90, August 1976. Reprinted from Psychology Today magazine, Copyright © 1976 by Ziff Davis Publishing Co.

areas of her life. She may come to see herself as less than womanly or feminine. She may engage in active grieving because of her loss of such an important function, or she might compensate for the loss by developing other talents and abilities.

Men are also affected by infertility. A man may see fertility and virility as intertwined, each having to do with sexual prowess and think his inability to impregnate a woman is a decrease in his manhood. He may associate fertility with feelings of power, masculinity, and even aggression. A man who is infertile may lack self-confidence, and this may lead to impotence, lack of assurance in other spheres of activity, and as with women, a general decrease in self-esteem. Or he might compensate by surging ahead in business or professional matters or by turning to other forms of creativity. With both men and women, a physical lack in one area of life can affect the rest of it either positively or negatively depending on the kind of person he or she is.

The marriage is bound to suffer as a result of infertility. Each partner openly or privately may blame himself or the other. Even after the cause of infertility is established, either or both partners may continue blaming the other or feeling guilty. A spouse who is infertile may feel guilty for not "proving" his or her own fertility before marriage and may fear the other will want a divorce but might not want to discuss it openly. Or the infertile partner might offer a divorce in a sort of sacrificial way because of feelings of inadequacy as a spouse. Or either spouse could be secretly glad, if he or she had had ambivalent feelings about wanting a child, because the childlessness can be attributed to physical circumstances rather than to a choice with which the other does not agree.

It is unlikely that both partners in any marriage desire a child with equal intensity. Depending on many factors including emotional and financial circumstances, one partner or the other is probably more desirious of having a child at any given time. Regardless of the intensity of desire for a child, and regardless of who wants one more at the time infertility is diagnosed and the cause established, the marriage will be affected. Even a strong healthy one will experience a serious crisis. A shaky marriage may fall apart because it might not be able to withstand accusations, blaming, and recriminations that may be expressed verbally or left unsaid. The honest expression of feelings and exchange of intimacy are generally a desirable goal in marriage, but the matrimonial bond needs to be strong to bear up under the verbalization of the kinds of feelings infertility engenders. The wise couple will seek help if they cannot work through their difficulties alone. An observant nurse, when she comes in contact with an infertile couple or the husband or wife separately, will recognize sources of strain or the potential for it and will investigate further to find out what the couple's level of communication is, how open they are with each other and toward the problem, and whether they feel the need for crisis intervention or some other form of counseling.

If the couple decides to resolve the problem by artificial insemination, it is important to realize that some physicians require that they meet psychologic criteria. Those characteristics most often sought are a stable, mature relationship and evidence of free and open communication. In the case of AID both the husband and the wife must come to terms with his infertility and with the fact that he will not be the baby's biologic father. He must accept the role of social father, and in many cases it is deemed desirable that he be willing to legally adopt the child to prevent any future questions of legitimacy. These criteria are by no means universally required, yet they raise an interesting ethical question: if a couple who conceives naturally does not have to conform to any criteria, why should such be imposed on couples who seek artificial insemination? There is no clear answer except that as is the case with adoption, artificial insemination is a procedure one must request because it is not free or available to everyone automatically. The physician who performs AID wields a kind of power over an infertile couple's ability to bear a child. A physician who requires that a couple meet his criteria is in effect saying to them that they must be worthy to receive what he can offer. This may seem a harsh view of the power implicit in the health care system, but when it is examined in the context of the paternalism involved and the situation is compared to that of the couple who must meet no criteria to conceive naturally, this view seems more realistic. Most physicians who practice artificial insemination do not exercise this degree of power over their infertile clients, for their goal is to help a woman become pregnant, but they do have the power and could exercise it if they chose to.

After the artificial insemination has been accomplished, strong psychologic factors can operate during pregnancy and in the years that the child is growing up in the family. The husband or wife may have a change of mind after the fact, perhaps because they were not entirely certain that the choice was correct in the first place, because the woman suddenly feels adulterous or feels she does not want to carry another man's child, or because now that the pregnancy is actually on its way or the child has been born the husband realizes he cannot accept or deal with the fact that he is not the biologic father. Perhaps the couple realize they do not want a child as much as they thought. If these feelings do not pass and they are certain about their change of mind, abortion is a possibility, although aborting a fetus that was conceived after such duress and effort is not an act to be considered lightly. It may place a heavy strain on the marriage, especially if, as is likely, only one partner has a change of mind.

More often than not it is the husband who decides he does not want the child, especially if it was conceived with AID, and thus jeopardizes his relationship with the child and with his wife. He might resent the child, ignore it in some way, or even physically abuse it. He might disown it psychologically and attempt to do so legally, and if his feelings are very strong he might simply walk away from his family.

One cannot always predict one's own or another's reactions to major life events, but in the case of artificial insemination sufficient evidence exists that some people do experience negative feelings when unqualified joy might be expected instead. The physician who discharges the client couple as soon as pregnancy is established does them a disservice. They require continued care and observation, if only so that they know they have someone to speak to should they experience unexpected negative feelings that confuse and frighten them. The nurse is in an excellent position to accomplish this. If she works with a physician who specializes in infertility, she can concentrate on the human aspects of the couple while the physician attends more to the physiologic problem. If she is alert to the couple's dynamics and their ways of relating to her and to each other, she should have an inkling of problems to come and can take action before a crisis erupts. The nurse is in a position to assess the situation, find out if the couple acknowledges potential problems, and see what they plan to do about it. She can refer them to crisis intervention therapy or to groups of other couples who have experienced artificial insemination. Probably the most important nursing function in this regard is the recognition and continued observation of a couple who find themselves developing unexpected emotional problems.

There are also psychologic implications for the child. Should he be told that he was conceived by AID, or is that not necessary? Could he somehow be traumatized by this knowledge, or does the idea that ignorance is bliss make a better policy? Somewhat of a parallel can be drawn between the situations of an AID child and an adopted one. The former can know his mother but not the biologic identity of his father, the latter neither. Studies of adopted children have shown that it is better to reveal the fact of adoption as soon as the child is old enough to understand than to delay the revelation or not to tell the child at all. Secrecy and deception can only weaken family ties because the deception blocks lines of communication and because the fear of eventual revelation lurks behind all family relationships. Parents fear divulging the fact of AID because of embarrassment or a reluctance to let a problem as private as infertility be known. There is, however, no need for deception and secrecy. They generally do not lead to good parenthood or successful family relationships, and AID has become common enough that the woman and child are not viewed by the public as experimental subjects.

Attention is seldom paid to the psychology of donors. A man goes into a private room in a physician's office, masturbates, hands his semen to the physician or even an office worker, is thanked, and goes home. Except for his sperm, which are no longer part of his body, his part is over forever or until his next donation. But is it? Does he simply masturbate and give no thought to what happens to his sperm? Or years later does he look at children who resemble him in some way and wonder if he is the father? If the donor is married, how does his wife react to the fact that her husband is father to children that are not also hers? Should she be told? Is it better to choose donors who are married or those who are single? "Experience has led many physicians to believe that a donor should be both married and a father, so that his personality and progeny have some 'proof in the pudding.'"[5] This position makes little sense either psychologically or biologically. A simple sperm count is sufficient to show a donor is adequate; he need not have fathered his own children. It is difficult to understand how and why his personality would be any more or less desirable as a donor simply because he had children. All manner of men with every conceivable personality trait father children and do not father children.

One further psychologic factor should not be overlooked, although it occurs only rarely: the "relationship" of the infertile woman to the donor. Does she fantasize about him, wonder what he looks like, imagine herself in an adulterous relationship with him, want to find him and possibly even make love with him? Does this sound preposterous or far-fetched? Leach[6] has reported an instance in which a

French woman learned the name of the donor and left her husband to join him. Another woman bore a remarkably beautiful child and began to press the physician for the name of the donor, whom she said she wanted to marry. These situations, however, are not common and are reflective of a woman whose personality is less than strong and fully integrated. The possibility of this happening nonetheless makes a good case for some sort of psychologic screening, no matter how informal, before AID is performed. A physician who views an infertile couple as *people* rather than a physiologic problem to be solved will be less likely to see this kind of aftermath to AID.

STORAGE OF SPERM FOR THE FUTURE

Sperm bank A. I. D. is now fairly common. When one thinks of the logistic problems of A. I. D. the reason is obvious. Without a bank the donor has to provide his specimen to order, probably on 2 successive days each month, perhaps for several months on end; and it has to get from donor to doctor, in secrecy, within thirty minutes. This is a strain, so few donors will donate for more than about a half a dozen patients. This means that A.I.D. doctors are for ever having to search for willing donors and screen them medically and genetically. Some admittedly do not do this as well as they would like. There is also the husband-matching problem. With a donor shortage it is not always possible to get a healthy, high I.Q., genetically cleared donor who also matches the husband's physical characteristics.*

This description makes the solution to the problem seem obvious, uncomplicated, and desirable. Simply walk into a room filled with rows of neatly tagged vials of semen arranged according to physical characteristics, IQ, and perhaps even personality traits. One envisions the same sort of calm, efficient atmosphere as in a blood bank. In many respects the concepts are similar, although the ethical issues differ.

Sperm banks could have a variety of uses. A man could deposit his sperm for future use if he planned to have a vasectomy or if he thought he might in the future marry an infertile woman. A future-oriented purpose of a sperm bank is the protection of semen from mutation by exposure to radiation. A man's semen could be collected early in his life and frozen for use when he decided to have children. This idea might not be popular and would probably be considered only by men who worked in places with a high risk of radiation damage to spermatogenesis, such as nuclear power plant employees, astronauts, radiologists, and the like. As another purpose, a couple for eugenic reasons might want to use the sperm of someone with particular physical characteristics. This also might not be popular and would have to be mutually decided by the couple after long and serious deliberation. One of the strongest yet most psychologically questionable uses of a sperm bank is the artificial insemination of a widow with her dead husband's sperm, a kind of link with the dead that many health professionals would view as emotionally unhealthy and a retardant to grieving.

There are distinct advantages to a sperm bank. The bank can operate with much more efficiency, control, and economy than an individual physician. Donors would all be screened according to the same criteria, and various chromosomal and genetic

*Leach, Gerald: The biocrats, New York, 1970, Mc Graw-Hill Book Co., p. 81.

tests could be run on all samples of semen. The secrecy of identities is more likely to be secure, for the physician performing AID perhaps hundreds of miles away would have no reason or way to learn the identity of the donor. Sperm banks established in various locations throughout the country or the world could be connected by computer to establish the number of times a particular donor's semen is used and also to determine whether a new donor has already given sperm and has been identified and screened at another bank.

There are also disadvantages and dangers in the use of sperm banks. One of the most serious is the possibility of a genetic disaster. The first sperm bank child was born in 1953[6] and was normal, but as the number of these children increases, so does the possibility of genetic damage. Not all sperm can be expected to survive being frozen without damage, and so far no test has been devised to determine that sperm have not been damaged in the process.

Sperm samples from different donors vary enormously in their ability to withstand the freeze-store-thaw process. There is also intense selection within any one sperm sample from whatever donor. Since "freezability" must in some way be a genetic trait it is extremely likely that it is connected with other genetic traits that matter—like disease resistance, stature, intelligence and so on. So sperm with these traits will tend to survive and the traits be passed on.*

With a large-scale establishment of sperm banks and a national computer network a political danger arises. What is to prevent a government from stepping in by either direct control or the establishment of a regulatory agency and setting up all sorts of guidelines and criteria? The possibility exists that a government might substitute the sperm of donors of the government's choice, perhaps the sperm of people of a particularly passive nature or semen from which all the gynosperm had been removed to increase the percentage of males born. Could a commercial operator as well as a government be as unscrupulous as he wished and use the bank for his own purposes? Could an operator or government enact some incredible political fantasy, a bank filled with the sperm of men with certain physical traits and a certain passivity of character? The bank might refuse to sell sperm unless the recipient met certain physical and emotional characteristics; perhaps she also would have to be a rather pliant person and resemble the donor. This possibility is frightening, but because the percentage of children conceived by AID through a sperm bank is negligible unless coercion is involved, it is not likely to occur.

Sperm banks could change the nature of the way we reproduce. In theory any woman could be impregnated by the sperm of any man. The time/place nature of reproduction would be altered; that is, the emotional and sexual relationship of a man and woman—husband and wife—need not be present. A woman could be completely autonomous in her reproductive capacities. Her husband need not contribute to her decision; she would not even need a husband. The resulting child could be *her* property and responsibility; even if she is married, if her husband had no part or a minimal part in her decision to reproduce, he might not feel much

---

*Leach, Gerald: The biocrats, New York, 1970, McGraw-Hill Book Co., p. 82.

love or attachment to the child. Feminists may be tempted to applaud this state of affairs, for at first glance it might seem desirable for a woman to have that degree of control over her reproductive powers. But if the idea is examined further, one might wonder what would be gained by the acquisition of this much personal power. Although the structure of the American family is changing rapidly, one cannot assume that all changes are beneficial. If all women *could* choose to bear children by artificial insemination with sperm from banks, although of course not all would want to, the nature of male-female relationships might be unalterably affected. The emancipation of women might be total, but in this case emancipation may or may not be equated with freedom. The political and social consequences might be enormous, for it is not reasonable to expect that men would react positively to the tossing aside of their sexuality.

Some interesting and complex scenarios can be imagined to follow the advent of sperm banks. Suppose in the year 1980 a husband donates sperm to a bank in anticipation of having a vasectomy or for some other reason. In 1981, still not having made the decision for vasectomy, the couple have a child conceived through sexual intercourse. The next year the husband has a vasectomy, and several years later in 1985 the couple decide they wish to use the sperm on deposit in the bank. They do so, a child is conceived and born, and all proceeds normally. What is the birth rank of the children? One might automatically say that the child conceived naturally is the firstborn, but what is the legal status of the child conceived and born after his father has been sterilized? Can it be *proved* that the sperm deposited in the bank in 1980 is the same sperm thawed and used in 1985? Can it be proved that even if it is the same sperm, it has not been genetically altered by the freezing or thawing process and thus contains genes no longer identical to those of the husband? Is the husband then the real father?

Another possibility is a man contributing his sperm to the bank and then dying. His widow is impregnated with her husband's sperm and while pregnant remarries. Is the second husband legally responsible for the child? Even though it can be proved that he is not the biologic father, he is the husband of the mother and therefore might have some responsibility, especially if he knew the situation before he agreed to marry.

If a woman could persuade a physician to perform AID without her husband's consent (there are probably some physicians who would do this) with sperm from a bank, would the husband be in any way responsible for the child? What if a married woman stole a sample from a sperm bank and simply impregnated herself? Who would be the legal father of the child? If she chose not to tell her husband, there might not be cause for him to question her pregnancy, but if she did tell him, what legal remedies would be available to him? Would he have grounds for divorce? Would he have to support the child? If a husband refuses to give his consent for AID, can the wife demand to be impregnated anyway and legally release her husband from responsibility? These situations may seem like flights of fancy, but they are all possible, even probable, as sperm banks become more frequently used. The proliferation and increased use of them seems to be a trend in the United States.

IN VITRO FERTILIZATION

In vitro ("under glass") fertilization is the process by which an ovum is removed from the body, placed in a petri dish filled with a sterilized growth medium, and then covered with healthy motile spermatozoa. One sperm then pentrates the ovum in the normal manner, and growth of the blastocyst begins. After a period of time, usually 10 to 14 days, the blastocyst is implanted in the woman's uterus via the vagina by means of a syringe, and the pregnancy proceeds normally. The first human born after in vitro fertilization (IVF) was Louise Brown, born in England in 1978 as a result of the work of Edwards and Steptoe. Louise's birth was the medical media event of the year. What is not generally known is the amount of experimentation and unsuccessful attempts that preceded her birth.

It is not known exactly when research began, but as early as 1878 Schenk of Germany unsuccessfully attempted IVF with rabbits, and for about 50 years thereafter various scientists experimented with mammalian fertilization. In 1940 Rock claimed to have fertilized human eggs; some of them had actually divided but all died. In 1950 Shettles claimed to have advanced IVF techniques to the point where an actual embryo, in the form of solid mass of cells, existed. There was much skepticism about the validity of all this work, but in 1959 Chang of the United States succeeded in impregnating a rabbit with an ovum fertilized outside the body. The rabbit gave birth. The procedure was interesting in that the ovum was removed from one rabbit, fertilized with sperm recovered from the uterus of another rabbit after coitus had taken place, and then implanted in yet another rabbit. Four rabbits, three female and one male, were needed for the procedure. Chang's experiment was replicated several times in succeeding years. In 1961, Petrucci of Italy claimed to have fertilized a human ovum that then lived for 29 days. He destroyed it because it became deformed (this set off a wave of moral furor and is discussed later in the chapter). Petrucci's work could not be validated because he took no photographs of the embryo, and he was accused by the scientific community of fraud. Animal experimentation continued through the 1960s, and in 1969 Edwards and Steptoe of Cambridge University began working with human IVF.[7] They perfected a method of obtaining large numbers of human ova from women volunteers who had been injected with gonadotrophin, which caused them to mature many ova per menstrual cycle instead of the usual one. Thirty hours after the injection the women underwent a laparoscopy in which a suction tube and a sophisticated optical device were inserted into the ovary and the mature ova were isolated and aspirated into the hollow tube. This provided fresh, undamaged ova for experimentation. The eggs were put in the presence of the woman's husband's sperm. None of their initial attempts were successful, and during the next few years fertilization experiments continued in a variety of ways. Some used ova matured inside the women's bodies, and in some the ova matured in vitro. Various growth media were used and subjected to all kinds of environmental conditions. After 9 years the work resulted in Louise Brown.

The greatest physical danger in this kind of experimentation is that the manipulation of the ovum, the sperm, or the blastocyst will damage it to the extent that a deformed fetus results. The embryo could in theory be karyotyped, that is, have a chromosomal examination. For this to be done it would have to be removed from its petri dish, subjected to further manipulation, and thus endangered even more.

IVF is seen by some as a positive research step in the ultimate achievement of surrogate procreation; others see it only as a medical technology to alleviate barrenness; and still others view it as dangerous tampering with natural human life.

Future developments

It was exactly 100 years from the first unsuccessful attempts to fertilize rabbit eggs to the birth of Louise Brown. What will the next century bring? The speed at which technology is advancing is increasing, and therefore in the next century the leaps forward will come faster and go further than in the last. Many scientists think that the next logical step is the creation of an artificial uterus, thus eliminating the need for human bodies in procreation (except for producing ova and spermatozoa). If a human conceptus can be grown to the blastocyst stage in vitro, why not continue for another $8\frac{1}{2}$ months of fetal development?

The technologic problems in developing an artificial uterus are great but not insurmountable. During the course of experimentation, however, fetuses would die or would have to be sacrificed at all stages of development. If the ethical issue of abortion is then raging as violently as now, consider the issues and feelings involved in the development of an artificial uterus, the deliberate planning of artificial life, and in many instances the killing of that life. It is likely that public sentiment would prevent funding of such experimentation, but many think there are definite reasons to proceed with the development of an artificial uterus: fetology would be advanced because scientists could watch fetal development and learn how many congenital abnormalities develop; corrective surgery could take place or the fetus could be immunized against a variety of diseases while still in utero (in this case in vitro); tissue samples could be taken from the fetus, frozen and stored for injection in the event the person required organ transplantation in future; an artificial uterus would be kept in an absolutely safe and sterile environment, and thus the fetus would be protected from infection, radiation, and other environmental hazards; a fetus in an artificial uterus would not be exposed to the effects of smoking, alcohol, drugs, or an unbalanced diet; mutations could be bred out of the human race and selected genetic traits could be bred in (see Chapter 3); if the use of artificial uteruses were universal, the concept of illegitimacy would cease to exist, as would spontaneous abortion and all other problems associated with in utero gestation.[7]

Most of these reasons to procede with the development of an artificial uterus can also be seen as reasons to ban this development. Those who disapprove of any form of reproduction that is not completely natural could be expected to protest loudly. Women, who would be most affected, will be divided. The very concept of motherhood would be forever altered. Physical pregnancy could become rare though as with many forms of technology, a couple need not choose this option but could conceive and carry the fetus naturally. The relationship between men and women would be altered.

Once a woman has no more difficult or lengthy role in reproduction than a man (or not much more difficult or lengthy: she will still have to undergo laparoscopy once, when several dozen eggs will be collected and put into cold storage), she will find that society does not expect her to have a special relation to her offspring that takes up years of her life, and also she will not expect it of herself. Too, a society that can grow fetuses in a laboratory will be more disposed to have meaningful day- and night-care centers and communal nurseries on a large scale, for the state, being a third parent, will wish to provide for the maintenance and upbringing of its children.*

This inevitable alteration of the mother-child relationship may or may not be ultimately beneficial; one could speculate endlessly about what would happen to other aspects of society in an attempt to determine the psychosocial implications of the development and common use of an artificial uterus. One thing is certain: the nature of sexuality, when intercourse is no longer necessary for procreation, will change. Homosexuality might increase, and the purpose for which sex is used might change the *way* in which it is used. Since intercourse would no longer be necessary to have children, it might no longer be seen as the most normal form of sexuality, and taboos about other forms of sexual gratification might disappear. Altering the way we procreate might have as far-reaching evolutionary, social, cultural, and psychic effects as a major alteration in the way we breathe or the way our heart beats. The nature of humanity would be changed, and we might have to redefine what we mean by a person. It seems almost inevitable that sooner or later (sooner if national priority and funding is given to the research) an artificial uterus will be developed. This kind of research might be suppressed for a while, as it was in the United States with in vitro fertilization, but the human need to know, develop, and invent will outlast those who wish to suppress research.

Ethics of in vitro fertilization

The artificial uterus lies in the distant future. Louise Brown is alive and well now and has already been followed by other babies who are the result of IVF. Although speculation about the distant future is endlessly fascinating, the ethical dilemmas of the present and near future are more important here. Credible, logical arguments appear on both sides of the issue of IVF.

In 1975 the federal government banned grants for research on IVF, and without funding research all but ceased in the United States. The ban was instituted because of moral and religious qualms about tampering with natural reproduction and because it involved research on embryos, which politically was too close to the abortion issue. In 1979 the Ethics Advisory Board of the Department of Health, Education, and Welfare urged lifting the ban after it had held extensive public hearings in which the testimony of lay people as well as theologians and scientists was heard. The board recommended four safeguards when the ban is lifted: (1) the public must be informed if research reveals an increased incidence of abnormal children as a result of IVF, (2) research should be funded only if it seeks informa-

---

*Grossman, Edward: The obsolescent mother: a scenario. In Wertz, Richard W., editor: Readings on ethical and social issues in biomedicine, Englewood Cliffs, M.J., 1973, Prentic-Hall, Inc., p. 98.

tion that cannot be obtained in other ways and if it seeks to increase the safety and effectiveness of embryo transplants, (3) embryos shall be implanted only for lawfully married couples, and (4) research should be limited to embryos in the first 14 days of development, the length of time implantation takes naturally.[8] This report is controversial because it involves the use of public funds for research of which a large segment of the public disapproves.

The ethical issues of IVF range far and wide. One of the most important is the risk of damage to the embryo that would result in an abnormal baby. During the period before implantation when the conceptus is still a blastocyst and has not yet become an embryo, cells are still undifferentiated; that is, each cell has much the same function as each other cell. These undifferentiated cells have a greater ability to regenerate than more fully developed cells. Thus if a blastocyst is damaged during the manipulation that it must undergo, the risk of an abnormal fetus forming is relatively slight. The questions, of course, involve how slight the risk is, how it compares with damage that occurs in normal implantation, and whether it is worth taking. The first two questions have not yet been definitively answered; the latter would seem to be up to the couple who is contemplating IVF. A complicating factor is that the couple cannot make an informed decision about the risks they are willing to take if they have incomplete information. Thus until more research is done, their decision will be a more or less blind one. Even though the risk of damage is small, it does exist. One debate centers on the question of whether human interference may increase the risk of damage that does or does not occur in nature. Many scientists and moralists believe that even the smallest risk of damage is morally unacceptable. The counterargument is that it should be the couple's decision, after they have been informed of the possible danger, whether they wish to take the risk and whether they see it as acceptable. The decision in this situation parallels that in a recent incident in the United States. In March and April, 1979, during the nuclear power plant accident on Three Mile Island, Pennsylvania, when radiation was leaking into the atmosphere, pregnant women and preschool children were advised to leave the area immediately adjacent to the power plant. Although there was considerable debate at the time about the amount and quality of information given to the public, the decision to stay or leave was left to the individual after warnings had been issued about the possible dangers of exposure to atmospheric radiation. An interesting legal issue arises: if a child who is born as a result of IVF has congenital abnormalities, can he sue for damages either his parents or the physician who performed the procedure? Could it be proved that the abnormality occured as a result of IVF, or could the defense rest its case on the likelihood that it would have occurred in nature?

A question of rights is involved in IVF: a barren couple has the right to take action and to use available technology to counteract that barrenness. If a woman's fallopian tubes are blocked and surgery cannot correct the problem, as was the case in Louise Brown's mother, her only recourse is IVF. This view implies that IVF is a therapeutic procedure rather than an experimental one and should be available to anyone who wants it and can benefit from it. A physician treating an infertile couple generally has the right to use any procedure he thinks will help as long as he has received informed consent from the couple. What right, then, does the state or any other institution have to interfere with this exercise of human rights? An argument can be made that the rights of the couple and physician can be abrogated if the rights of society in general or a significant group of individuals have been infringed on in the process. This argument has been used by religious factions to say that the experimentation involved in IVF infringes on the rights of the embryo, an entity that is seen by some to have rights from the time of fertilization.

There are other objections to continuing IVF research. Some consider the research procedures involved to be ethically questionable and say that they should be subject to boards of review. The way one looks at this issue depends on whether IVF is seen as research or a therapeutic procedure or a combination of both. A review process should be concerned with documentation of informed consent for the couple submitting to the procedure. However, unless a blastocyst is considered an entity that can claim rights, one wonders what ethical violation could occur in IVF research. Some people would ban research on the basis that no one knows where it might lead. These same people would ban artificial insemination for similar reasons and in all likelihood might wish to prohibit all forms of research concerning reproduction or any other natural life process. They have been successful in stopping various kinds of experimentation for short or long periods of time, but it is unlikely that the research process will be permanently halted just because of a generalized fear for the future. It would be more profitable to raise the public's consciousness about life research by instituting a program of public education and awareness of research trends than to direct efforts at suppressing the urge to know.

In any event, if in vitro fertilization becomes a stratightforward low-risk procedure, banning it by legislation out of ill-defined fears of the future will merely deprive a whole class of currently barren women of their chief hope; and it will, as a result, encourage the development of "black market" or "bootleg" in vitro fertilization operations. In short, in vitro fertilization is a good case in which to refrain from legislative paternalism.*

Another question is whether limits should be placed on a couple's desire to have a child. In other words, how much research should be permitted to satisfy the essentially personal and selfish need to bear a child? If a child is born deformed because of IVF that was either properly or improperly done, who should bear the burden of caring for the child and paying for the care—the parents because they wanted it so badly and knew the risks they were taking, the physician who performed the procedure because he may have inadvertantly caused the defect, or society because it approved and paid for the research in the first place?

The Del Zio trial. Probably the most famous case involving IVF prior to the birth of Louise Brown was the Del Zio trial. Doris and John Del Zio were married in 1968 and tried unsuccessfully for several years to have a child. After a variety of tests were performed, a hysterosalpingogram revealed that Mrs. Del Zio had a blocked fallopian tube. The couple was referred to Dr. William J. Sweeney, a spe-

---

*Toulmin, Stephin: In vitro fertilization: answering the ethical objections, Hastings Center Reports 8(5):10, October 1978. Reprinted with permission of The Hastings Center. © Institute of Society, Ethics and the Life Sciences, 360 Broadway, Hastings-on-Hudson, N.Y. 10706.

cialist in infertility at New York Hospital–Cornell Medical School. Dr. Sweeney operated to remove the obstruction, and Mrs. Del Zio became pregnant but had a spontaneous abortion. Two further operations were unsuccessful, and in 1972 Dr. Sweeney suggested IVF. Mrs. Del Zio was excited at the prospect and consented to the procedure presumably after having been told the risks and being informed that it had never been successfully performed with a human being.

Dr. Sweeney called in Dr. Landrum Shettles of Columbia University College of Physicians and Surgeons, who had been doing IVF research since World War II. Ova were removed from Mrs. Del Zio at New York Hospital and given to her husband, who took them to Presbyterian Hospital (associated with Columbia University College of Physicians and Surgeons) and gave them to Dr. Shettles. Mr. Del Zio masturbated in a hopital men's room and handed his semen to Dr. Shettles, who combined the two specimens and put the container in an incubator.

Dr. Shettles told a colleague about the procedure, and word of it eventually reached Dr. Raymond Vande Wiele, Chairman of the Department of Obstetrics and Gynecology at both Columbia's hospital and medical school. Dr. Vande Wiele conferred with his superiors, who told him to halt the procedure. He and Dr. Shettles had a conversation in which the latter stated that he did not feel he needed approval for the experiment because it was "simply a surgical procedure" and had been done at another hospital. Dr. Shettles offered to discard the fluid, but Dr. Vande Wiele asked that it be frozen and preserved as a "document." Apparently it still is in a freezer somewhere in Presbyterian Hospital, although its contents have not been fully examined.

When informed that the procedure had been halted Mrs. Del Zio was most distraught. Afterwards she had a number of physical and psychologic problems and claimed to have lost interest in sex. The Del Zios filed suit against Dr. Vande Wiele, Columbia University, and Presbyterian Hospital for terminating a voluntary procedure undertaken by another physician and for intentionally causing Mrs. Del Zio undue emotional stress. Dr. Vande Wiele's defense depended mainly on the incompetence of Drs. Sweeney and Shettles and the view that his stopping the procedure prevented Mrs. Del Zio from incurring serious infection. The jury, however, awarded the Del Zios a total of $50,000 from the hospital, the medical school, and Dr. Vande Wiele.

The trial was emotional and bitter and in it the professional competence of the physicians was depicted as less than adequate. The ethical issue, not emphasized at the trial, involved the conflict between Mrs. Del Zio's intense desire to have a baby and Dr. Vande Wiele's obligation to observe the hospital's three-stage review process on all experimental procedures. It is ironic that although hospitals and other health institutions usually are reluctant guardians of experimental subjects' rights, this time the hospital and medical school found themselves protecting Mrs. Del Zio (and their federal funding for research) more than she wanted to be protected.[9] The Del Zios won their case, but a precedent was not established. It can be expected that further IVF dilemmas will end up in court.

Research protocols in that case were so haphazard that they could be considered nonexistent. Even if the procedure were considered therapeutic rather than experimental, it was carried out in a highly unusual way: two hospitals were used, and Mr. Del Zio carried his wife's ova from one hospital to another in a taxicab. In the future there will be more legal wrangling about IVF, and it is hoped that ethical issues will play a greater role in the courtroom.

SUMMARY

Artificial insemination is the process by which semen obtained through masturbation is introduced into a woman's cervix or uterus during ovulation. It is hoped that fertilization and implantation will take place naturally and the pregnancy proceed to term. Ther are two kinds of artificial insemination: homologous, artificial insemination by the husband (AIH), and heterologous, artificial insemination by a donor (AID). The former is more common.

Legal complications involving AID involve several basic issues. Is AID a modified act of adultery and thus subject to criminal prosecution? If it is considered adultery, what is the legitimacy of the child and what is the subsequent legal and financial responsibilty of the woman's husband for the child?

The two major ethical and social considerations involved in artificial insemination are (1) the nature of sexuality and breeding and the concept of parenthood and family, and (2) the question of how much technology of artificial insemination should change the way we reproduce.

AID has become a solution for single women who want a child without having a relationship with a man. Objections to single women availing themselves of AID are strong even though single-parent families are increasingly common in the United States. Objection are raised on several levels. The strongest belief is that the traditional two-parent family is the most socially acceptable and that a single woman who uses AID is insulting the institution of marriage. It is probably easier and more practical to begin a family in the usual way, but one cannot say that it is any more or less moral. In addition, the notion that a woman neither wants nor needs a man in her life is disturbing to many people.

Religious objections to AID, voiced mainly by the Catholic Church and conservative Protestant and Jewish theologians, are concerned mostly with the idea of adultery and the danger to the sanctity of the family and also see AID as a dehumanization of physical sex. The Church feels that AID is adultery, although this is not a popular view. Not many people equate placing a semen-filled syringe into a vagina with a physical act of sex. Furthermore, the aura of secrecy and deception that surrounds adultery is missing in AID. Children born of AID, however, might be considered illegitimate because they were conceived in an adulterous manner. The Catholic Church does not forbid AIH but prohibits masturbation, making the collection of semen difficult and painful. Moral theologians have countered the Church's position with several arguments based on scientific, technologic, and humanistic principles.

There are many views about social policies in AID. One concerns the possibility of inadvertant incest if one donor fathers so many offspring that the children might marry and reproduce without knowing that they are biologically related. The problem could be easily controlled by computerized matching of donor and recipient and accurate record keeping.

Opponents of AID fear that too much power might be placed in the hands of physicians and scientists who might misuse it. This fear is mostly unfounded because the percentage of children conceived by AID is negligible when compared with the total number of conceptions in the world. The only opportunity for genetic manipulation in AID is in predetermination of gender when gynosperm and androsperm can be separated in a sample of semen. The implications of a world numerically dominated by men are far-reaching and would affect every aspect of society and culture. Most of the predicted changes would be extremely negative to women.

The human aspects of artificial insemination cannot be ignored when one deals with technology and ethics. Being infertile has a profound psychologic effect on both men and women. People tend to believe that if they cannot reproduce naturally, they are somehow inadequate as human beings. This lowered self-image spills over into other spheres of life, most notably marriage, which can be destroyed or badly damaged by the stress of infertility. It is a crisis that can be effectively dealt with, especially if an observant and sensitive nurse recognizes it and intervenes so the couple can confront and work through their feelings and conflicts.

It is not uncommon for a husband or wife to have a change of mind for various reasons after artificial insemination has taken place. Abortion could be considered, but it is likely that the feelings are temporary and similar to the heightening of ambivalence that all husbands and wives feel when pregnancy becomes a reality. Strong negative feelings, especially on the part a spouse who might abuse or ignore the child, can be predicted. Again, an observant nurse can help avert disaster. Parents often feel confused about whether to tell a child that he was conceived by AID. The general consensus of experts in the area is that the child should be told. Truth is easier to deal with than deception, and secrecy is not a healthy foundation for family relationships.

Storing frozen sperm in banks for the future is becoming more common and is likely to continue. There are advantages and disadvantages. A sperm bank could operate efficiently, safely, and economically by using accurate records and statistics. The semen of men who wished to undergo vasectomy could be collected and stored to be used later. A possibility of genetic damage does exist when using frozen semen; not enough research has been done to prove that the freeze-store-thaw process is entirely safe.

Political and social dangers exist in that sperm banks might be taken over by a government or private citizens for their own purposes. The popular use of sperm banks could change the way we reproduce and would surely affect the nature of sexuality.

In vitro fertilization (IVF) is the process by which an ovum is removed from a woman's body, mixed with the sperm of her husband, and placed in a growth medium. Fertilization then occurs, the blastocyst is inserted into her uterus for implantation, and the pregnancy proceeds as usual. The procedure sounds simple, but experimentation went on for a century before the first baby conceived by IVF was born. The greatest physical danger in IVF is that the blastocyst will be damaged during physical manipulation, resulting in a deformed child.

Many scientists feel that the next technologic step in reproduction is the development of an artificial uterus in which fertilization, implantation, and the entire pregnancy would occur. The developmental problems are not insurmountable; the technique could become a reality within the next century. The ethical issue concerns whether an artificial uterus should be developed and used. There are advantages and disadvantages to development of an artificial uterus, and the ethical dilemmas would seem endless and insoluble. In 1979 the Ethics Advisory Board of the Department of Health, Education and Welfare recommended that a 1975 ban on funding for research on IVF be lifted. Not everyone agrees with the propriety of this recommendation; some feel that IVF research should be halted. IVF is still so new, however, that one cannot know what future danger exists.

Another issue involves the right of a couple to expose an embryo to risk because of a personal desire to bear a child. Does the embryo have rights? It presently has no legal rights, but many moral theologians feel that it should be protected from the time of fertilization. If a defective child is born, who is responsible for its care, and can the child eventually bring suit for damages against his parents or the physician who performed the procedure? What responsibility does society have?

REFERENCES

1. Francoeur, Robert T.: Utopian motherhood: new trends in human reproduction, New York, 1970, Doubleday & Co., Inc.
2. Campbell, Colin: The manchild pill, Psychology Today, p. 86, August 1976.
3. Westhoff, Charles F., and Rindfuss, Ronald R.: Sex preselection in the United States: some indications, Science 184 (4127):633-636, May 10, 1974.
4. Postgate, John: Bat's chance in hell, New Scientist 58(810):12-16, April 5, 1973.
5. Fletcher, Joseph: Morals and medicine, Princeton, N.J., 1954, Princeton University Press.
6. Leach, Gerald: The biocrats, New York, 1970, McGraw-Hill Book Co.
7. Grossman, Edward: The obsolescent mother: a scenario. In Wertz, Richard W., editor: Readings on ethical and social issues in biomedicine, Englewood Cliffs, N.J., 1973, Prentice-Hall, Inc.
8. Yes to test-tube babies, Time, p. 89, April 2, 1979.
9. Powledge, Tabitha M.: A report from the Del Zio trial, Hastings Center Reports 8(5):15-17, October 1978.

BIBLIOGRAPHY

Baby gender choice studied, The Baltimore Sun, p. A3, September 6, 1978.
Campbell, Colin: The manchild pill, Psychology Today, pp. 86-91, August 1976.
Etzioni, Amitai: sex control, science, and society, Science 161:1107-1112, September 13, 1968.
Fletcher, Joseph: Morals and medicine, Princeton, N.J., 1954, Princeton University Press.
Francoeur, Robert T.: Utopian motherhood: new trends in human reproduction, New York, 1970, Doubleday & Co., Inc.
Gould, Donald: The children of the dead, New Statesman 94:48, July 8, 1977.
Gould, Donald: Not just doctors' dilemmas, New Statesman 95:74, January 20, 1978.
Grossman, Edward: The obsolescent mother: a scenario. In Wertz, Richard W., editor: Readings on ethical and social issues in biomedicine, Englewood Cliffs, N.J., 1973, Prentice-Hall, Inc.
Leach, Gerald: The biocrats, New York, 1970, McGraw-Hill Book Co.
Lappé, Marc: Ethics at the center of life: protecting vulnerable subjects, Hastings Center Reports 8 (5):11-13, October 1978.
Postgate, John: Bat's chance in hell, New Scientist 58(810):12-16, April 5, 1973.
Powledge, Tabitha M.: A report from the Del Zio trial, Hastings Center Reports 8(5):15-17, October 1978.
Ramsey, Paul: Manufacturing our offspring: weighing the risks, Hastings Center Reports 8(5):7-9, October 1978.

Robertson, John A.: In vitro conception and harm to the unborn, Hastings Center Reports 8(5):13-14, October 1978.

Smith, Harmon L.: Ethics and the New Medicine, Nashville, 1970, Abingdon Press.

Steinfels, Margaret O'Brien: In vitro fertilization: "Ethically acceptable" research, Hastings Center Reports 9(3):5-8, June 1979.

The Torah, Philadelphia, 1967, Jewish Publication Society of America.

Toulmin, Stephen: In vitro fertilization: answering the ethical objections, Hastings Center Reports 8(5):9-11, October 1978.

Westhoff, Charles F., and Rindfuss, Ronald R.: Sex preselection in the United States: some indications, Science 184(4127):633-636, May 10, 1974.

Yes to test-tube babies, Time, p. 89, April 2, 1979.

6

Contraception and sterilization

The modern birth control movement may have begun in 1798 when Thomas Malthus, an Anglican clergyman, wrote his famous essay, "On Principles of Population as it Affects the Future Development of Society." Malthus was concerned about population increasing faster than the capacity of resources to support it. He did not advocate contraception but instead recommended late marriages, no marriage, or abstinence within marriage. No wonder the population kept increasing! Ironically, Malthus in developing his reasoning ignored intercourse that did not occur within marriage, though in England at that time many illegitimate children were being born.

Women have sought ways to prevent pregnancy since they first connected the act of sexual intercourse with pregnancy. At first the most commonly used method was the insertion of various items into the vagina, usually sponges or cloths soaked with herbs or mineral salts, to prevent semen from flowing into the uterus. Some were ineffective, some were quite caustic and painful, and some worked either by mechanical blocking or because of the potency of the substance used. Sometimes objects were put into the vagina, but these were less effective and tended to anger men who found their way blocked. This trick is said to have originated with caravan drivers in the Sahara who used to place peach or apricot pits into the vaginas of camels to prevent them from becoming pregnant in caravans that took months to cross the desert. All these methods, as ineffective and potentially harmful as they were, circulated quietly among women who often felt a desperate need to control their bodies but who were living in an era that saw the primary purpose of womanhood as motherhood. The contraceptive failure rate was high, as was the death rate from complications in pregnancy and labor.

In the United States during its first century and a half no effective and safe forms of birth control existed. Many women were relatively isolated, and dissemination of even inaccurate information was difficult. Pioneer women frequently did not see each other for weeks and were encouraged by men to bear as many children as possible to populate the West. Physicians had only slightly better knowledge of human reproduction than the public, and because of society's thinking at the time it did not occur to them to help women prevent pregnancy. The first step was not taken until 1822 when Dr. Charles Knowlton, a Massachusetts physician, published a tract called "The Fruits of Philosophy; or, The Private Companion of Young Married People," for which he eventually was fined and jailed.[1] The piece sold exceptionally well despite repeated legal attempts to ban it for the birth control information it contained. During the period from 1863 to 1893 Charles Bradlaugh and Annie Besant published in England a magazine called the *National Reformer* in which they advocated planned parenthood; in 1877 they were tried for selling Knowlton's book. The resulting publicity only served to increase sales.

From then on the birth control movement was on its way, and the journey from total ignorance to complete freedom from fear of pregnancy is still not complete. The trip has been a rocky one, with storms of protest involving issues that range from the morality of preventing conception to the purpose of womanhood. Those who advocated birth control were once slandered by the press, scorned by society, physically assaulted, arrested, fined, put on trial, and even imprisoned. The Woman's Suffrage movement in the late nineteenth and early twentieth century, although it concentrated mostly on voting rights, began to help women look at their lives, functions, and societal roles. It was at about this time that women began to demand more freedom of control over their bodies, including effective methods of contraception.

Probably the greatest pioneer in the American birth control movement (and as a result, in the liberation of women) was Margaret Sanger. Her work as a public health nurse convinced her that being able to limit family size was essential for social and economic progress. She began her birth control campaign alone. In 1915 she was indicted for sending birth control information through the mails and the next year was arrested for operating a birth control clinic in Brooklyn. Women clients, however, supported her and flocked to her clinic in enormous numbers. Gradually she won public and legal support, and the Margaret Sanger Clinic that she opened in 1923 in New York City is still operating and is a leading force in birth control information and research.

The federal government, however, by its policy of noninterference and its refusal to fund research for safe and effective birth control, held back progress. It was not until the 1963 amendments to the Social Security Act (concerning improving maternal and child health services for high-risk, low-income families) that funding was made available for family planning services. The Child Health Act of 1967 stipulated that 6% of all funds allocated for maternal and child health services *must* be used for family planning services that are to be offered to all families receiving Aid to Dependent Children. In 1971 the Family Planning Services and Population Research Act (Public Law 91-572) authorized $30 million each for research and services, though only $6 million was ultimately appropriated.

Today all states sponsor some type of family planning service, and there are hundreds of privately owned and operated clinics that are both independent or associated with hospitals. Many are run exclusively by and for women who increasingly are demanding to control their reproductive processes.

ETHICS OF CONTRACEPTION
Freedom to control one's body

The major underlying ethical question about contraception concerns whether individuals have a right to control parenthood, and if so, what means are permissible. A second question, which cannot be separated fully from the first, concerns *who* has the right to that control. Is it the woman's right because it is her body that is used for reproduction since the man's presence is not required after the act of intercourse? Is it a right of both the man and woman because they have joint responsibility for the resulting child? If the latter is correct, does either partner have a greater right to exercise control over reproduction? Can a man forbid his wife to use contraception because he wishes to exercise his right to fatherhood? Does a woman have a moral right to secretly take birth control pills even though her husband wants to have a child? Does a man have a right to impose birth control on a woman, for instance, by refusing to have intercourse unless he is wearing a condom? How much control of one's own and one's sexual partner's reproductive functions should an individual be permitted to have?

The issue of control is also an issue of natural law, the idea that human beings do not have a right to interfere with whatever nature intends. Natural law is invoked in many areas of human endeavor, but nowhere is it more assiduously applied than in the realm of sexuality. Proponents of natural law state that God or nature intended pregnancy to result from sexual intercourse and that any interference with that cause-and-effect relationship is a violation of natural law and thus a sin. This is a fatalistic approach to human destiny, and some believe it is neither moral nor humane. Many believe that the true moral stature of human beings involves their acknowledgment of natural circumstances and how they control those circumstances. We take steps to prevent or control many events that occur in nature. Tall buildings in California are built to withstand earthquakes, fire department rescue squads are trained to rush to the side of heart attack victims to save their lives, dams are built to control the natural ravages of flooding. One might wonder if building a concrete dam to protect people's homes from the uncontrolled and natural rush of water is any more or less moral than inserting a rubber diaphragm into one's body to prevent an uncontrolled and natural rush of children. Both are natural occurrences, both can have devastating effects on the lives of people, and both can be controlled by technology with similar principles although on far different scales.

The ancient Greeks and early Christians thought of natural law as simply the will of God or an interpretation of right and wrong in the universe, the process by which people developed rationality and a sense of ethics and morality to cope with the natural world. Natural law did not pass judgments about physical law or physiologic occurrences. *Natural* to the Stoics meant what was true or ideal, not what was physical or material. The word was bound to cause confusion, and natural law came to mean the physical laws about what was observable in nature, including such things as gravity, the movement of stars in the heavens, tides, and all physiologic processess of animals and humans.

Natural law today is generally defined as a "higher law," as opposed to the positive law of a state. The rules of natural law were considered universally valid and discoverable only by rationalism. The term has lost much of its ethical meaning, but some Christian theologians and moralists have assigned ethical values to things that occur in nature, thus complicating the issue even further. To establish standards of what is right and wrong about what exists factually in natural human physiology is as illogical as saying that the rotation of earth in one direction is more moral than if it were to rotate in the other direction.

Even if one were to base morality only on what nature intended by a physiologic process, the human reproductive physiology could not be seen as being well designed for reproduction. In a 28-day menstrual cycle only about 5 or 6 days are near optimum for conception, and a woman's need and desire for sexual intercourse continue well beyond the time when she is able to reproduce. Human beings desire and are capable of intercourse at any time, not just during the woman's fertile period, and thus it would seem that nature's design was to give humans the opportunity for sexual pleasure at times when conception is not likely. On the basis of time percentages it appears that pleasure is as much or more important than reproduction in nature. Intercourse is necessary for reproduction, which is one of its major purposes. But why does it feel so good? One answer is that nature made intercourse so pleasurable that we would have not only a source of physical delight but also another way of communicating love, affection, closeness, and intimacy. It can be seen as nature's way of permitting us to share our physical selves with other human beings. It is pleasurable apparently because nature intended us to have intercourse for reasons other than procreation. Sexual intercourse is not simply a prescription for pregnancy.

Control of one's body is part of the control of one's destiny; to be a morally or ethically developed person is to have the ability to make choices about how one uses one's internal and external environment. Technology has given us the gift of freedom of choice in being able to control our reproductive environment. Many believe that exercising that choice is an exhibition of a higher level of morality than is subjecting oneself to the whims of chance and simply accepting whatever pregnancies happen to occur. A moral human being is not a helpless reed swaying in the wind of chance. Human beings have evolved to the point where they can exercise some control over their lives. If evolution is seen as natural, not using our evolutionary capabilities and behaving as though we cannot control ourselves would be against natural law. Natural law can be used to support a variety of points of view.

To prohibit choice in the matter of reproduction is to prohibit freedom, and permitting uncurtailed access to birth control does not mean that anyone is necessarily obligated to use it—one merely has the freedom to make the choice to do so or not. Even in matters that unlike birth control may be physically harmful, this kind of choice is left to the individual. Cigarettes and alcohol are harmful to our bodies, but they are readily available; one is perfectly free not to buy them. If violence on television is disturbing, one is free to turn it off. Nonetheless one has the choice to smoke, drink, or watch television and the freedom not to. Preventing choice by law or a variety of social sanctions is less moral than granting it. This does not imply that the *use* of contraception is any more or less moral than the non-use; I refer only to the availability of choice. If human beings are rational creatures, we must embrace an ethic of responsibility rather than accept a form of determinism. If, as is often said, the brain is the most important sex organ, then it should be used in reproduction at least as frequently as the actual organs of copulation.

How much freedom to control one's body should exist? At first the answer might seem obvious, especially to women: total and absolute freedom. But is it this clearcut? The issue is correctly raised in terms of women's bodies, for women bear all the physical burden and usually most of the social and emotional responsibility of childbearing and childrearing. How much control should a man have over his wife's reproductive capabilities? The following example will illustrate the issue. Amanda and Larry had been dating for several years and assumed they knew each other well. When the relationship developed to the point where marriage became a possibility, they discussed children. Amanda was adamant in not wanting children; she did not particularly like them, and the idea of motherhood was not part of her self-concept. Larry wanted children very much and refused to marry unless Amanda agreed to change her mind. She refused, and with great reluctance they parted. They were unhappy apart, and Larry decided to change his approach. Instead of giving Amanda an ultimatum, he negotiated by saying that all she had to do was bear the child, and he would assume most of the parental responsibilities, the role ordinarily assigned to women. She could have as much or as little contact with the child as she wished. Amanda agreed, and they were married. Shortly after the wedding Amanda decided to go to veterinary school and succeeded in persuading Larry to postpone starting a family until after she received her degree. He agreed reluctantly. The further she went in school, the more she realized that she did not want to have a child at all, and she told her decision to Larry. He was angry and claimed that she was now morally obligated to bear a child because those were the conditions under which he married her and to which she had agreed. He claimed that the agreement was as binding as any legal contract and that he had a right to expect her to bear a child.

Did he? Was Amanda morally obligated to keep her part of the bargain even though she clearly did not want to use her body in the childbearing process? If marriage is seen as a social partnership and division of responsibility, and if a woman is forced by biologic circumstances to take all the physical responsibility of pregnancy, should the decision therefore be completely hers? If the husband is to have a reasonably equal role in the social responsibility of fatherhood, and since that role lasts about 20 times as long as pregnancy, should he not have equal choice in the decision? A woman, if she is careful and knowledgeable, has the ultimate physical control over her body; that is, she can take contraceptive pills or have an IUD inserted without her husband's knowledge and if desired can have an abortion without telling him. She holds the physical trump card. Does this place a greater burden of moral obligation on her to seek her husband's equal participation in the decision, or should she interpret it as simply an accident of nature that she can use to her advantage?

How can a woman achieve control over her body as she relates to the health care system, most notably to the physician who prescribes contraception? The ethical issues depend on a number of variables: the woman's age, her capacity to learn and desire to know about her body, physiologic factors that might preclude one or another form of birth control, and factors involved in her sex life. For example, if a woman has a history of phlebitis and her physician tells her why contraceptive pills are contraindicated, can she nevertheless demand a prescription? Most physicians would not prescribe them, but there are many who would think that as long as the woman knows and understands the risks, she is free to do as she chooses. If the woman then developes serious vascular consequences, who would be morally and legally responsible?

How much control can a woman exercise when she does not know what it is that she should be controlling? In other words, if a woman is almost totally ignorant of the reproductive process and knows only about the cause-and-effect relationship of intercourse and pregnancy, she cannot begin to know what to do to take control into her own hands. In a small city in the East there is a program for pregnant adolescents that consists of a full-time school, health and social services, and day care for infants. The program was designed and established to prevent adolescents from dropping out of school during their pregnancy and then never returning. The vast majority of clients come from inner-city poverty areas, and some are pregnant for the second or third time. The program is reasonably successful in that many of the girls finish it, thus ensuring themselves of adequate prenatal care, and some do return to regular school after the baby is born. Routinely during the 6-week postpartum examination an IUD is inserted if the girl's mother consents, even though the state has an emancipated minor law (an emancipated minor, legally considered an adult, is a girl who has had a child or a boy who has fathered one). The girl is told what will happen and does not have a choice in the matter unless she protests strongly; no one is *forced* to have the IUD inserted.

Several ethical issues are involved here. Those who favor this procedure say that the IUD is the best method of contraception for these young women who are unlikely to use another method, because it can be inserted and then left alone. They also maintain that some girls do not care whether they use contraception or not and give little thought to the consequences of unprotected intercourse for themselves and society, and therefore society is obligated and permitted to protect itself by inserting the IUD. The program director states that no one is being harmed because the girls are free to engage in sexual intercourse and are not forced against their will to submit to the IUD. Proponents of the procedure claim that the clients do not exhibit much interest in their own bodies and would not voluntarily use birth control no matter how many times they were encouraged to do so. For this reason they see the IUD as an ideal solution. The procedure *is* explained, and most of the girls accept it as passively as they seem to accept other aspects of their lives and as they had accepted what they saw as inevitable pregnancies.

Those who are opposed to this procedure say that no matter how effective the IUD is and how logical a choice for birth control it may be in this situation, the clients have little *actual* choice and thus have almost no chance to exercise control over their bodies. They also point out the questionable legality of having the mother of an emancipated minor sign the consent form. This allows the client to be even more passive about what is inserted into her body because *she* does not need to read the consent form before signing. Her mother may or may not explain what is going on; she is not legally bound to do so.

When a woman consults a physician for some form of birth control, she frequently has an idea of the method she might like because she knows her personal preferences and the nature of her sex life. The physician has a choice in the way he practices medicine, and he may not choose to prescribe the method the client wants. Thus conflicts exist in the locus of control. For instance, a woman may know she cannot take birth control pills because of serious side effects and may have decided on an IUD as the next best thing. The physician says he does not believe in IUDs and instead measures her for a diaphragm. She says she does not want a diaphragm and probably will not use it, he still refuses the IUD, and they are at an impasse. Who should have control, and what rights are involved? The physician has a right not to insert the IUD, but he also has an obligation to explain his reason to the client. To simply say he does not believe in them does not meet the client's need to know; perhaps he has information that would benefit her. The client has a right to effective contraception, but she also has a right to complete and accurate information about what will be put into her body. Does she have an obligation to explain why she would not use a diaphragm, thus providing the physician with more complete information about her? She can, of course, obtain an IUD from another physician, but she must pay the first even if she leaves the office without contraception, and as well she has no guarantee that she will receive satisfaction from the next.

What can the physician and client do about resolving their conflict? One may assume that the office nurse has observed all or most of this exchange and that she is the ideal person to open lines of communication between physician and client, to encourage the physician to give more information, and to ask the client why she is opposed to a diaphragm. Perhaps a compromise could be arranged, and perhaps the locus of control will not have changed at all, but information will have been exchanged.

Many "nurses" in gynecologists' offices are not nurses at all but merely receptionists in white uniforms who are assumed by clients to be nurses. Their task is to keep the office running smoothly, but the client is deprived of a professional nursing service when she may need it most. Those physicians who employ professional nurses, however, provide their clients with a health educator and an advocate even if the physician may not have had those functions in mind when the nurse was first employed. The professional nurse in a gynecologist's office, if she is to consider her behavior ethical, will meet clients' needs as they arise and would confront the previously described conflict in a way that benefits the client and raises the consciousness of the physician.

Emancipation of women

The word *emancipation* means freedom from restraint and is usually used in the context of political bondage or slavery. Although *slavery* is too strong a word to use in referring to women's lot in life in the United States, political bondage is more accurate, especially in the area of human reproduction. It is not appropriate here to delineate how society over the years has placed women in certain roles and behaviors, a phenomenon that has been excellently described elsewhere in books on the history of women, but the emancipation of women should be discussed as it relates to contraception and sterilization. Society has assumed an interest in the reproductive powers of women, as well it should because it is dependent on those powers for survival. Since only women can bear children they are obligated to do so, but to what degree? On the other hand, society has an interest in the number of people it can care for adequately and comfortably. Again, women have a more basic control over the number of children they bear; are they thus obligated to control that number, and what degree of obligation exists? How much control should society have over the reproductive powers of an individual woman?

This question is frequently raised in economic matters such as bank loans, eligibility for public housing, and employment, as the following example indicates. Gwen and George had been married for a few years and had one 6-year-old child, who was in first grade. They decided to buy an expensive house and applied for a mortgage. Both Gwen and George were professionals and earned good salaries, but both salaries were necessary to pay the mortgage. Gwen had decided that she would have no more children but had not chosen the permanence of sterilization. She had been taking birth control pills for several years, had had no side effects, and planned to take them indefinitely. The loan officer at the bank raised the possibility of further children. Although Gwen felt that her reproductive life was none of the bank's business, she wanted the loan and thought that cooperation with the officer was the best policy. She said she did not intend to have more children and thought that reply would suffice. The loan officer insisted on knowing how she could be certain she would not become pregnant, what method of birth control she was using, and what she would do if she did become pregnant. Gwen refused to answer these questions but assured the officer that she fully intended to keep working and that the presence or absence of children in her life would not affect the couple's ability to repay the loan. The officer said he would have to "look into the matter further" and let Gwen and George know the bank's decision in a few days.

One can understand the bank's concern about the security of a loan, and one would also expect them to investigate the borrower's ability to repay it. A bank can be expected to refuse a loan to a person who is a poor financial risk, but how far does Gwen or any woman have to go to prove she is a good financial risk? How much of her personal life must she divulge to meet the bank's requirements? In this example, Gwen's ability to earn money was not in question, but the continuation of that ability was. The banker thought that if Gwen became pregnant, she would stop working at least temporarily and her income would cease. Thus the bank's money would be in jeopardy. This is not necessarily true. In all likelihood Gwen would not become pregnant, but if she did, she could elect either to abort the fetus or to have the child and continue to work. But should she have to speculate about these personal matters to a stranger when conducting a business arrangement? The feminist, ethical, and humanitarian answer is no: she should be able to keep private matters private. Furthermore, the bank should be equally interested in her husband's ability to earn money, for there are possibilities that he might lose his income too, such as through a serious accident or death. Her reproductive capacities have nothing to do with her earning ability.

Many states now have credit laws that prohibit just this kind of situation. A woman's sexual and reproductive life may not be used as a criterion for withholding credit.

Emancipation of women can be viewed as freedom from physiologic bondage as well as from that imposed by societal values. This concept is complex: how can one be freed from the conditions of one's body? Fletcher expresses the view that people are inextricably tied to nature:

> It is not our thesis that in order to be moral a person must be *independent* of nature. He is, on any realistic and humble view, still a creature of nature, however highly developed his spiritual faculties may become as compared to the rest of the animals. He may be *of* the order of grace (as theologians say) but he is also *in* the order of nature. Human control does no imply human autonomy.*

He goes on to say that freedom does not exist in controlling nature and being independent of natural laws but in knowing the laws and making them work to one's advantage. "Freedom of the will therefore means nothing but the capacity to make decisions in the control *over ourselves* and over external nature."[1,p.67] This is simply another view of the natural law argument.

Emancipation from nature in this sense could mean controlling our reproductive capacities to the extent that we benefit. Women *could* free themselves from natural rhythms by having their uteruses removed or by not engaging in sexual intercourse. Both actions would be liberating in the sense that no pregnancies would occur. Nature would indeed be thwarted. But would the woman benefit, and would she be controlling nature by altering it (by hysterectomy) or ignoring it (by denying her natural need for sex)? She would benefit only insofar as she would not bear children, but the attendant discomforts would outweigh the benefits. How much better to acknowledge the body's natural rhythm and thwart only that which is necessary to achieve the desired goal. Emancipation should not be from nature itself but from the helplessness to control nature. Hurricanes are a part of nature; They are seen as evil because we have no way to protect ourselves against them. If we could build fortifications against the wind and water, we would view a hurricane as no more menacing than a severe thunderstorm. So it is with the menstrual cycle: if we can protect ourselves from unwanted pregnancies, we can view the cycle as a natural aspect of our bodies that is no more threatening than the cycle of eating and eliminating.

Religious views

Chapter 4 on population control discussed the position of most major religions on individual birth control and societal population control. It is, however, interesting to examine contraception as a moral issue in religion. In the Western world the

---

*Fletcher, Joseph: Morals and medicine, p. 66. Copyright © 1954, 1979 by Princeton University Press; Princeton Paperback. Reprinted by permission of Princeton University Press.

Catholic Church has given more consideration to isssues of contraception (even with papal encyclicals) than any other religious body. The Church has also had an enormous influence on the morality and attitudes of Western society, perhaps because of the sheer number of Catholics in North America and Europe or because of the political influence of the Vatican. For this reason only the Cathoic view of the morality of contraception will be examined here.

Jesus himself said little about the morality and ethics of sex. He did not discuss who did what with whom, how many chidren resulted from sexual intercourse, how large families should be, or what might be done to prevent conception (even in Jesus' time there were various reasonably effective contraceptive methods). In its attitude toward sexuality and contraception Catholicism may seem based more on an interpretation about Jesus rather than on his actual words.

The Catholic tradition of making judgments about sexual matters probably began with St. Paul, who in his First Letter to the Corinthians (after the death of Jesus) made the following assertions: (1) it is better to marry than to be "aflame with passion," (2) sexual access to a marriage partner is a conjugal right, and (3) sexual abstinence in marriage must be mutual and then only for short periods of time. Fletcher[1] comments that St. Paul also advised "race suicide" by celibacy since he believed the world was to end shortly. The idea that the apocalypse was at hand soon passed, but the ideal of virginity or celibacy remains in the Church today. Although the Church acknowledges the need for intercourse within marriage, it is sometimes thought less spiritual than celibacy. Those who do not opt for celibacy by taking vows may be seen as less than spiritually perfect, perhaps because they choose not to inhibit their sexual urges.

In the Protestant Reformation one of Martin Luther's revolts was against celibacy. He maintained that other ways of living, including parenthood, were proper and could be classified as true Christian vocations, and the Council of Trent reaffirmed that view by stating that virginity was not a higher state than marriage.

Conservative Catholic moralists of today still believe that the only way to control conception is by periodic abstinence from intercourse and that the principle of self-control for preventing conception supersedes spontaneity and the fulfillment of sexual need. Catholics do not object to birth control *per se* but to artificial means to prevent conception. The only two methods of preventing conception acceptable to the Church are complete sexual abstinence and refraining from intercourse during the time a woman is likely to be most fertile (commonly referred to as the rhythm method). Thus the morality of contraception concerns not the end itself but the means used to achieve that end, the method rather than the result.

This places a specific ethical slant on the issue. It is interesting to note that St. Augustine opposed even the rhythm method and believed that the only purpose for copulation was procreation. Catholic moralists are in a difficult position since they look to St. Augustine for moral guidance in other areas. The moral quality of any choice or action is determined by the intention or desired end and the means used to achieve that end. Since the Church does not believe that birth control as an end is wrong, the moralists must then demonstrate that certain means to achieve that end are wrong. This they have tried to do by banning artificial means to control a natural phenomenon. This argument may seem illogical since the Church approves much medical technology that is used to control natural processes.

It has already been shown that nature apparently intends us to use our sexuality for purposes other than procreation, but the Church makes no statement about the pleasures of sexuality. It does not say, "Do it, but don't enjoy it." The Church approves of intercourse during nonfertile periods and thus acknowledges that sex serves more than a reproductive purpose. Thus the Church has not shown that contraception is immoral simply because it is unnatural.

Another reason for the Church's proscription against contraception is that it is seen to make intercourse merely masturbatory; that is, if the outcome of a possible pregnancy is eliminated, then the couple having intercourse are committing the sin of onanism (see Chapter 5) by "spilling the seed," or using semen for an unlawful purpose. No definition of masturbation, no matter how judgmental, includes sexual intercourse; equating the two is preposterous. Another argument, which is taken more seriously, is that artificial birth control may involve a kind of murder. This argument is based on the fact that spermicides kill spermatozoa, possibly ova, and possibly a fertilized ovum. Other contraceptives that do not use chemicals but work by preventing the union of sperm and egg are banned because they eliminate the potential for fertilization. The charge of murder is still applied. Catholic theologians agree that a life is at stake, but is it? Does a sperm or egg or even a freshly fertilized ovum have a life? The argument can be countered by pointing out that nature allows an ovum to be wasted each month by menstruation.

Increasing numbers of Catholic theologians do not support the Church's official doctrine even though they still believe that the act of sexual intercourse is essentially a creative one. They think that what is created does not necessarily have to be a human life. Each act of intercourse does not have to be "open to the transmission of life" (the phrase is from Pope Paul VI's 1968 encyclical "Humanae Vitae"). In the early 1960s Catholic moralists began to question the Church's position on oral contraceptives and other methods of artificial birth control. According to Dedek,[2,p.59] the majority conclusion was that "in ethical terms it does not matter what method or technique is used for birth control." These moralists think that the link between sexual love and parenthood must remain unbroken in principle but that decisions about the number and spacing of children should be made unselfishly and with regard for the quality of life created.

This position opposes the Church's official view that the method does matter and that the means to the end are as important as the end itself. These Catholic moralists support their view by saying that respect for human life also means respect for the quality of that life in terms of the ability to feed, house, clothe, and educate children born into a family. The more elusive aspectof loving and caring for.those children who are wanted is not specifically stated but must have been in the minds of those Catholic theologians debating the issue. They could not have ignored the mounting body of evidence showing an incidence of neglect and abuse that is higher with children who are not wanted than with those who are. The health of the mother was also a consideration in this shift away from the traditional view. It is irresponsible to force a woman to bear more children than she is physically, mentally, and emotionally capable of doing; this too is seen as part of a respect for human life. The problem of overpopulation was also in the minds of those who broke away from official Church policy.

Many Catholic theologians, or at least those who have spoken publicly and published their views on Church dogma, are priests who are not personally and directly affected by whatever position the Church takes on any issue of sexuality. But their deliberations have a tremendous affect on the daily lives of ordinary Catholics who might feel themselves relieved of a burden but who might also be thrown into a state of confusion about Church dogma in this moral issue. The nature of Catholic religious education is that doctrine is learned rather than debated. Think of the confusion of a woman who has believed for 30 years that she must take no artificial steps to prevent conception and has perhaps lived her sexual life with her fingers crossed. Now suddenly her parish priest says it is permissible to use artificial birth control, and she is not certain what to do. The priest, whom she trusts, says to follow her own conscience, and the Pope, whom she reveres, says to do only what the Church officially sanctions. It is a difficult dilemma for many Catholics. Even though matters of sexuality are not part of papal infallibility, they are authentic noninfallible doctrine, which means they require serious consideration and respect though the possibility of error is not ruled out and serious legitimate dissent is allowed. Nonetheless, encyclicals and opinions that originate with the Pope tend to have an authority that cannot be taken lightly. If a parish priest advises individual judgment in matters of birth control, he may be regarded at the same time as a heretic and a savior, but if this priest is suddenly replaced by one who adheres more rigidly to official Church doctrine, what happens to the practice of individual Catholics? It may be tempting to conclude that since the Church is in conflict over the issue, each Catholic should decide for himself the most morally correct course of action. But usually agreement with the papal position is encouraged, and the decision is not left so completely to the individual. Some liberal Catholics will act independently in the choice of birth control methods. Most of the rest will be in turmoil.

Ethics of some birth control techniques

Most people agree that birth control in general is desirable, ethical, and beneficial to the public and private good. However, some aspects of the means to achieve contraception may not be ethical, desirable, or beneficial to the individual. Any drug or device consumed or inserted into the body with a positive effect can also have a negative effect that may equal or outweigh the positive one. Health hazards are the most obvious negative effect, and one immediately thinks of the various side effects of the contraceptive pill and complications from improperly inserted IUDs. The moral issue involves whether the known and potential risks are worth taking when compared to the consequences of pregnancy and to the effectiveness and desirability of other methods of contraception.

Informed consent is a major issue as always. Everyone would agree that a woman should be informed of the major and minor side effects of contraceptive pills, but must she be told every discomfort ever reported? A purist would say yes, definitely. A more pragmatic person might think that the long list of side effects would frighten the woman, causing her either to look for symptoms or to interpret every minor mood change as a result of the pill. She might then stop taking it without using an alternative method of birth control, thus increasing her risk of pregnancy. The pragmatist would surely agree that she should be told of major symptoms that are warnings of serious side effects; the problem is deciding which symptoms to disclose. If a physician or a nurse tells a newly married woman who is taking contraceptive pills for the first time that some women find that they become depressed while on the pill, how is this woman to differentiate between any depression caused by the pill and the letdown she may feel after the excitement of her wedding and honeymoon? She would then face the dilemma of waiting to see how she feels in a few weeks and risking an increase in depression or discontinuing use of the pill and possibly becoming pregnant before she is ready.

> The mere introduction of the idea of danger may immediately induce psychological reactions unfavorable to the success of the therapy. Few people can regard themselves as subject to average statistical chances, and the statistically correct information that there is one chance in 30 thousand of a fatal accident with the pill may well result in a quite erroneous subjective appreciation of the chances.*

This physician's view of the dilemma raises a pragmatic issue that is a major part of the informed consent dilemma: how much information should be given to a client about a drug or treatment? The view that each physician or nurse must according to the situation make a judgment about what side effects to disclose sounds like a morally correct compromise, but what if the judgment is erroneous? The professional could leave the client in so much doubt about what to expect that she might not report serious symptoms, or if the judgment is made differently she might leave the office with such a long list of side effects that she is unable to stop worrying.

The women's movement has begun to help women take this matter into their own hands. Networks of women's information services are springing up all over the country, and books written by women about the functioning of their bodies are directed specifically toward women and are written in everyday language. (The most famous is *Our Bodies, Our Selves* which was written by the Boston Women's Health Collective, produced originally on newsprint, and distributed through women's groups at a cost of 35¢. It is so informative and became so popular that a major publisher bought the rights and expanded its content, and it is now on sale in bookstores.) Clinics that provide a wide range of gynecologic and reproductive services are staffed by women physicians, nurses, and counselors; the policy of most includes full disclosure of all treatments and prescriptions. Questions and discussion are generally encouraged. Some clinics manage this freedom better than others, but the number and popularity of this kind of clinic should indicate to the health care establishment that many women feel their needs have not been met by traditional modes of care.

---

*Taylor, Howard C.: The ethics of the physician in human reproduction. In Visscher, Maurice B., editor: Human perspectives in medical ethics, Buffalo, N.Y., 1972, Prometheus Books, p. 180.

The ethical considerations of various contraceptive techniques can be viewed in direct relation to the permanence of the method and the degree of risk usually associated with it. For example, use of a condom is completely impermanent, lasting only through one act of intercourse, and generally has no side effects. Therefore, except for explaining the pitfalls regarding the use of a condom, one could probably ignore the ethical issues, if indeed there are any. On the other hand, the contraceptive pill is permanent for as long as a woman takes it, and the effects frequently last long after use is discontinued. Some of the risks are considerable, up to and including death from emboli. Thus the use of the pill involves ethical issues: deliberately altering a natural body function so that physiologic mechanisms operate as if the body is pregnant so it will not become pregnant; subjecting women to the risk of serious side effects to prevent a condition that is not life threatening (pregnancy); placing a drug on the mass market that has not been sufficiently tested to determine long-range effects; the possibility of teratogenic effects; and the question whether pregnancy itself or the use of the contraceptive pill causes a greater health hazard.

Other birth control techniques such as the diaphragm and jelly, IUD, and various other far less effective methods also involve ethical issues. The IUD, for example, provokes a theologic debate. Because the exact mechanism of action is not known (the most common theory is that the IUD prevents the fertilized ovum from implanting on the endometrium, probably by causing minute wave-like contractions of the uterus), it must be considered an abortifacient rather than a contraceptive; that is, it kills a fertilized ovum instead of preventing the union of sperm and egg. This creates a more complex issue: has a woman by consenting to insertion of the IUD thus consented to participation in continuous abortions, perhaps every month? Or could she be said not to have aborted because the phenomenon occurred before she was aware she was pregnant and because she took no conscious and deliberate action to remove an embryo she knew was there? Those who feel that human life begins at the moment of conception are morally opposed to the IUD if they are unconditionally opposed to abortion. The use of an IUD is considered by some religions to be a more serious breach of the ban on artificial contraception than the use of the birth control pill.

Several years ago a dilemma occurred involving the use of a particular IUD, the Dalkon Shield. The shield had been in use for several years when in the summer of 1974 evidence suggested that the Dalkon Shield had caused septicemia during pregnancy, more than 100 spontaneous abortions, and even several maternal deaths.[3] The FDA stated that the Dalkon Shield should be removed from the market and no new ones inserted. The FDA also recommended that the shield not be removed from women who were wearing them successfully and had developed no problems. The latter recommendation produced the dilemma: if a woman were to become pregnant while wearing the Dalkon Shield (as many did), what should be done? Should the shield be removed, thus terminating the pregnancy? Should nothing be done, thus subjecting the woman to possibilities of infection, septic abortion, and possibly even death? Even if no maternal damage occurred, should the shield be left in place when there might be risk to the fetus? The FDA's official recommendation was that if a woman became pregnant while wearing the shield, she should have an immediate abortion. This solved the FDA's problem and that of the manufacturer of the Dalkon Shield, but it did not resolve the ethical dilemma. One wonders why women were not advised to have the Dalkon Shield removed and replaced with another kind. If a woman could wear the Dalkon Shield successfully and if an IUD continued to be her contraceptive method of choice, it could reasonably be assumed that she could wear another IUD equally successfully. On the other hand, if removal of the Dalkon Shield involved a greater risk than leaving it in, the woman was placed in a position of having to choose between two evils, and the ethical dilemma worsens. Should women who were wearing the shield have been informed of the possible dangers, and how could their confidentiality be protected if family members were not aware that the IUD was in place?

ATTITUDES TOWARD SEXUALITY

The choice of contraception and the way it is used, misused, or not used depend to a large extent on one's attitudes toward and beliefs about sexuality. Sexual attitudes and ethics are affected by many variables such as the sexual climate of the society in which a person develops (a woman who had matured in Victorian England would have an outlook far different from that of a woman coming of age in San Francisco in the 1960s), the sexual mores and practices of the family (a child who never sees his parents display physical affection will grow up differently from one whose household is filled with hugging and kissing), religion (a conservative Catholic will have values different from those of a liberal Protestant), and general ethical codes.

The shift from moral absolutes to relative moral values may contribute to confusion, ambivalence, guilt, and fear regarding sexuality and intimacy. Furthermore, an existing societal paradox adds to a personal conflict. On the one hand, American society values individualism, and changes do take place regarding sex roles, yet an opposing force—that of conformity to group pressures and adherence to certain kinds of sex-role behaviors—coexists and is still rewarded.*

Another variable is the priority one gives to sexuality and to the fulfillment of sexual needs. A person who generally meets as they arise is likely to view sexuality differently from the person who has sex rarely and only when all other obligations and needs are met. If sex is an important part of a couple's relationship, they will probably feel more responsible about contraception than a couple who give sex a lower priority. The commitment partners have to each other makes a difference in their choice of contraceptive, as does the length of time the relationship is likely to last. A person who engages in isolated sexual encounters or relationships that last only a few weeks is more likely to use an ineffective and impermanent form of birth control than one who feels a long commitment to the sex partner.

Age is another variable. Adolescents are likely to be unprepared for sex and

---

*Mazurkewicz, Dolores T.: The family. In Fromer, Margot Joan: Community health care and the nursing process, St. Louis, 1979, The C. V. Mosby Co., p. 236.

often seek spontaneity, which they interpret as romantic. An older person is more liable to take responsibility for the eventuality of sexual intercourse. A high school girl may go to the prom without worrying that the drugstores will be closed after the dance; a more mature woman tucks her diaphragm into her purse before meeting a new beau for dinner.

One's self-knowledge and the acknowledgment of one's sexual needs and values play an important role in the ethics of sexuality and contraception. The urgency of the need to use contraception and the consideration of the consequences of pregnancy can determine the birth control method used. In inner-city poverty areas young girls and women frequently have sex with little thought given to birth control because if pregnancy results, the community mores will be supportive; the action may not be seen as unusual, and the baby may simply be accepted into the family. In upper-class suburbia a pregnant adolescent is a subject of gossip; major alterations may be made in future plans, and the family may be disrupted to a much greater extent.

The contraceptive method itself has much to do with the way it is perceived and therefore used. Asking a physician for contraception implies an active sex life, and thus making this request is difficult for some people, especially those who view sex as an intensely personal matter. A trip to the gynecologist involves a vaginal and rectal examination that is unbearable for many women who feel embarrassed or ashamed about another person viewing or touching their genitals. These women may simply buy whatever is on the drugstore shelf—and even this experience can be acutely embarrassing—or depend on sex partners to provide condoms. A woman who has a negative attitude about her genitals and dislikes touching them will not choose a contraceptive method that involves self-insertion, for example, a diaphragm or spermicidal foam, but may be a good candidate for the pill, which will not disturb her in this way.

Those couples who practice cunnilingus and for whom the taste of spermicidal cream or jelly is unpleasant may find a diaphragm impractical because it causes an interruption when it has to be inserted between cunnilingus and intercourse. For them the pill or an IUD might be a more practical choice. Those who feel that sex should always be completely spontaneous and who do not like to prepare in advance for the eventuality of sex will most likely be poor users of contraception and may depend on the partner to take full responsibility, for example, a woman who expects the man to be equipped with condoms and a man who thinks the woman should take care of contraception.

A woman who takes the pill or wears an IUD may suffer from the often justified anxiety that a particular man or men in general will think she is always ready for sex because she is always protected against pregnancy. Such a woman may say she feels under some obligation to engage in sex even though she may not want to because she cannot use the excuse that she is afraid of pregnancy. She may not yet have been able to make the switch from "I'm afraid I'll get pregnant" to "I don't want to."

Every effective method of contraception has some side effects or drawbacks that can be seen as a rationalization for not using that method (the pill may cause blood clots, the IUD may give one severe menstrual cramps, a condom may decrease sensitivity, a diaphragm may be a nuisance, and so on) or any contraception at all. "I can't be bothered" and "It won't happen to me" are statements that reflect feelings about responsiblity toward sexuality. Can a person who uses contraceptives only sporadically or not at all be said to be immoral or unethical? Assuming that nonuse is not related to religious convictions but is related to a variety of other factors, one *could* see the risk of unwanted pregnancy as immoral, although the many psychoemotional factors make it difficult to separate morality from fear, anxiety, or years of misinformation. If the morality of an action depends on the intent involved and the means chosen, one has to look closely at all the factors.

Margaret, a 24-year-old graduate student who had had an abortion a year ago, was primarily a lesbian although she had not foresworn men entirely. Her primary sexual attraction was to women, and her desire to make love with a man decreased sharply after the abortion. Thus she felt no need to do anything about contraception. Sometime later, however, she formed a relationship with a man that eventually led to sexual intercourse. The affair was continuing several months later when she noticed that her period was late. It turned out that she was not pregnant, but the scare forced her to think about contraception. She did nothing about it, however, because she thought of herself as a lesbian and of her affair with Karl as a temporary situation. Was Margaret behaving unethically, irresponsibly, stupidly, or all three?

To say she was stupid is too harsh, although her perception of her sexual preferences was probably not as realistic as she believed. One could say she behaved irresponsibly because even after her fertility had been established and she had had another scare she still chose to do nothing about birth control. But is she unethical? If one equates irresponsibility with an immorality of intent, then she could be considered unethical. But Margaret did not seem to be deliberately or consciously seeking pregnancy and did not use her affair with Karl to achieve the goal of pregnancy. Therefore she could not be considered unethical. On the other hand, she knew where unprotected intercourse can lead, and because of this knowledge her refusal to prevent pregnancy, for whatever reason, can be seen as a conscious and deliberate attempt to ignore the consequences of her actions. Therefore her behavior could be seen as unethical. All negative behavior and all behavior that results in negative consequences cannot be said to be immoral, but this situation is open to debate.

Adolescent sexuality

The ethical issues of adolescent sexuality differ widely from those of adult behavior, although there are some similarities. Of 21 million teenagers between ages 15 and 19, 7 million males and 4 million females are reported to be sexually active, and most do not have a reliable means for contraception.[4] Almost half the adolescent in the United States are potential parents, and still the controversy about teaching sex education in school is raging.

Because, as many think, the consequences of adolescent pregnancy are more harmful to society and the people involved than those of adult pregnancy, should adolescents receive special education about contraception? Is it ethical not to teach adolescents about contraception merely because half of them have no current need for the information though the other half needs it badly? About half of all sexually active adolescent women are receiving no birth control services, and the bulk of unwanted pregnancies occur in this age group.[4] There are several reasons for this lack of services. Funds are limited, probably because of community resistance and legal restrictions, although many states now legally permit contraceptive advice and prescription as well as treatment for venereal disease for minors without parental consent. Clinics may not be located in areas where most adolescents need them. In large inner cities there are usually several city- or state-supported clinics for disadvantaged adolescents, but the affluent suburban adolescent is in a different position. Her access to transportation may be limited, and she may not know how to select a gynecologist; she may not know about existing free services and might not feel comfortable going to such a clinic. Thus she uses no contraception or relies on her boyfriend to provide a condom, which he may or may not do.

Only about half of the colleges and universities in the country provide birth control services for students,[4] and although no figures are available it could be assumed that only rarely do high schools provide such services. Is it any more or less moral to provide adolescents with birth control information than to provide adults the same? At what age is it moral to begin having sex? If we know that people are sexually active, is it ethical to withhold information from them merely because we think their behavior is inappropriate? If adults ignore the contraceptive needs of 16-year-olds because they are too young, have these adults contributed to an unwanted pregnancy? Many who disapprove of adolescent sexuality take the position that adolescents should not behave in adult ways unless they are prepared to take adult responsibility. Is this counterproductive attitutde ethical? There is no specific age at which it is morally permissible to have sex, although society has some strong but poorly defined feelings about adolescent sexuality. Most states have a law about the age of sexual consent (usually 16 or 18, although New Jersey has recently introduced a bill to lower the age to 14), but this law is practically unenforcable except in cases of rape or kidnap and conflicts with the law that allows a minor to receive birth control or VD treatment without parental consent. Society seems to be saying to the adolescent, "You can obtain a device to prevent you from becoming pregnant and we will help you if you catch a disease that is sexually transmitted, but don't have sex." No wonder adolescents are confused by the adult world.

Those who oppose giving birth control information to adolescents think that access to knowledge about sex will increase the chances that they will become sexually active; this is also a reason for opposing sex education in school. The fact is that young people already have ideas about sex, but many of them are erroneous. Accurate information could help correct their misconceptions, resulting in a decline in unwanted pregnancies. Other people oppose giving birth control information to adolescents because they feel they *should* not need it, that they are too young to handle it responsibly. This also is incorrect; adolescents do need the information, and it might increase the responsibility with which they handle their sex lives.

The ethical issues inherent in adolescent sexuality can be summarized as follows:

1. How competent or mature must an adolescent be to engage in sexual activity, give consent to procedures that affect sexuality (birth control, abortion, and so on), understand the information involved in giving informed consent, and participate in sociologic research that either invades their privacy or affects their sexuality, even if nothing is done to their bodies?

2. Adolescent women seem to bear most of the burden in regard to sexuality: having to decide whether to engage in sex (common belief holds that it is usually up to the girl rather than the boy to decide whether to proceed with sex), to protect herself against pregnancy or do most of the worrying about it, and to have the abortion or bear the child. Given the obvious biologic restrictions, adolescent men should be encouraged to accept more responsibility for sexuality, contraception, and prevention of VD.

3. Those organizations that provide some kind of sexually oriented services to adolescents (such as schools that teach sex education, community clinics that offer contraceptive counseling, abortion clinics, and municipal VD centers) face an ethical dilemma: to improve the service offered and to provide what adolescents specifically need, data must be gathered. Is it ethical to use clients of the service in gathering data, and if so should they be told? If an adolescent who may have been reluctant to come to the clinic in the first place is told that she is also to be a subject of research and is to be one of a number of statistics, even though her identity will not be revealed, she may be frightened into not returning and the original purpose of the service will be diminished. If the client is not told, have her rights as a research subject been violated even though no identifying characteristics will ever be published? The researchers know who she is; does she in turn have a right to know that they know and then make a decision about whether to continue attending that clinic?

4. When engaging in data gathering research, whose consent is required? There are three alternatives:

   seeking parental consent for survey research in adolescent sexuality acknowledges the vulnerability of the subject and recognizes legitimate parental interest and responsibility for their adolescent children. Seeking only subject consent accords adolescents an autonomy and maturity which implies that they represent their own best interests. Seeking no consent implies that the researchers regard their own precautions as satisfactory protections for adolescent subjects.*

   The latter choice is always dangerous, the first will destroy the privacy that adolescents seek at the clinic, and the middle choice depends on the judgment of the researcher in relation to what he knows about a particular adolescent and thus is also potentially dangerous.

---

*Lieberman, E. James, and Tannenwald, Carol B.: Ethical issues in adolescent health: proceedings of a conference sponsored by APHA, Institute of Society, Ethics, and the Life Sciences, and USPHS, Washington, D.C., December 6-7, 1976, p. 8.

5. For what purpose will research on adolescent sexuality be used? Most research in this area is directed toward formulation of public policy about contraceptive use and pregnancy.[4]

Should there indeed be public policies about matters involved in adolescent sexuality? If teenage pregnancy is considered mainly a health problem, what kinds of health policies would affect treatment? If it is mainly a social problem, in what ways would society need to change or adjust to decrease the problem, and how would public policy affect societal attitudes? Research about adolescent sexuality is threatening to some because it involves learning more than one wishes to know about the subject and that can be disturbing. In Woody Allen's movie *Manhattan*, the main character, a 43-year-old writer, has affairs with two women, one a 17-year-old high school senior and the other an adult journalist. The adolescent is portrayed as mature, responsible, and capable of communicating in a much more developed way than the woman journalist, who seems to live like an irresponsible adolescent. There was public sentiment about the portrayal of adolescent sexuality in the film even though the older woman displayed more adolescent characteristics than the younger one. Many parents prefer to ignore their children's sexuality for a variety of complex reasons and as well oppose research and services dealing with adolescent sexuality in general. Parental pressure is a strong influence on establishment of public policy.

DISSEMINATION OF BIRTH CONTROL INFORMATION

The obligation to provide people with information about contraception falls to health professionals; of all the professionals having access to both clients and sources of information, the nurse is in the best position to be of service. Although we wish that more men would take an active interest in contraception, women will always have a greater vested interest; therefore most of the research and services about contraception are directed toward women. Because most are women, nurses should be able to relate to the contraceptive needs of their clients on both a professional and personal level. A physician is likely to prescribe the requested contraceptive technique and perhaps discuss some of its side effects and disadvantages, but it is the nurse who can do the real teaching that is needed. For example, a woman requests a diaphragm from a gynecologist. He makes certain she has the correct size, and if he is conscientious he will require the client to insert and remove it once while she is in the office. She then walks out of the office with a new diaphragm, a tube of spermicidal cream, and many questions she may have been hesitant to ask. The nurse, if she is a professional, would bring her into a quiet private room and explain all the little but crucial complexities of actually using a diaphragm: how much cream to use, what position to assume when inserting it, how to make certain it is in place, how to care for it, what to do if it becomes dislodged during intercourse—the many doubts that might lead to her not using it if she has to figure them out for herself. This is the dissemination of information and knowledge rather than just facts. Physicians generally do not have the time, inclination, or personal experience to do this. A nurse who takes the time and trouble to explain the ramifications of a contraceptive technique is more likely to be asked then or over the telephone later if something is puzzling to the client, and that inquiry could prevent a pregnancy.

Nurses are also in a position to be helpful to women in a broader and more general way than simply on a one-to-one basis in a gynecologist's office. If they work in a hospital or community health agency, they are in a position to take a sexual history from clients as part of the assessment necessary to formulate a nursing diagnosis. A sexual history is not something nurses are used to doing, and many will not react well to the idea at first.

Health professionals usually do not hesitate to explore a client's urinary or bowel status, yet many have a great deal of discomfort at the thought of eliciting a sexual history. This response has no doubt been conditioned by the social prohibitions regarding the discussion of sexual matters. However, the consumer is becoming much more aware of sex and sexuality and frequently will present sexual concerns with a great deal of candor. This new-found openness creates the need for health professionals to be prepared to discuss sexual concerns as well as to educate and counsel clients.

Sexual assessment is a legitimate concern of the health professional and increasingly is integrated into general health assessments. The sexual history provides the professional with a data base on which to make diagnoses or inferences and to subsequently initiate a plan for education or counseling, or perhaps referral to another professional.*

Woods[5] offers the following suggestions and principles for taking a sexual history:

1. Privacy is an essential ingredient. This means not only closing the door or being away from other people but also that the client can trust the professional's confidentiality.
2. Taking a deliberate sexual history, as opposed to making a few offhand remarks, implies that sexuality is an important and appropriate concern and is an important part of general health. The client who sees that the professional is serious is more likely to respond seriously and honestly.
3. The sexual history may be therapeutic as well as a form of assessment; that is, it provides an opportunity for the client to air concerns and understand that the concerns are normal and acceptable when the professional responds in a serious manner.
4. Definition of terms is important, and the professional needs to use language the client can understand. Street language may be just as unfamiliar to the nurse, especially if it is geographically regional, as technical language is to the client. Asking about orgasm may produce a blank stare from a client who knows the phenomenon as "coming."
5. Moving from less sensitive issues to more sensitve ones as the interview progresses will tend to put the client more at ease. Stating question in non-judgmental and nonthreatening terms will tend to ensure a more open and honest answer than an evasion of the issue. For example, "How old were you when you first began to masturbate?" is more acceptable than "Do you masturbate?" The former question assumes masturbation is normal and ac-

---

*Woods, Nancy Fugate: Human sexuality in health and illness, ed. 2, St. Louis, 1979, The C. V. Mosby Co., p. 77.

ceptable and so common a practice that the health professional thinks everyone does. The latter gives the client no information to put him at ease and forces him to choose between telling the truth or lying.

6. In any approach the interviewer must be careful not to assume certain practices or behaviors of the client, such as assuming that everyone masturbates or is completely heterosexual.

7. The professional's attitudes are easily communicated while taking a sexual history; thus the interviewer must remain nonjudgmental but not so passive that the client feels as if he is talking to a robot. The health professional needs to be an interested but nonjudgmental human being.

The client's choice of contraceptive should be part of the sexual history, and frequently the client will relate how a particular method either enhances or impedes sexual expression. We have seen that contraceptives affect and are affected by attitudes toward sexuality. Woods[5] describes how each method influences sexual behavior:

1. A condom may reduce sensitivity and cause annoyance at having to put it on prior to intercourse. It can be used to help maintain a faltering erection, however, and putting it on can be incorporated into sex play with the woman's participation. It can help prevent some sexually transmitted diseases, although if either partner has VD he or she should not engage in sex. Some men and women prefer to use a condom when having sex with strangers, and it is ideal for people who have an aversion to having the penis come into contact with the vagina, although this may be a serious psychologic problem for which one should seek counseling.

2. Use of the diaphragm requires some planning, but its insertion can also be incorporated into sexual activity. Many men and women object to having intercourse during menstruation, and a diaphragm can hold back the flow to some extent.

3. The IUD disturbs some men who claim that during intercourse they can feel the plastic string that protrudes from the cervix into the upper part of the vagina and are irritated by it. Heavier menstrual flow could disturb some, although not everyone views the added wetness as negative.

4. Spermicidal foams have an unpleasant taste for those who engage in cunnilingus. They require planning, but they can be inserted also as part of sex play.

5. Oral contraceptives are so disassociated from sex that many women report a feeling of great freedom; others, as described previously, feel men may think they are always ready for sex. Some women report a decreased sex drive while taking the pill; this should disappear after the first few months. If it does not, a brand change should be considered.

6. The rhythm method and other forms of abstinence can be both frustrating and pleasurable. It is frustrating because the need of human beings for intercourse may not coincide with the safer days; it is pleasurable because it can encourage the couple to explore alternate methods of sexual gratification. Both partners need to be committed to the success of the method, and if

intercourse is seen as the only acceptable mode of sexual expression, this method of contraception will be difficult.

7. Coitus interruptus has almost nothing beneficial about it. It requires more self-control than most people have during sex; the man is required to remove his penis from the vagina exactly when he has the strongest need for deeper penetration. Repeated acts of coitus interruptus will probably lead to a diminution of sexual desire, and as a contraceptive method it is ineffective because of the concentration of sperm in the few drops of Cowper's secretions during sexual arousal.

One might wonder what these descriptions have to do with the ethics of contraception. But if health professionals have a moral obligation to disseminate information, they also have an obligation to know what they are talking about and to be able to relate to their clients in a knowledgable manner. The principles of informed consent in the area of contraception are the same as for brain surgery or any other health procedure. It is not sufficient for a health professional simply to say, "Here's your prescription for birth control pills. Take them as directed and you won't get pregnant." The client may take them, but she will have no idea how they work and what effect they might have on her sexual functioning. That behavior from a health professional would be similar to an anesthesiologist saying to a client before an operation, "Sign the permission form. We're going to put you to sleep and you'll wake up when the operation is over." No real information has been given, and the client blithely assumes that the "sleep" referred to is the same kind that occurs in bed at home.

Under what circumstances can a health professional disseminate information about birth control to someone who does not want it or initiate the subject if the client has not? Some groups of people are less enthusiastic about contraception than others. Blacks comprise about 11% of the American population and are more concentrated in some areas of the country than others. (Most blacks live in urban centers; few live in rural areas, and the black population in suburbia is small but growing.) Many black leaders feel that racism will increase if the percentage of blacks in the population decreases. They may see the efforts of the health care establishment, which is mostly white, to encourage blacks to practice birth control as an attempt to keep the black population small. Some have even referred to this as genocide, an overstatement that is perhaps understandable in view of American history. Some of the accusations are undoubtedly true, because racism exists among health professionals to the same degree as in the rest of the population. But it cannot be said that every nurse and physician who recommends contraception for black clients is doing so for racist reasons.

Thus there is a dilemma: when should a health professional broach the subject of contraception to a client, and when should she remain silent? A nurse on a postpartum unit who is caring for a young woman with three small children and a new baby can face this decision. As an ethical and responsible health professional she wants to give the client the opportunity for making choices in her life. At the same time she does not know if the client has made an informed choice to have so many children. In addition, if the client is black, she does not want to appear racist.

Instead of saying "You have a lot of children for someone so young," which might put the woman on the defensive and cause her to tell the nurse to mind her own business, she might say, "Four children must be quite a handful." This gives the client the opportunity to say whether she had planned on such a big family, and it opens the door for the client to ask about contraception.

There is another kind of situation a nurse may face. Perhaps she is treating a 19-year-old black man for gonorrhea, and when she explains that the use of condoms can sometimes prevent the spread of VD, he says he will not use a condom because it would prevent him from impregnating his sex partner. He feels politically motivated to help increase the black population and thinks that if a woman with whom he has intercourse does not want to become pregnant, it is her responsibility to prevent it. In addition some men, white or black, relate their sense of manhood to their sexual prowess. The nurse may see the man's behavior as immoral and irresponsible, though he may see it as important. In this case the nurse should weigh the alternatives. What effect would her information about birth control, no matter how nonthreatening her manner is in giving the information, have on him? Might he avoid returning to the clinic if he contracts VD again because he does not want to be subjected to another talk on birth control? The dissemination of information in this instance may be counterproductive, and perhaps the most the nurse could hope for is that the man's sex partners will come to the clinic.

Are there people who should be discouraged from using birth control? Consider this example. A couple who had been married for a year and who had decided not to have children came into a gynecologist's office. Jonathan and Assa were both extremely intelligent, with IQs well over 150, and both worked in professions that required maximum use of their intellectual capabilities. Their decision not to have children was not absolute, so they chose birth control pills instead of sterilization. When the physician, who was also very bright and had four children, learned of their choice, he tried to convince Jonathan and Assa to have as many children as possible to add their intelligence to the gene pool. He argued that people like them were morally obligated to reproduce to keep the IQ level of the population from falling. The couple argued that they had no guarantee of intelligent children and that since they had no intention of leaving heirs, they were not particularly interested in what happened to the world's gene resources after they died. The physician refused to prescribe birth control pills because he felt that doing so would be irresponsible. Jonathan and Assa left the office angry and went to another gynecologist to obtain the contraception they wanted.

What the physician did was counterproductive, but was it ethically correct? A physician does have a right to refuse to treat a person as long as he is not endangering that person's life or health, but does he have the right to refuse a requested treatment when he knows it will not place a client in jeopardy, when the client thinks he will benefit from the treatment, and when the refusal is made for purely personal reasons? If the physican were acting as a private citizen or layperson he could refuse to help someone or withhold advice outside his field of expertise, but in his practice as a physician does he have that right? Those who are proponents of physicians' professional autonomy would argue that he does have a right to refuse treatment under the circumstances described, especially if the client is requesting something that he morally opposes. Consumerists and client advocates might disagree, saying that the needs of the client are or should be of prime concern to the physician or any health professional and must be met as long as no harm is done. Jonathan and Assa did eventually have their contraceptive needs met, but they were put to some trouble and added expense in doing so. Another interesting ethical issue concerns whether they are obligated to pay the physician if he refused to treat them.

Mandatory contraception

Should contraception ever be mandatory? This ethically controversial question has been discussed and debated concerning certain groups of people, such as those on welfare who produce children to be supported by tax money, women who have had so many children that their health or life is in danger and their children in jeopardy of being motherless, carriers of genetic diseases, adolescents who are not yet mature or responsible enough to assume the role of parent, and those with a history of child abuse. All these groups are seen by one segment of society or another as being unfit for parenthood or somehow undeserving of the opportunity to bear children. Several ethical principles can be used to debate the issue.

Utilitarianism. The principle of utilitarianism is commonly used to defend various actions in health care. Utilitarianism is a familiar moral theory that has often been erroneously characterized by catch phrases such as "the end justifies the means," "the greatest good for the greatest number," or "what is right is that which is most useful" (utility is commonly thought to mean usefulness). Beauchamp and Childress have pointed out that utilitarianism is much more complex and sophisticated, as

the moral theory that there is one and only one basic principle in ethics, the principle of utility. This principle asserts that we ought in all circumstances to produce the greatest possible balance of value over disvalue for all persons affected (or the least possible balance of disvalue if only evil results can be brought about).*

Achievement of balance is a much more complicated way of solving a problem than simply counting numbers of people who will or will not be benefitted by a certain action. One of the difficulties in applying the principle of utilitarianism to the solution of actual problems involves the concept of values that tip the balance of the outcome in any direction.

Utilitarians agree that ultimately we ought to look to the production of what is intrinsically valuable. That is, what is good in itself and not merely what is good as a means to something else ought to be produced. . . . We really ought to seek certain experiences and conditions in life that are good in themselves without reference to their further consequences, and that all values are ultimately to be gauged in terms of these intrinsic goods.*

---

*Beauchamp, Tom L., and Childress, James F.: Principles of biomedical ethics, New York, 1979, Oxford University Press, pp. 17 and 18.

An intrinsic value is something we want for its own sake, not for something it will produce. Honesty is a characteristic or value that is desirable because it is intrinsically good rather than because it will keep us out of trouble or away from other uncomfortable positions.

One could say that contraception is in itself good because it gives people choices in the area of reproduction and because choice generally leads to happiness and fulfillment. According to the principle of utilitarianism it could be seen as wrong to mandate contraception because choice would then be removed from reproductive functioning and contraception would then be an evil. Balance would be tipped toward disvalue for the individual. "What is intrinsically valuable is what individuals prefer to obtain, and utility is thus translated into the satisfaction of those needs and desires that individuals choose to satisfy." [6,p.24] This view of utilitarianism avoids the necessity for measuring the intrinsic worth of values by permitting individuals to measure their own values in terms of a hierarchy of need or choice.

Deontology. Another principle that could apply to mandatory contraception is that of deontology, which holds that the features of an act rather than its consequences make it right or wrong; rules and acts are right or wrong in themselves. The difficulty in applying deontologic theories to life situations comes in making judgments about which rules or acts are right or wrong. Moralists *do* make these judgments, basing them on divine revelation (for example, the Ten Commandments), natural law, intuition, common sense, social contracts, or common morality. Deontologic theories can be divided into monistic or pluralistic theories. The monistic theory "holds that there is one single rule or principle from which one can derive all other rules or judgments about right and wrong. Thus, one could affirm basic principles such as love and respect for persons and derive other rules such as truth telling and fidelity from them." [6,p.34] A prime example of monistic deontology is the Categorical Imperative postulated by Kant (see Chapter 2), the universal maxim by which all actions can be tested. Pluralistic deontology is a more popular and easily applicable principle that holds that there are more than one basic rule or principle, such as beneficence, fidelity, or justice, that can be applied to an ethical dilemma. There is, of course, difficulty when rules or principles come into conflict. Some principles take precedence over others, but rules do not exist for establishing the priority of one over another. Some moralists maintain that the decision rests on intuition or perception.

While we intuit the principle . . . we do not intuit what is right in the situation; rather we have to find "the greatest balance" of right over wrong. If a pluralistic deontological theory does not provide some ordering or ranking of its principles and rules, it offers little guidance in the moment of decision making.*

In applying pluralistic deontology to the issue of mandatory contraception, one runs into difficulty. If the three principles mentioned above—beneficence, fidelity,

---

*Beauchamp, Tom L., and Childress, James F.: Principles of biomedical ethics, New York, 1979, Oxford University Press, p. 21.

and justice—are chosen, (the ones most commonly applied to health care situations) it cannot be determined which will benefit most from mandatory contraception: the client, who is deprived of liberty but who is relieved of the responsibility of difficult motherhood, or society, which perhaps relieved itself of some responsibility but has also deprived *itself* of liberty. If a society mandates contraception, is it being faithful to its promise of providing individual liberty to its citizens? In the matter of justice, is society perhaps justified in easing its own burdens by not having to support welfare children or to educate and treat those with genetic diseases by depriving a citizen of choice? Is the principle of justice to be given priority over utility, and is justice the appropriate deontologic principle in deciding the issue? Would perhaps nonmaleficence (see below) be better? Using monistic deontology or the Categorical Imperative to solve the issue of mandatory contraception is impossible because everyone could not agree on one universal maxim that could be applied to every situation; too many variables and individual differences exist.

Nonmaleficence and beneficence. The principle of nonmaleficence stems from Hippocrates, is incorporated into the Hippocratic oath ("I will use treatment to help the sick according to my ability and judgment, but I will never use it to injure or wrong them") and generally comes from the Latin maxim *Primum non nocere*, translated as "above all, do no harm." Some philosophers separate it completely from the principle of beneficence, and some see it as a negative form of that positive principle; that is, doing harm is the opposite or the absence of doing good. It is difficult to separate nonmaleficence from beneficence, both in ordinary life and in providing health care. For example, it is wrong to push someone into the street in front of a truck, and it is also wrong not to try to rescue him if he is already in the street. But which is worse—pushing the person or not rescuing him—and which is the higher duty or greater principle? Most people would say the former (nonmaleficence) because in the latter situation the person wandered into the street on his own; rescuing him would be an act of good (beneficence) but would also depend on a number of variables (such as how much danger to himself the rescuer would be risking). This automatically places beneficence lower on the scale of duty than nonmaleficence, which is a moral absolute. Since the principle of nonmaleficence revolves around the concept of harm, it is necessary though difficult to define harm.

Some definitions of "harm" are so broad as to include injuries to reputation, to property, and to liberty. For example, if the object of harm is always an *interest*, it is possible to have various interests that could be violated or damaged, such as health, property, domestic relations, and privacy. Then it would be possible to distinguish trivial and serious harms by the order and magnitude of the interests involved.*

Nonmaleficence as a principle is useful when considering mandatory contraception. What harm would be done, and to whose interests? We could compile a list of obvious harms: (1) a woman would be harmed because her right to privacy,

---

*Beauchamp, Tom L., and Childress, James F.: Principles of biomedical ethics, New York, 1979, Oxford University Press, p. 22.

liberty, and choice are abrogated; (2) her mental health might be harmed because of interference with personal convictions; (3) her happiness and sense of purpose in life might be harmed if she had a strong desire for more children and saw her primary role or function as motherhood; (4) her marriage might be harmed because of stress; and (5) society would be harmed because the deprivation of liberty to one individual affects and changes the nature of the society that caused the action. More possible harms could be added, but even with this abbreviated list it can be seen that mandatory contraception would be causing an intentional harm. Thus if one believes that the principle of nonmaleficence has a higher priority than the principle of beneficence, then no matter what good or benefit might accrue to the individual or society (even if a list of benefits is as long as the list of harms), mandatory contraception would be considered immoral and wrong. Intentional harm is always prohibited, except under very special circumstances such as self-defense.

Justice. The principle of justice, perhaps one of the most arbitrary and confusing moral principles, is the final one to be applied to mandatory contraception. Justice is what determines how social responsibility and benefits are allocated. However, in this complex society applying the principle of justice is no simple matter. A moral person has a sense of intuition about what is just and what action is more fair than another, but intuition alone is not sufficient to make justice work to solve moral problems. To use a principle, it is necessary to understand its shades of meaning. There are several different types of justice:

1. Distributive justice refers to the fair and proper distribution of social benefits and burdens. Taxation and a military draft are social burdens and responsibilities, whereas the fire department and national defense are social benefits. Benefits and responsibilities are never in precise balance, but the principle of distributive justice should serve to ensure that the balance does not tip too far in one direction.

2. Comparative justice involves persons competing for the same claim; determination of whose claim is just is made by society depending on how much or what benefit a person is due. The competition for research grants and scholarships is an example of comparative justice, as is transplantation of scarce donor organs.

3. Formal justice (a principle generally attributed to Aristotle) states that equals ought to be treated equally and unequals unequally. This does not mean that the persons have to be equal but only the *respects* under consideration. In other words, one person should not be treated differently from others despite any differences between that person and others, unless the difference is relevant in respect to the considered treatment. Formal justice is most easily explained when it is applied to law. If two persons are accused of committing the same crime in almost identical circumstances, the punishment for both should be the same no matter what differences exist in the persons in other respects. For example, two men forcibly rape two women on separate occasions. Both crimes are committed on a dark street at night, and in both cases the victim is unknown to the assailant. Both men are judged mentally competent to stand trial. The punishment should be the

same for both even if one is a white architect and the other a black laborer. These differences are not significant with respect to the crime or the circumstances under which it was committed. Now imagine the same crime and the same circumstances, and make the two men the same race. The difference now is that one is an off-duty policeman and the other a severely mentally retarded man who wandered off the grounds of a state institution. Punishment now might be different because the differences in the men are significant with respect to the crime. The major problem with formal justice is that it is often difficult to determine what differences are relevant to a particular situation.

Let us look at the issue of mandatory contraception using the principle of distributive justice. Beauchamp and Childress[6] have described a list of different principles of distributive justice that I shall apply to the determination of the morality of mandatory contraception:

1. To each person an equal share. Will a woman have her equal share of freedom and liberty if she is prevented from bearing the number of children she chooses? If she contributes too many children to society, will she be receiving more or less than her share of society's benefits?

2. To each person according to individual need. Will a person's needs be met if society enforces mandatory contraception in some circumstances? The answer at first glance might be an emphatic no, but will another individual be prevented from having his needs met if a neighbor has that extra child?

3. To each person according to individual effort. This principle is difficult to apply because effort in childbearing and childrearing is subjective. Is the welfare mother of four contributing less effort to society than the working mother of three? In terms of contribution to society, one might say that the working mother is contributing more, but how can the contribution of the welfare mother to the effort of raising her children be measured?

4. To each person according to societal contribution. Compare a welfare mother with two children to a Nobel Prize–winning scientist. Two of his four children are hemophiliacs; their combined treatment costs about $30,000 a year, which the scientist cannot afford alone. Who is contributing more to society; who should be compelled to practice birth control?

5. To each person according to merit. The determination of who deserves to continue reproducing and who does not is an entirely arbitrary decision based on the standards and values of a society or that segment of a society in a position to make such decisions.

STERILIZATION
Reasons for voluntary sterilization

One might think it unnecessary for there to be discussion about sterilization beyond the statement that one becomes sterilized because one has made a decision to have no further children. Unfortunately nothing in health care ethics is quite that simple. Various ramifications and opinions about voluntary sterilization do exist; in fact, it is quite a heated issue.

Sterilization originally simply meant amputation and was done only to men (amputation of a woman's uterus would surely have resulted in her death). Throughout history men have been castrated as punishment for rape. American slaves were castrated to make them more docile and devoted field hands (it was thought that they would not think about sex). In the Mideast men were castrated to guard harems, and in other areas it was done to young boys to keep their voices clear and high for singing hymns. Warriors castrated men in the lands they conquered and occupied, and some religious sects used castration as a sacrifice. It is no wonder that many men today feel fearful and squeamish when contemplating vasectomy; possibly they associate it with castration. Present methods of sterilization are more civilized and involve cutting only the vas deferens or fallopian tubes to prevent transport of sperm or ovum, respectively. The emotional arguments have changed in nature over time, but they have not decreased in intensity.

There are several basic reasons for voluntary sterilization. The first is a matter of choice; a person decides he or she wants no more children and requests the surgery, which is not always as obtainable as one might assume. The woman described in Chapter 5, who became pregnant when she was 37 years old, had made a conscious decision many years before to have no children. When she was about 26 she first sought sterilization. Her request was rejected out of hand because she was young and unmarried and because the physician was certain she would change her mind "when the right man came along." She tried several times in the next 11 years to obtain a tubal ligation, but the response was always a variation on the same theme: the request was refused because of her life circumstances. Ironically she was finally able to obtain sterilization at the same time she had the abortion. The physician, not knowing the previous history, agreed immediately.

Other arbitrary and capricious decisions are made about requests for voluntary sterilization. Veatch[7] reports sterilization being used with the 120 rule. A woman who had been born in Puerto Rico was denied sterilization in a New York City hospital clinic because she did not conform to the 120 rule, the hospital's policy that for a woman to be sterilized her age multiplied by the number of children she had already borne must equal at least 120. The woman in question was 28 years old and had two children; she was denied sterilization even though she could not face another Caesarean section and was certain she wanted no more children.

Sometimes decisions are made on the whim or personal convictions of a single physician and are not the result of planned policy. Several years ago when I was with students in the obstetric department of a teaching hospital, we cared for a client for 3 months. When we first met her she was 6 months pregnant and bleeding vaginally. She was mostly in the hospital for the next 3 months, and during that time she and I had several long talks. She was quite happily married and had two school-age children, and although she wanted the baby she was carrying, she was alternately angry and worried about the bleeding that would not stop. She intended to have a tubal ligation immediately after delivery; her husband concurred with the decision. She expressed her desire to the physician who refused to entertain her request seriously, saying that she would change her mind as soon as events turned out positively. She did not press him. The delivery went well, and the child was beautiful and healthy. The next day her husband and I were both in the room when she asked her physician when he had scheduled the tubal ligation. He patted her leg and said, "Don't be silly; you're a wonderful breeder," and strode out of the room.

Men are also victims of this arbitrary behavior. Many urologists require that men be subject to a psychiatric evaluation before they undergo vasectomy, especially if the man has fathered "too few" children or is seen as "too young." Men do have an advantage over women in terms of the permanence of sterilization. Although the surgical procedures are equally permanent (research has been done in reanastamosis of fallopian tubes and vas deferens, but it is still neither practical nor guaranteed and thus sterilization should be considered permanent), a man can deposit semen in a sperm bank in the event he may want children after his vasectomy.

Another reason for voluntary sterilization is therapeutic, the removal of a diseased organ of reproduction. The most common procedure of this type is hysterectomy, performed for a variety of reasons ranging from dysfunctional uterine bleeding (a kind of vague catch-all diagnosis that is used the when the cause is uncertain) to carcinoma. Sometimes the woman's life is at stake; more often it is not, and frequently the surgery is not medically necessary. Male organs of reproduction (penis and testes) are not removed unless cancer is definitely present.

Another reason for voluntary sterilization is to prevent abortion. Worldwide, abortion is the most common method of birth control, whereby 40 million pregnancies are terminated purposefully each year.[8] Whatever one's moral position on abortion, using it as a means of birth control is inappropriate. If sterilization were more widely available to people who have made a firm decision about childbearing, the number of abortions could be drastically reduced. In the United States a large percentage of abortions are performed on married women with children, many of whom have most likely tried to obtain sterilization.

Another reason is eugenic, to prevent the birth of a child who will most likely be defective. People who are carriers of genetic diseases or traits are encouraged by health professionals to seek genetic counseling and are informed of the statistical chances for bearing a child with the disease or trait. Whether people take this risk is a matter of personal choice, complicated as always by ethical considerations. If they choose not to take the risk and want assurance that pregnancy will not occur, sterilization is the logical answer.

Voluntary sterilization for eugenic reasons can be manipulated by health professionals to become less than voluntary. Again we have an example from Veatch[7]: a 24-year-old woman with sickle-cell disease almost died in the process of having a child. She had periodic sickle crises during which she was incapacitated by severe pain. Recent research pointed up the very negative aspects of pregnancy in women with sickle-cell disease: about 50% terminate in spontaneous abortion, stillbirth, or neonatal death, and about 10% of the mothers died some time during the pregnancy or postpartum period. The research advocated sterilization or abortion for those who conceived. The woman in question refused to be sterilized even though her physician had painted a clear picture of the likely consequences of another pregnancy. The physician did not want to give up trying to convince her and thought he eventually could if he were dramatic enough.

The physician in this case seemed to be confusing medical facts with his own values and those of the client. The physician saw a 10% risk of death as not worth it to the client if she risked another pregnancy. But there might be sound reasons in the client's values for her to become pregnant again: she may have felt siblings are desirable and have been acting out of a commitment to her present child, or the possibility that the physician's judgment was affected by racism may have been present in her thinking. The physician's values can also be questioned: he thought he was acting in the best interest of the client, but his position of power over her might have influenced her behavior: the issue of coercion, although it is not blatant, cannot be ignored.

Voluntary sterilization is elective surgery, although it is not judged as necessary or unnecessary by the usual medical criteria for elective surgery. Not all clients who voluntarily sign the consent form remain pleased with their decision. The three factors found to contribute most to later regret are (1) being very young, (2) deciding under duress, and (3) having the procedure suggested by the physician rather than the client.[9] Various kinds of subtle coercive techniques are used to increase the likelihood that a woman (usually young, unsophisticated, poor, and perhaps black) will voluntarily consent to sterilization: asking her to sign the form either immediately before Caesarean section or immediately after delivery when she is undergoing considerable emotional stress, describing laparoscopic tubal ligation as "Band-Aid surgery" and thus minimizing its importance, and avoiding use of the word *operation* if the incision is made vaginally. McGarrah[9] describes two other phenomena that tend to increase the coercive aspects of voluntary sterilization. The first is the fact that surgical residency programs in most teaching hospitals reward residents for the number of operations they perform; rewards increase as the technical difficulty of the surgery increases. Thus sterilization is encouraged, and hysterectomy is encouraged even more. The second reason is that there are fewer ward or service clients for residents to gain experience with, and thus they feel obliged to push even harder for sterilization consents. Obviously the more pushing that is done, the more women will consent. As a result of continued sterilization abuses, the Department of Health, Education and Welfare established guidelines of safety and voluntariness for persons being sterilized in federally funded programs.

Religious aspects of voluntary sterilization

Only the Catholic Church opposes sterilization as a means of birth control, for the same reasons it opposes all other forms of artificial contraception.

For the present, then, the position is that sterilization is permitted by Catholic morals only as a right of self-defense in cases of what our Supreme Court calls "a clear and present danger." Catholic moralists will not allow any moral justification of sterilization as a preventive measure of self-defense or as a practice in preventive medicine on a principle of "clear and *future* danger."*

This means that an organ of reproduction may be removed with an outcome of sterilization only if it is diseased and would place the health or life of the person in jeopardy. No other Christian doctrine prohibits sterilization. The Catholic ban is a moral interpretation of Scripture or natural law and is widely ignored by the Catholic populace as are bans on other forms of artificial birth control.

Involuntary sterilization

Fletcher states the following as the crux of the issue of coerced, forced, or punitive sterilization:

> Our courts of law in this enlightened country will not knowingly grant a decree for an insane, feeble-minded, or otherwise unfit person to adopt a child. Their objective in such cases would rest upon moral grounds: a child has a right to a minimum standard of care and security, and parents, whether natural or adoptive, are obliged in conscience to possess the competence necessary to render to their children their dues. In this view of the obligation of parenthood, we cannot avoid asking the question: if the law will not permit unfit persons to adopt a child, why should it permit them to conceive and bring forth a child?*

The logic of this argument seems inescapable; Fletcher's position, if followed to its conclusion, would have society determine which adults have the competence and conscience to "render to their children their dues." Considering the number of cases there have been of enforced and coerced sterilization, this is not simply a theoretical issue; it raises serious questions. What would be the criteria for a fit parent, who would establish the criteria, who would determine the application of the criteria, what are minimal standards of care and security, what is due a child, and how much much of it, and would the child have recourse if he felt he was not receiving his due? Debates over these issues are never-ending; it does not seem possible to reach a practical solution to the dilemma posed by Fletcher.

Punitive or compulsory sterilization is regarded by most Americans as a drastic procedure that is unwarranted in any but the most extreme circumstances. Abuses of compuslory sterilization laws or mandates would be too tempting; we remember too well the sterilization of non-Aryans by Nazis. Our tradition of liberty in the way we use our bodies is strong, and too many people are alerted to abrogation of civil rights of individuals or groups to permit compulsory sterilization without a hue and cry. It would remove an aspect of sexual freedom that is part of personal liberty. Sterilization enhances freedom of sexual expression without fear of pregnancy only when it is voluntary.

One proposed reason for punitive sterilization is the punishment of criminals either in direct retaliation for sex offenses or to prevent incorrigible criminals from reproducing. The proposal is counterproductive for several reasons, although it

---

*Fletcher, Joseph: Morals and medicine, pp. 157, 141. Copyright © 1954, 1979 by Princeton University Press; Princeton Paperback. Reprinted by permission of Princeton University Press.

might provide society with some psychologic satisfaction. Rape, the most common form of sexual assault, is not a sexual act. It is instead an act of physical violence, with the penis used as the weapon of aggression. Men who rape women do so not out of a desire for sexual contact with them but out of their hatred for women and their need to hurt them. Sterilizing rapists by castration (vasectomy is not the punishment generally recommended for rapists) would not quell their anger toward women; they might simply vent their possibly increased anger with another weapon, probably a far more lethal one.

In the case of incorrigible criminals, one would need to prove that criminal behavior results *solely* from genetic causes and that the genetic trait could not be circumvented by environmental changes. To date no proof exists that criminality is genetically caused, although there has been suspicion that men with an XYY chromosomal configuration tend to be more criminally aggressive. It can be acknowledged that rehabilitation and major changes in the behavior of hardened criminals have been mostly unsuccessful, but is not likely that sterilization will prove to be a better deterrent to crime.

Legal precedents for another kind of involuntary sterilization, that involving the mentally retarded, have been divergent, with courts ruling both for and against. Clarification is needed, and the issues are complex and emotionally laden. Informed consent is a major part of the issue. Two questions need to be answered regarding sterilization of the retarded: is the person to be sterilized capable of understanding what is to happen and how can this be proved, and if the person is not capable of consenting, will the proxy have the best interests of the client at heart? Committees can be established to ponder the questions, but a definitive answer is not easy. If a physican is legally liable for performing a sterilization without valid informed consent, why would a committee be necessary? If there is a question in the physician's mind about the mental competence of the client, he is morally and professionally obligated to obtain a second opinion. It is true, as discussed earlier, that physicians are sometimes more eager to sterilize people than they are to ensure that client's rights are enforced, and fear of a malpractice suit is not always a deterrent to ignoring informed consent, especially when relatively unsophisticated clients are involved. But a review committee for every proposed sterilization of a questionably competent person could be seen as a constraint on voluntary sterilization, and it would be a cumbersome procedure. It might be more practical to restrict committee review to institutionalized people or to those with no family.

In what situations could a court override a person's fundamental right to reproduce by ordering involuntary sterilization? This could be done perhaps only if a court could prove that a person's childbearing would harm society and could thus rule that sterilization would be in the best interest of society. To do so, the state would need powerful justification; that is, society would have to be clearly endangered. The conditions considered dangerous to society vary widely and do not necessarily involve berserk criminals firing rifles into crowds. The presence of genetic defects that would prevent a child from growing into a responsible adult is considered reason enough by some, as is presence of proven inheritable criminal behavior, although it is questionable whether due process of law would exist in such circumstances. It is generally the poor, uneducated, and unsophisticated who are involuntarily sterilized. The vast majority of these operations are done on women; one almost never hears of involuntary vasectomy. As long as the law is unclear and precedents have not been firmly established, the obligation falls on health professionals to protect people from involuntarily giving up their right to reproduce.

SUMMARY

The central ethical question in contraception concerns whether people have a right to control their own reproductive powers, and if so, what means of control are permissible. Do men or women or both have the right to determine parenthood? The issue of natural law is invoked in matters of sexuality in general and in contraception in particular, the idea that no one but God should have a right to control the results of sexual intercourse. Conservative Catholic moralists object to contraception for religious reasons; their thinking is based almost entirely on the foundation of natural law. The Catholic populace, however, is not generally disposed to obey Rome on this issue, nor are many liberal Catholic theologians and parish priests who tend to advise people to follow their own conscience in matters of family planning. One can see contraception as a matter of personal choice in the way one uses one's body; to prohibit contraception is to withhold liberty and freedom in sexuality. Should any amount of freedom be abrogated? Can a husband or wife claim any degree of control over the reproductive functioning of the other spouse?

The locus of control in deciding which form of birth control is appropriate is another issue: should the health professional or the client decide? Various factors and ramifications affect the decisions, such as the person's attitude toward sexuality, how much she knows about various contraceptive methods, physicians' biases and how they feel about contraception in general and a certain client in particular, and the nature of a person's sex life and the kinds of sexual relationships formed.

Nurses can play an important role in helping the client understand contraception and have greater control in contraceptive use; this usually results in more successful contraception.

Each birth control method has its own particular ethical considerations, and its risks or negative effects must be weighed against desirable outcomes. Clients must be informed, as fully as possible, about the risks so that they can make an intelligent choice. The degree of risk is usually associated with the permanence of the method, as is complexity of the ethical issues.

Attitudes toward sexuality have a great deal to do with contraceptive choice, but adolescent sexuality is more charged with emotionality and ethical dilemmas than is adult sexual behavior. Almost half the adolescents in the United States are sexually active, yet many people question the morality of providing them with contraceptive information. Others believe it wrong to withhold contraceptive advice and services from adolescents who need it, because consequences of an adolescent pregnancy can be much more serious and far-reaching than an adult's.

Health professionals are obligated to disseminate birth control information to people who want it; nurses can be especially useful in this area, particularly by incorporating a sexual history into the nursing diagnosis. Under some circumstances it might be appropriate for the health professional to initiate the subject of contraception even if the client does not; other circumstances might preclude a conversation about birth control.

Are there groups of people for whom contraception should be mandatory? That dilemma is examined by the application of various ethical principles including utilitarianism, deontology, beneficence, nonmaleficence, and justice.

The ethics of sterilization to a large extent parallel the ethics of other forms of artificial contraception, although because the method is permanent, the issues are possibly more important. Voluntary sterilization is usually done because a person makes a choice to have no more children, because a particular part of the reproductive anatomy is diseased (in which case sterilization is not the primary reason for surgery), or because one desires to prevent the birth of a child with a hereditary defect or trait or to prevent future abortions. Voluntary sterilization could tend to be coercive, especially if the person is young, uneducated, and relatively unknowledgable about health procedures.

Involuntary sterilization involves so many issues that criteria for deciding who should be sterilized and for what reasons could never be established or enacted. Legal precedents for involuntary sterilization are divided, and the guidelines for action are incredibly complex.

REFERENCES

1. Fletcher, Joseph: Morals and medicine, Princeton, N.J., 1954, Princeton University Press.
2. Dedek, John F.: Contemporary medical ethics, New York, 1975, Sheed & Ward, Inc.
3. Steinfels, Margaret O'Brien: An IUD and the question of safety (case studies in bioethics, case 427), Hastings Center Reports 4(6):10, December 1974.
4. Lieberman, E. James, and Tannenwald, Carol B.: editors: Ethical issues in adolescent health: proceedings of a conference sponsored by APHA, Institute of Society, Ethics, and the Life Sciences, and USPHS, Washington, D.C., December 6-7, 1976.
5. Woods, Nancy Fugate: Human sexuality in health and illness, ed. 2, St. Louis, 1979, The C. V. Mosby Co.
6. Beauchamp, Tom L., and Childress, James F.: Principles of biomedical ethics, New York, 1979, Oxford University Press.
7. Veatch, Robert M.: Case studies in medical ethics, Cambridge, Mass., 1977, Harvard University Press.
8. Davis, Joseph E.: Birth control by sterilization. In Frazier, Claude A.: Is it moral to modify man? Springfield, Ill., 1973, Charles C Thomas, Publisher.

9. McGarrah, Robert E., Jr.: Voluntary female sterilization: abuses, risks and guidelines, Hastings Center Reports 4(3):5, June 1974.

BIBLIOGRAPHY

Aranoff, Gava, and Sidel, Victor, W.: Case studies in bioethics: comment on case # 427, Hastings Center Reports 4(6):13, December 1974.
Bayles, Michael: The legal precedents, Hastings Center Reports 8(3):37-41, June 1978.
Beauchamp, Tom L. and Childress, James F.: Principles of biomedical ethics, New York, 1979, Oxford University Press.
Davis, Joseph E.: Birth control by sterilization. In Frazier, Claude A.: Is it moral to modify man? Springfield, Ill., 1973, Charles C Thomas, Publisher.
Dedek, John F.: Contemporary medical ethics, New York, 1975, Sheed & Ward, Inc.
Donovan, Patricia: Sterilizing the poor and incompetent, Hastings Center Reports 6(5):7-8, October 1976.
Fletcher, Joseph: Morals and medicine, Princeton, N.J., 1954, Princeton University Press.
Lieberman, E. James, and Tannenwald, Carol B., editors: Ethical issues in adolescent health: proceedings of a conference sponsored by APHA, Institute

of Society, Ethics and the Life Sciences, and USPHS, Washington, D.C., December 6-7, 1976.

Mazurkewicz, Dolores T.: The family. In Fromer, Margot Joan: Community health care and the nursing process, St. Louis, 1979, The C. V. Mosby Co.

McGarrah, Robert E., Jr.: Voluntary female sterilization: abuses, risks and guidelines, Hastings Center Reports 4(3):5-7, June 1974.

Peck, Susan L.: Voluntary female sterilization: attitudes and legislation, Hastings Center Reports 4 (3):8-10, June 1974.

Pepper, Anita Golden: History of the health care system. In Fromer, Margot Joan: Community health care and the nursing process, St. Louis, 1979, The C. V. Mosby Co.

Steinfels, Margaret O'Brien: An IUD and the question of safety, Hastings Center Reports 4(6):10-12, December 1974.

Taylor, Howard C.: The ethics of the physician in human reproduction. In Vischer, Maurice B., editor: Human Perspectives in Medical Ethics, Buffalo, N.Y., 1972, Prometheus Books.

Veatch, Robert M.: Case studies in medical ethics, Cambridge, Mass., 1977, Harvard University Press.

Woods, Nancy Fugate: Human sexuality in health and illness, ed. 2, St. Louis., 1979, The C. V. Mosby Co.

7

Abortion

PHILOSOPHIC HISTORY

Abortion is the expulsion of a fetus from the uterus prior to 28 weeks' gestation, the arbitrarily established time of viability—the point at which a fetus could reasonably be expected to survive outside the uterus. A natural (spontaneous) abortion, commonly called a miscarriage, may occur for a variety of reasons, but induced abortion requires intervention by the pregnant woman herself, or more commonly, a health professional. This chapter is concerned only with induced abortions.

Abortion methods depend mostly on the time of gestation; the uterus is invaded with a variety of instruments and the products of conception are removed. Any gynecologic text will describe the procedure. Abortion performed by a competent health professional in an aseptic environment is a physically safe procedure, and the morbidity and mortality are lower in the United States than for childbirth at term. In Chapter 6 it was noted that abortion is the most widely used method of birth control in the world; in many countries more pregnancies are aborted than continue to term.

Women have chosen to have abortions since the beginning of recorded history. In ancient Greece and Rome abortion was used to control population; the gods did not forbid it, and the fetus was not protected by either Greek or Roman law. Most Greek philosophers applauded abortion or at least did not condemn it. The Pythagoreans, however, disagreed because they believed that the embryo became infused with a soul at the moment of conception. Hippocrates was a follower of Pythagorean philosophy—hence the sanction on abortion in the Hippocratic Oath. This proscription was widely ignored, and Greek and Roman physicians performed abortions for all women who requested them.

At the height of Greek and Roman civilization Judaism had been flourishing for 2000 years and Christianity was beginning to develop. Early Jews and Christians forbade abortion on practical as well as religious and philosophic grounds. The Decalogue is specific: Thou shalt not kill. God's injunction to be fruitful and multiply was obeyed literally. A human life, even a potential one, was viewed as valuable and something to be saved. The Old Testament command to love thy neighbor as thyself and to do justice was followed by the New Testament concept of sacrifice of self for the sake of another, based on the ultimate self-sacrifice of Jesus. Jesus

205

commanded his followers to love one another and to value human life; from this example Christians developed the valuation of human life, which they believed began at the time of conception.

Secular and religious philosophers have long debated about abortion. All conflicts stem from the way one determines the humanity or personhood of an individual. If we accept Fletcher's view of personhood (see Chapter 1), abortion is morally permissible. The concept of ensoulment, the time at which an embryo or fetus is infused with a soul, is central to the morality or permissibility of abortion. St. Thomas Aquinas placed ensoulment at about 3 months, or when the fetus became recognizably human. The Catholic Church today, however, believes that ensoulment occurs at conception and that the embryo or fetus is a human being simply at a stage of development different from that of a human being who has already been born, in the same way that a child is at a stage of development different from that of an adult. The Church sees no moral difference between infanticide and abortion.

According to the Talmud, the Jewish interpretation of oral law and of the first five books of the Old Testament (known as the Torah), a fetus is not a human being until the head emerges from the body of its mother. Even so, abortion is not permitted in Orthodox Judaism unless the mother's life is threatened. Reform and Conservative Judaism take a more liberal view of abortion.

In discussing the philosophic history of abortion it is almost impossible to separate secular from religious or theologic ethics. Carney[1] defines theologic ethics (also known as moral theology) as a critical reflection about belief in God as a basis for understanding moral life. Moral theology usually exists within the context of a systematized religion. Carney goes on to say that three types of normative judgments are basic to theologic ethics, the judgments of obligation, virtue, and value. When these judgments are discussed in terms of abortion, one might ask the following questions. (1) To whom is obligation owed—to the fetus, the pregnant woman, or even to society? (2) What qualities are there in a person or act (the pregnant woman, the physician, or the abortion itself) that are worthy of virtue or are morally reprehensible? And (3) what objects, persons, or states of affairs are good or bad and to what degree? These three types of judgments are sometimes grouped together and called values or value judgments, a term that is commonly used to describe the good or bad nature of a person or action. Thus when one makes the value judgment that abortion is wrong or morally impermissible, one is saying something about the identification and assessment of specific moral components.

Summation of the three normative components does not necessarily result in a neat moral package; consequently we have individual and societal conflicts about the morality of abortion. For example, one might think that a greater obligation is owed to a pregnant woman than to a fetus and at the same time think that all forms of killing are morally reprehensible. A conflict is thus created before the third question is even addressed. The question of whether abortion (or the person performing it or having it performed) is good or bad then rests on resolution of the conflict already established.

Theological ethics shares these three types of normative judgment with philosophical ethics (or moral philosophy). What distinguishes the two enterprises from each other, therefore, is not a difference about the need to employ judgments of obligation, virtue, and value, but rather the orientation that is brought to their employment. Philosophical ethics may, but need not, assess the bearing of theistic beliefs and attitudes on the moral life, and to a very considerable degree proceeds today without doing so in European-American society. . . . Theological ethics, on the other hand, is committed by its very nature to the examination of the moral life from the viewpoint of theistic beliefs and attitudes. It characteristically seeks its orientation in inquiries about the appropriate human response to whatever is held to be God's nature, will, or activity, and examines and advocates theories of obligation, virtue, and value associated with that response.*

The essential difference, then, between moral philosophy and moral theology involves a leap of faith. If one does not acknowledge the existence of God, then the three normative judgments cannot be made with a view toward their theistic relationship. This does not mean that the philosophic problems and moral dilemmas are different but it does mean that they are examined from a different viewpoint. However, when one examines an issue or problem such as abortion from a moral theologic view, it still must be done in a rational manner. It is not sufficient to say, "Abortion is wrong because God forbids it." A theistic orientation to the solution of moral dilemmas is more complex than simply falling back on what one *believes* God has commanded.

The historic development of an orientation predicated on belief in God (called a theistic orientation) implies that human beings are required to make some sort of response to God. This may take the form of pentinence, prayer, fasting, pilgrimage, or a life that pursues human excellence. The last is the highest response and the most difficult to achieve. One can explore various positions on the way to achieving this excellence. The first is that God is responsible for universal order and human beings must respond by understanding and abiding by that order. The implication is that happiness and fulfillment will be achieved by so doing, but the difficult task is the process by which one comes to understand God's order. The Catholic Church does it by defining and adhering to natural law, and Hindus achieve it through karma, by which a person is and gets today what he deserves because of his past and will recieve in the future results from his actions today.

The second position (or theistic orientation) assumes that God has intervened in human history and has entered into a new relationship with humanity. One must then respond to this event by making it central to his life and relating an understanding of his own existence in relationship to it, thus creating a divine-human relationship with attendant duties and obligations. For example, when God gave Moses and the Israelites the Ten Commandments after God had provided for an exodus out of the land of Egypt, this event, the granting of freedom and providing

---

*"Theological Ethics" by Frederick S. Carney. Reproduction by permission of The Free Press, a Division of Macmillan Publishing Co., Inc. and The Kennedy Institute of Ethics, Georgetown University. From Encyclopedia of Bioethics, Warren T. Reich, Editor in Chief. Volume 1, pages 429-430. Copyright © 1978 by Georgetown University, Washington, D.C.

of a route to Israel, created a perpetual debt of obligation and gratitude in the Jew, who must strive for human excellence to pay the debt to God.

A third position emphasizes the attributes or characteristics of God as they are perceived by the believer. These attributes are to be imitated if they are loving or revered if that is more appropriate. There is no place for attributes that viewed on a human scale could be interpreted as negative, such as vengeance, anger, or wrath. The Christian responses of faith, hope, and charity are examples of the emulation of God's attributes, as is the Islamic tradition of justice, for example, chopping off the hand of a thief.

Relationships between moral theology and philosophic ethics can be examined and described in terms of the morality of abortion. In a historic relationship a particular moral concept has its roots in an early religious tradition. Through social and psychologic evolution this moral concept may have come to prominence in modern Western thought, though it might just as easily have lost popularity and died out (for example, priestly celibacy is an idea that has gained and lost popularity and practice several times between the time of St. Peter and the present.)

A logical relationship is one in which a certain moral judgment is derived from a theistic orientation and is very similar to a historic realtionship. The logical can, however, differ from the historic in that moral judgments are justified by a theistic orientation. This requires faith to show that a theistic orientation is necessary to establish the validity of a moral judgment. For example, in a logical relationship we can make the moral judgment that abortion is wrong only if we can prove that God disapproves of killing in all circumstances. If doubt exists, then a logical relationship cannot be established.

A psychologic relationship provides a motivation for doing one's duty mandated by a theistic orientation and can result in development of worthwhile values and improvement of one's character. Since values and character always are tested in action sooner or later, one needs some sort of motivation for their development or they will collapse when called into action. A psychologic motivation would prevent a woman from having an abortion if she were morally opposed to it but tempted to do so for practical reasons.

An epistemologic relationship (epistemology is the study of knowledge and how things are known) rests on the claim that a theistic orientation is known to contribute to morality. This means that certain basic moral truths are not generally known except through a theistic orientation; it depends quite heavily on faith and the love of God, which figure prominently in most Western religions. But this leap of faith is too wide a gap for people who discount the epistemologic relationship. Some believe that all people have or can be taught a rational knowledge of morality and that no one has absolute knowledge of a theistic orientation, with the possible exceptions of some of the old Testament patriarchs who spoke directly to God and of Jesus Christ, Mohammed, Buddha, and perhaps a few saints. The epistemologic relationship can also flow in the opposite direction; that is, the knowledge and practice of morality can add to our knowledge of God.

One frequently sees the term *ontology* in discussions and essays about abortion.

Ontology involves important concepts that can be difficult to understand because of their highly theoretical nature. Ontology is usually defined as the theory of being *as* being and sometimes is referred to as the concept that the fact of being (as existence) is sufficient unto itself to continue being. In other words, I am and shall continue to be *simply because* I am. No other reason for my existence need be set forth except that I do now exist. Since many people feel that all existence arises from God, an ontologic relationship maintains that the existence of moral obligations, virtues, and values is connected with the existence and activity of God; that is, morality cannot exist without God. This also requires faith and is a difficult connection to make. We see evidence of morality, but it is more difficult to say that we see evidence of God.

These relationships rest on what modern philosophers term a "slippery slope"; in trying to cast one's mind back and forth between moral philosophy and moral theology, one feels one is playing catch with a cake of wet soap. You think you have the concept, then it slips from your mental grasp. It is, however, more important to know that a history of these analogies and relationships has been made than it is to fully understand all their ramifications. Abortion, like euthanasia and other bioethical dilemmas, slides back and forth between the theologic and the secular because it deals with taking a potential or actual human life. Stepping back and forth between the realm of the divine and the human produces conflict.

It is necessary to comment on the use of words and terms that figure prominently in the abortion debate. Since the issue itself is emotion-laden, words connected with it are also. Because an abortion involves fetal death in almost all instances, a verb must be used to describe the action that results in death. The two most common are *kill* and *murder,* which are not synonymous although people tend to use them interchangeably. The verb *kill* means to deliberately end a life; it can refer to bacteria, plants, people, cockroaches, rats, and fetuses, anything that has life. To murder is also to kill, but *murder* is generally used to refer only to human beings and to killing of an innocent person, as with a murder victim. The word *kill,* although its aura is more negative than positive, does not necessarily mean a negative action. Many instances of killing can be seen as positive or at least as appropriate: killing termites that are chewing up your house, killing the rattlesnake whose open jaws are close to your ankle, killing enemy soldiers in battle, and for those who favor abortion killing a fetus. Those who are in favor of abortion, however, tend to avoid *kill* in favor of *abort, remove,* or some other more neutral word.

They never refer to abortion as *murder,* which is the word used by those opposed to abortion. *Murder* has an entirely negative connotation and is used almost exclusively to refer to innocent human beings. (A person I know who is much opposed to hunting refers to hunters as murderers of defenseless animals, thus anthropomorphizing the animals to create guilt in the hunter.) One speaks of *killing* soldiers in war and *murdering* civilians, thus making a value judgment about whom it might be appropriate to kill and who should not be killed. Whether *murder* is a correct word to use in regard to abortion depends on whether a fetus is considered a human being, an issue discussed in detail later in the chapter.

Another set of words important to the abortion debate includes *life, potential life,* and *alive.* Few argue whether an embryo or fetus is alive or is a potential human life. What is more arguable is that a fetus *is* a human life rather than an entity that *has* life. To say that a fetus is a life is to imply that it is a separate and unique being, already an individual, even though it is still physically attached to its mother. This is the picture painted by antiabortionists. Proabortionists acknowledge that a fetus has life but do not view it as a separate individual. The issue becomes even more complicated during the latter part of the second trimester when the fetus's chances of surviving outside the uterus begin to increase.

Another confusion of terms occurs between the words *fetus* and *embryo.* An embryo becomes a fetus when it assumes recognizably human form, in the first trimester. *Fetus* is more emotionally laden than *embryo.* When we envision the latter we generally think of a jumble of cells or some indefinable shape vaguely reminiscent of a baby chick. The word *fetus,* however, conforms more closely to our idea of a baby person; some even conjure up an image of the Gerber baby snuggled inside its mother's belly taking a nap. The idea of harming the fetus in this image jars our sensibilities more than with the image of a kind of free-form being floating in nothingness. Although an embryo and a fetus are not the same physically or symbolically, the word *fetus* will be used here for ease of readability, and it will be assumed that the reader understands that in most first-trimester abortions it is an embryo that is expelled.

In defining words or terms that have some emotional impact, a line can be drawn between the abstract concept of the word and the reality. An example is the word *starvation;* we understand the physiologic process that occurs when a person starves to death, and we might even understand the economic and social conditions that lead to starvation. But as we push our grocery carts through supermarkets full of food, we cannot *feel* the concept of starvation. We can understand the impact of the reality only if we have seen the haunted eyes, heavy bellies, and matchstick limbs of a person scratching in the dirt for grains of wheat.

So too with abortion. It is not emotionally threatening to sit at a desk and write about the ethical ramifications of abortion, and it is only slightly less so to stand before a class of nursing students and guide them through an intellectual discussion of abortion ethics. It is far less threatening to discuss the issue than to be a participant or the partner of one.

I will remember always the emotional impact the first time I saw an aborted fetus. It was the result of a saline instillation at about 22 weeks of gestational age. I did not expect to see it, and when my eyes strayed to the counter next to a sink I was using, I felt the impact almost as a physical assault. It was quite perfectly formed, although its color was very blue and dead looking. It was in a stainless steel basin, unattended, with no cover or label and nothing to indicate from whom it had come. I was alone in the room and stayed there for a long time, simply staring at it. I can see it as clearly today as I could at the time, over 10 years ago.

No matter how emotionally charged the words and concepts involved, it is still possible and desirable to debate the ethics of abortion on a rational and intellectual level.

Methods of debate

In all discussions of ethics one uses metaphors and paradigms to support or argue a point. One can construct situations from which analogies can be drawn, although any hypothetical situation can never precisely mirror the situation in reality, particularly in the case of abortion. The following example can work as an analogy. Noonan[2] reports the case of *Depue v. Flateau* (Minnesota, 1907) in which Orlando Depue, a cattle buyer and dinner guest of a farming family, the Flateaus, asked if he could remain in the Flateau home overnight because he felt sick and faint. The Flateaus refused and turned him out into the cold January night. Depue lost his fingers to frostbite and sued the Flateau family for damages. The Court stated that the Flateaus were under no contractual obligation to minister to Depue although they had a legal and humanitarian responsibility not to expose him to elements in which his survival would be in doubt. The American Law Institute stated that a host has a duty not to place a guest (or even a trespasser) in a position in which he will be endangered. Although Depue obviously had more resources and physical protection at hand than a fetus, the analogy could be made that the pregnant woman (host) has the same obligation not to endanger her fetus (guest). Opponents of abortion maintain that once a woman becomes pregnant, she is obligated to provide a safe environment for the fetus until it is sufficiently developed to cope with the external world, just as the Flateaus had a moral obligation to provide a safe environment for Depue until he felt well enough to venture out into the cold Minnesota winter.

The circumstances of horror and hardship that might surround a pregnancy— for example, pregnancy as a result of rape, a fetus that is known to be suffering from Tay-Sachs disease, or a pregnant woman who has a history of severe child abuse—could be generalized into a principle: any pregnancy that might cause emotional or other distress to the mother or an incapacity or inconvenience to the future child can be terminated at will. This principle can also include pregnancies resulting from poor planning or lack of concern about contraception. In general, any reason the woman has for not being pregnant is seen as a justifiable cause for abortion; this concept has given rise to the phrase *abortion on demand*. This position is used both by those in favor of abortion, who see it as justification for putting the needs and rights of the pregnant woman ahead of those of the fetus, and by those who oppose abortion, who see it as a moral argument to sanction placing the life of the fetus ahead of the woman carrying it. The term *compulsory pregnancy* has been used in comparing maternal and fetal rights. To those who believe that a fetus is a human being, it is an unacceptable principle. To those who see the fetus occupying a gray zone between that which is definitely and recognizably human and that which is definitely not human, the principle is acceptable because the rights of the pregnant woman, who is assuredly human, take precedence over this gray-zone entity.

Status of the fetus

The central issue in the abortion dilemma involves whose rights take precedence, the fetus's or the pregnant woman's. To make any headway at all in resolving this question, one must address the ontologic status of the fetus, that is, the question of to what extent it can be considered a person.

Thus, by ontological status I shall mean certain general categories of being, such as being an inanimate object, being a mere animal, being a fully developed self conscious human person. With regard to the question of abortion, this is the issue of whether the fetus shows itself to be something to which one owes obligation in the sense one owes obligations to persons.*

Engelhardt goes on to state that the dilemma or argument cannot be resolved on rational grounds and should for the purpose of clarification be divided into two poles, the ontologic and the operational. The ontologic refers to the meaning of a human person, of human life; the operational refers to measurable criteria to justify the statement that a person now exists where none existed previously. The latter is based on proof of a physical body; the former is analogous to proof of an existing soul. Engelhardt tries to draw distinctions and make comparisons to provide more rational grounds for deciding the status of a fetus.

The first distinction is metaphoric, linguistic, and complex. It involves a concept of what we visualize a person to be and what characteristics we ascribe to that person. Engelhardt uses the analogy of a clubfooted man. One can describe him as a man with a clubfoot; his affliction likely has played a large role in his life. But at death the fact of the clubfoot makes no difference; neither would it matter to the man if he were lying in a coma waiting for a heart transplant. By inference the clubfoot did not matter to the man when he was a fetus. It had no relevance because there was no personhood to his life as there is no personhood after death. One does not assign gender to a fetus and refer to it as "he" or "she"; in so doing one would be assigning societal roles and functions, thus conferring personhood on the fetus, which engages in no interaction with society.

One could object to this distinction by comparing the fetus to a person who is asleep; that is, during sleep one plays no societal role and is owed no moral obligations. One could even question whether a person is present during sleep, especially if it is a deep, dreamless one. What difference exists between a sleeping person and a fetus?

The difference is suggested by the fact that the potentiality of the sleeping person is concrete and real in the sense of being based upon the past development of a full-blown human person. Unlike the fetus, the sleeping person has secured the capability of being fully human and has exercised it in the world. Far from a promisory note, the potentiality of the sleeping person to awaken is presented in concrete actuality in the physical substratum of that person, in his intact and functioning neocortex.*

The fetus has not demonstrated past neocortical or functional ability and thus cannot be considered an intact person. The sleeping person is merely taking a break in a fully developed life; a fetus has never actualized its potential and therefore cannot be viewed in the same way as a sleeping person.

Medicine has made a distinction in the ontologic status of a person in regard to

*Engelhardt, H. Tristam, Jr.: The ontology of abortion, Ethics 84:218, April 1974. Copyright © by The University of Chicago.

death; that is, it distinguishes between a person who is fully human and one who is irreversibly comatose although not quite dead because certain life processes are being kept alive artificially. Although an individual in such a coma cannot be compared biologically or rationally to a fetus, an ontologic comparison can be drawn. If the essence of humanity has departed the comatose individual, it could be said that it has not yet appeared in the fetus; thus because the fetus has no characteristics of personhood, no moral obligation is owed it. Those who speak of the fetus as a human being do so because of its potentiality, not because of its actuality. It is so obviously not *not* human (that is, it is not any other living thing) that to label it human seems the only reasonable course of action.

Another distinction concerns whether the fetus is ensouled or unensouled. Aristotle believed in a sequence of three souls: the vegetative, animal, and rational. The last occurred at birth, but the appearance of the first and the shift to the second are what is generally meant by ensoulment of the fetus. Aristotle believed that first fetal movement occurred at about the 40th day for a male and the 90th day for a female, the time at which animal ensoulment took place. St. Thomas Aquinas referred to this change as mediate animation as opposed to immediate animation and stated that abortion after animal ensoulment was forbidden but abortion prior to that was regarded as birth control.

The jump from Aquinas to modern Catholic dogma, which places ensoulment at conception, is a matter of historical shift in interpretation that may have been arbitrary. The birthday of the Blessed Virgin already had been determined as September 8, but the Church thought it needed to set a date for the day of her ensoulment which, following Aristotle and Aquinas, would have been 6 months earlier. But in 1708 Pope Clement XI set the date as December 8, thus suggesting that her conception as a person occurred at the time of biologic conception. In 1854 Pope Pius IX officially proclaimed the doctrine of Immaculate Conception and declared that Mary was free of original sin from the moment of conception. This in effect removed the distinction between an unensouled and an ensouled fetus and reversed Aquinas's doctrine.[3] Thus we have the concept of the ensouled fetus, a human being from the moment of conception.

Ensoulment does not necessarily mean that the fetus is a rational animal; it shows none of the characteristics of rationality or personhood. Therefore the presence of a soul does not confer personhood, if indeed one believes that the fetus is ensouled before birth. The concept of a soul is so amorphous and its origins are so uncertain that it is sheer speculation to theorize ensoulment at any point on a continuum. How do we even know that an individual is ensouled at birth? How do we know that a neonate is ensouled? Its rationality is no more developed than it was a day or two previous when it was still a fetus.

One is faced with the difficulty of distinguishing between biologic human life (as in a fetus or an irreversibly comatose individual) and personal human life to which are owed moral obligations. One could say that obligations are owed to the comatose individual by virtue of the person he *had been*; it is clearly more difficult to cease being obligated to someone than it is to begin. Here I refer again to the ontologic status of a person. If an ontologic position implies that a person is defined as such because he exists, then that existence also implies his entitlement to moral obligations owed him by others. If he is not yet a person (fetus) or has ceased to be one (a comatose individual), this principle does not apply and moral obligations are not owed.

Human life is a continuum from the formation of a zygote to mere biologic existence to development of a rational human being to death. Where on that continuum does personhood begin and end, and when is the individual to be treated as a human being to whom obligation is owed? At what point does the ontologic status change?

The criterion or concept of viability is often cited as a turning point on the continuum. Viability is a biologic fact, the point at which certain physiologic functions are sufficiently developed and stable to allow for probability of extrauterine life without such extraordinary measures that the fetus might as well be back in the uterus. The crucial issue involves what occurs at viability, a change that is more like a short continuum itself than a specific point. While the fetus remains in the uterus, nothing happens except that with each passing day it becomes more capable of extrauterine life. When it is born, its status (legally, if in no other way) changes from that of a fetus to that of a human being to whom moral obligation is owed. Its death at the hand of another would be termed infanticide rather than abortion, even though its age of existence from conception onward has not changed. Viability in and of itself confers no social status; personal interaction has not suddenly begun. The biologic fact does not imply moral obligation. The event of birth is what changes the ontologic, social, and legal status.

When discussing lack of rationality or ensoulment as a criterion for abortion, Engelhardt states that rationality does not appear until some time after the child's second birthday—but this does not lead to an argument favoring infanticide. Therefore we could conclude that rationality has nothing to do with the morality of killing.

> The question of the time of the emergence of a human person has, thus, received two answers. First, a human person in the strict sense of a self-conscious rational animal is not present until somewhat late in infancy. Second, there is a social category of child into which one allows newborn infants to enter as one brings them within the social context and schema of the family. . . . Further, the social criterion of viability places the fetus with regard to the obligations of medicine and sets a time in the ontogeny of man for the infant to emerge as a person to whom medicine has obligations. . . . In short, the first answer concerning the strict definition of a person establishes the rationale for liberal abortion laws, and the second answer concerning the social category "child" gives a basis for the proscription of abortion on demand beyond the point where viable birth is possible.*

In addition to the ontologic status of the fetus, we must examine the concept of humanity. Is humanity simply the presence of biologic human life, that is, those genetic characteristics that distinguish a human being from all other species, or is humanity

---

*Engelhardt, H. Tristam, Jr.: The ontology of abortion, Ethics 84:218, April 1974. Copyright © by The University of Chicago.

life that is definitely human, that is, those characteristics that are the essence of humanity or personhood? The definition of a person as defined by Fletcher was discussed in Chapter 1; briefly, they are consciousness, self-consciousness, the ability to reason and act on that ability, the capacity to communicate with other persons, moral capacity, and rationality. If one assumes that a fetus develops on a continuum of ontologic status, or humanity, from no status at all to full humanity, one is then faced with the decision of when on the continuum the fetus should be given human status, thus prohibiting abortion. Using the idea of ensoulment at conception to determine the morality of abortion is to abide by a decision made by Church officials and is a method unacceptable to many. The ancients used quickening as a turning point in ontologic status, and many modern thinkers use the age of viability, neither of which can be precisely pinpointed. The least problematic are the polar views that the fetus has no ontologic status of any importance during any part of fetal life and that the fetus has full ontologic status during its entire intrauterine life.

One may develop whatever ontologic theory about the status of the fetus one chooses, but according to Beauchamp and Walters[4] the theory must be clear in two crucial matters: (1) it must be specified that what is under consideration is the ontologic status of either a person (human being) or some other category of life and (2) regardless of the point at which the line is drawn, it must be argued that the line can justifiably be drawn there and that the theory is not simply an arbitrary one.

The question of the rights, or moral status, of a fetus has been endlessly debated. If one chooses to grant any moral rights (rather than legal rights) to a fetus, the problem of which ones to grant arises. Conservatives believe that a fetus has full moral status, that is, the same rights as a person who has already been born, and liberals believe that a fetus has no moral status. To some it might seem useless to argue about the moral status of a being that has no developed sense of morality, but the debate is important insofar as rights are inextricably connected to obligations. If one assigns no moral rights to a fetus, then no corresponding obligations are assigned and one may do with it what one pleases. However, if it is assigned full moral rights, then one is obligated to protect and care for it as any other human being. It is easy, then, to determine one's moral position on abortion on the basis of one of these two divergent views. The ethical issue arises when it must be decided which rights exist and when they take effect. A moderate view is that a line is drawn during fetal life between the time when a fetus is genetically human but not a member of the moral human community and the time when it should be granted full moral rights. Viability is the most popular point at which this line is drawn.

The moral battle over abortion is often fought on the "right to life" field; the issue at stake is whether the pregnant woman's right to legitimately kill the fetus ever overrides the fetus's right to life, and if so, under what circumstances. Is abortion justifiable homicide, is it murder in the first degree, or can it be considered killing in self-defense?

Even if the conservative theory is construed so that it entails that human fetuses have equal rights because of their moral status, nothing in the theory requires that these moral rights always override all other moral rights. Here a defender of the conservative theory confronts the problem of the morality of abortion on the level of conflicting rights: the unborn possesses some rights (including a right to life) and pregnant women also possess rights (including a right to life). Those who possess the rights have a (prima facie) moral claim to be treated in accordance with their rights.*

When these rights conflict, a moral dilemma is created. Many moderates feel that the fetus has some claim to protection against arbitrary actions of others, but they do not grant the fetus the same moral rights to life as possessed by a person already born. The ultimate justification for the morality of abortion lies in the determination of which rights and obligations take precedence over which others.

REASONS WOMEN CHOOSE ABORTION

The most common reason for a woman in the United States to choose abortion is that she does not want to continue the pregnancy or thinks that adding a child to her life would so complicate matters that the child's quality of life would be jeopardized. Because a first trimester abortion is relatively uncomplicated physically and because it involves so little time and money compared to other operative procedures, many people believe that women have abortions "just like that" with no thought to the kind of tissue removed from their bodies. Some have compared abortion with appendectomy in terms of its emotionality, but the vast majority of women who have an abortion do not view it as an emotionally neutral procedure. Although they may not verbalize their feelings, they are aware of the definite distinction between embryonic tissue and any other tissue that could be surgically removed. It is naive to believe that a woman who undergoes abortion, no matter how free her choice is and how morally justified she feels, experiences no strong emotional reaction.

It is important to differentiate between the reasons and justifications for abortion because they are not the same. A reason is usually a pragmatic consideration, whereas a justification involves ethics, morality, and frequently a rationalization. Those who oppose abortion do so on grounds of the justification, not the reason. For example, a 14-year-old girl who finds herself pregnant gives her age as the reason for requesting an abortion. The justification in this instance takes age into consideration but goes beyond that fact to include other moral aspects of the abortion issue itself.

A woman may choose abortion for many other reasons: she may be unmarried and not want the burden of raising a child alone, her marriage may not be as solid as she would like, she may already have all the children she wants or can afford, the fetus may have been exposed to some teratogenic substance, the father of the child may not be her husband, the father may not be a man she wants to marry, the pregnancy may have occurred as a result of rape or incest, she may have a

---

*Beauchamp, Tom L., and Walters, Leroy: Contemporary issues in bioethics, Belmont, Calif., 1978, Wadsworth Publishing Co., Inc., p. 193.

physical condition such as heart disease that creates a risk for her, she may have eugenic reasons such as wanting to prevent the birth of a deformed or retarded child, and so on. All these factors might explain why women seek abortion, but in the view of many people some or all these factors do not *justify* abortion. Even those who take the most liberal position on abortion do not feel it is automatically justified in every instance. A woman who is planning a summer-long camping trip and finds herself pregnant in April and has an abortion only because of the nuisance of being pregnant while camping might have a more difficult time justifying her abortion to liberal moralists that a woman who is a graduate student and already has two children.

The reasons or indications for abortion described above can be divided into four major categories: physical health, mental health, fetal abnormalities, and sexual reasons. The first could be classified as purely medical and usually involve some health risk to the pregnant woman. Severe heart disease is the most commonly cited justification because of the considerable strain on the heart caused by carrying a pregnancy to term and enduring either labor or the major surgery of caesarean section. Ectopic pregnancy and malignancy of the reproductive tract are also viewed as justifications for abortion. The Catholic Church permits abortion for the latter two reasons by invoking the rule of double effect; that is, the harmful effect (abortion) is considered an indirect but foreseen effect of an action, not the direct and intended effect (removal of a diseased or damaged body part to save life). In general, medical reasons for abortion carry the least degree of moral approbation.

The second classification involves the mental health of the pregnant woman and is morally controversial because in this classification are placed reasons with social or economic bases, which some see as reasons of convenience or personal preference rather than of mental health. Before the 1973 Supreme Court decision many physicians would not perform an abortion unless the woman could present testimony from a psychiatrist that her mental health would be clearly jeopardized if she were forced to bear the child. This practice led to an enormous number of superficial psychiatric consultations and faked suicide threats and much fraudulent testimony. The lengths to which women were prepared to go to obtain an abortion for mental health reasons were an indication of how much they wanted the freedom to make the decision without moral interference from the medical or religious establishment.

A third major classification of reasons for abortion is a strongly suspected or demonstrated abnormality of the fetus. With the increasing sophistication of intrauterine and fetal examinations by amniocentesis, ultrasonography, and other methods, this group of reasons is growing and will continue to carry a heavy moral weight. Between 40% and 50% of all fertilized ova are aborted spontaneously even before implantation has been fully established. Nature cannot, however, rid itself of all malformed fetuses, and of those that remain many can be diagnosed in utero. Accurate diagnosis cannot be made until the pregnancy is well into the second trimester when abortion is a more medically complex and emotionally traumatic procedure.

The moral arguments about aborting a deformed fetus center on the many facets of the quality-of-life issue. Can an infant who is severely retarded or deformed attain a life that gives it a measure of satisfaction sufficient to justify bringing it into the world? One must consider the quality of life not only of the fetus but also of other family members. Ther lives will be permanently disrupted emotionally and financially from the moment the deformed baby is born. A conflict thus arises between the claims of the fetus to continue the life already begun and the claims of the family to continue living without the disequilibrium that a deformed baby would bring. To justify aborting a deformed fetus because a satisfying life would be impossible is to predict what that particular individual human being would consider a satisfying life. Since no such prediction can be made, the moral justification of abortion for this reason must be made on the basis of what the pregnant woman and her family prefer, not what the fetus would prefer. This is not meant to imply that aborting a deformed fetus is unjustified; it is, however, necessary to be clear about the locus of justification and the lines of reasoning used.

The fourth classification involves sexual reasons and is concerned with the circumstances under which the fetus was conceived. The two situations most commonly discussed are rape and incest, and with these the moral controversy tends to be less heated although some of the arguments are more emotional than rational. It is frequently argued that when intercourse is forced on a woman, she is likely to have intensely negative feelings toward the resulting child and should not be compelled to bear it. Only the most conservative deny a raped woman the opportunity for abortion. Experts in child abuse acknowledge that unwanted children, as well as those born with moderate defects (those with severe defects who must undergo prolonged and complicated treatment are an exception), are more likely to be neglected and abused than children who are both wanted and normal. A child with a known deformity may be as unwanted as a child conceived in a rape, but the moral justification for abortion in these two instances is argued on different grounds. The fetus conceived in rape may be perfect in every detail, but the woman carrying it will feel much better about abortion than the woman carrying a deformed fetus. Incest carries an even greater societal taboo, and the eugenic considerations complicate matters. Many incestuous acts of intercourse occur as rape but are frequently not reported because the woman feels an overwhelming sense of shame and guilt.

LEGAL CONSIDERATIONS

On January 22, 1973, Justice Blackmun of the United States Supreme Court delivered the majority opinion in the case of *Roe v. Wade*. The decision reversed the illegality of abortion in the United States and permitted, for all intents and purposes, abortion on demand in the first trimester. Because *Roe v. Wade* has such far-reaching implications, the majority decision[5] will be described in some detail.

First the Court described the reasons for the restrictive abortion laws enacted by most states in the nineteenth century (earlier than the mid-nineteenth century early abortion was not usually punished):

1. The laws were seen as a result of a Victorian social concern to limit sexual conduct.

2. Prior to the development of antisepsis, abortion was seen as medically hazardous, and the mortality was high. States argued that their main concern was to restrain a woman from submitting to a procedure that placed her life in jeopardy. The Court recognized that this consideration was no longer valid and that the high mortality at illegal "abortion mills" strengthens the state's position to regulate the conditions under which legalized abortion takes place.

3. The state had an interest or duty in protecting prenatal life (the argument rested in part on the premise that a new human life began at conception), which was to be sacrificed only when the pregnant woman's life was at stake. The Court maintained that the interest of the state need not stand or fall on acceptance of this or any other belief about when life begins.

Various parties challenged state abortion laws on several grounds. One was the contention that the purpose of these laws was to protect prenatal life. They pointed to the absence of legislation specifically to that effect and claimed that the laws were designed solely to protect women. But because medicine had advanced to the point at which abortion had become a low-risk procedure, women were no longer in jeopardy and thus the law was not justified.

The most persuasive ground for the challenge was the woman's right to personal privacy in matters concerning her body. The Constitution does not specifically mention any right to privacy, but sufficient precedent had been set by the Court to guarantee certain areas of privacy under the Constitution. Roots to those rights are found in the First, Fourth, Fifth, Ninth, and Fourteenth Amendments as they relate to personal liberty in matters of marriage, procreation, contraception, family relationships, and the like. The Court found that these rights to privacy are broad enough to encompass a woman's decision to terminate her pregnancy, although this right is not absolute. There comes a point during a pregnancy at which the state may properly assert itself to protect potential life. It was also noted that those federal and state courts that had considered abortion laws had reached the same conclusions.

The appellee argued before the Court that a fetus is a person within the meaning of the Fourteenth Amendment and therefore has all legal rights of personhood. If the Court had agreed with this definition, the case would have collapsed, but it did not. It held that if those trained in medicine, philosophy, and theology have been unable to agree when life begins, the Court was not in a position to speculate on the answer. Furthermore, except in areas of criminal abortion the unborn have never been recognized by law as whole persons and have no legal rights.

The Court further stated that the state has a "compelling interest" in the life and health of the mother and established that interest at the end of the first trimester because during the first 3 months of pregnancy the mortality from abortion is lower than that of normal childbirth. After the first trimester the state may regulate the circumstances under which an abortion is performed, but during the first trimester the state may not interfere. After the age of viability the state may proscribe abortion except when it is necessary to preserve the life or health of the mother.

Roe v. Wade was a victory for those who believe that a woman should not be legally prevented from having a safe abortion and a defeat for those opposed to abortion. For the time being, abortion is legal in the United States, and the number performed increased from 899,000 in 1974 to about 1.3 million in 1977.[6] In some large cities, such as Washington, D.C., the number of abortions has exceeded the number of live births each year for several years. Whether one views Roe v. Wade as victory or defeat, it must be acknowledged that the Supreme Court decision changed the reproductive practices of American women.

In 1976 the Hyde amendment to the Social Security Act cut off all federal funds for abortions, meaning that federal Medicaid money could not be used. However, the Center for Disease Control in Atlanta reports that the feared impact of the amendment has not occurred. Seventy-six percent of poor women seeking abortion live in the 15 populous states that have used state funds to make up for lost federal funds, and the other 24% have obtained private financial help or have gone to low-cost abortion clinics.[6] Athough the impact of the amendment was not as severe as anticipated, the intent remains the same—to deprive poor women of funds necessary to obtain an abortion. The constitutionality of the amendment was upheld by the Supreme Court in the spring of 1980, and there is reason to expect that individual states will follow the federal example and prohibit the use of public funds for abortion.

Prohibiting the use of public funds for abortion can be seen as discrimination by class and in some areas of the country also discrimination by race. All women who cannot afford the price of a private abortion can be considered poor, and many are in racial minorities. Even in those cases in which race is not an issue, the fact that access to abortion is denied to some women who want it is unfair and unethical. It is also impractical and short-sighted of these legislators who refuse to appropriate public funds for abortion. The children resulting from these "compulsory pregnancies" will most likely require some kind of public support that will ultimately cost the taxpayer more than an abortion would have. In addition, unwanted children are more likely to be neglected and abused than those who are wanted and may eventually become a societal burden in some direct or indirect way.

Like any legislation that has an impact on the lives of people, especially at such a fundamental level as their reproductive capacity, Roe v. Wade raises ethical questions. One is the concept of personhood. The Court specifically ruled that a fetus cannot be legally considered a person. One can see two major problems in arriving at this decision. If a fetus is not legally a person, one wonders whether the Court demonstrated an inconsistency by protecting or permitting individual states to protect this nonperson in the third trimester but not in the first two. If the fetus is not a person until birth, why bother to protect it at all? On the other hand, other nonpersons are protected by law; we may not kill animals whenever we choose, and even some endangered species of flora are protected by law. The assumption that a fetus is a nonperson does not mean that it cannot be legally protected. A fetus is considered by the Supreme Court to be a *potential* person in the third trimester. The Court does not explicitly differentiate between a potential person and a nonperson and may have been influenced by emotion on this point.

Another serious question raised by *Roe v. Wade* concerns the ambiguity of language. The Court granted women the "right" to an abortion and refused to "limit the number of reasons for which an abortion may be sought." At the same time the Court stated that abortion is primarily a medical decision to be "left to the medical judgment of the pregnant woman's attending physician." If the decision is primarily a medical one, what happens to the woman's rights? What if she chooses to abort for a reason that is somehow deemed unacceptable by her physician? Whose rights take precedence, the physician's because of his medical judgment or the woman's because of her right to privacy? In practice this has not proven to be a problem because if a woman encounters a physician who will not perform her abortion, she can find dozens who will. But today's permissive atmosphere surrounding abortion could change, and if the medical community in any area were to exert its collective judgment against abortion, *Roe v. Wade* might not provide a sufficiently clear path to allow a woman to exercise her right over that of physicians.

Another important legal and ethical landmark in regard to abortion, specifically concerning to whom the fetus belongs, was *Planned Parenthood v. Danforth* (428 U.S. 52, 1976) in which the Supreme Court struck down as unconstitutional the Missouri statute that required written consent of the woman's spouse unless a physician certified that the abortion was necessary to preserve her life. This decision granted women more political and legal control over their bodies. But *Danforth* did not resolve the ethical issue of individual rights as they conflict with the sanctity of marriage. Regarding *Danforth* the Supreme Court ruled that marriage is simply a state of legal cohabitation and that the individuals involved still have personal rights that cannot be limited by the status of marriage. The right to abortion is one of those personal rights.

It is not completely clear why the Court struck down joint consent to abortion when state laws require or do not prohibit joint consent in many other activities within marriage, for instance, the adoption of a child, the release of a child for adoption, and artificial insemination. One could suppose that an issue of personhood is involved here. In the matter of artificial insemination the intention is to create a person for whom both spouses will eventually be responsible, whereas abortion is the destruction of a nonperson that leaves neither spouse with a lingering legal responsibility. In Missouri as in other states prior to *Danforth*, a husband could veto his wife's abortion even if he was not the father of the fetus. Even if he were the father, is justice served if a woman has the right to destroy a fetus that is genetically half not hers? It could be argued that of the millions of cells that comprise a fetus the father contributed only one; therefore because the entire fetus resides in the woman's body, it thus belongs to her. The fetus is therefore hers to do with as she pleases. It could also be argued that without that one paternal cell the fetus would not exist and that by virtue of the equal role in physical creation the decision for disposition should be equally shared. The Court reasoned that a woman is more directly and immediately affected by pregnancy (she has no guarantee that her husband will remain with her to help protect and support the child); therefore the balance between spouses should be weighted in her favor. If one can arrive at a sense of justice in this matter, it would seem that a woman has the greater claim.

SOCIAL AND CULTURAL
IMPLICATIONS

A strong underlying framework of the abortion debate is Americans' ambivalent attitudes toward sexuality. The "sexual revolution" of the past generation notwithstanding, a good deal of puritanism is still evident in Americans' beliefs about sexuality. The tongue-in-cheek definition of puritanism—the fear that somewhere, somehow, someone is having a good time—seems well suited to contemporary attitudes about sexuality. Many people are opposed to abortion for punitive reasons; that is, a woman should be punished for having engaged in sexual intercourse. There is a strong feeling that if a woman is not prepared to be responsible for a child, she should refrain from intercourse. Some of this repressive attitude spills over to other forms of sexuality about which legislation exists in many states. Not only is extramarital intercourse forbidden, but so are sodomy and oral-genital contact (these two are prohibited in many states even within marriage). Therefore if a woman wishes to refrain from intercourse for fear of pregnancy, she is not permitted to fulfill her sexual needs with a man in any other way.

Another social consideration involves the access to abortion. Women who know about abortion clinics, who can afford the fees, and who are able to arrange for transportation are more likely to have abortions than those whose access is in some way limited. The ability to make moral choices about abortion implies that society has provided a means to act on whatever choice is made. For example, if sufficient antiabortion support is mustered in a community to prohibit the establishment of an abortion clinic, a pregnant woman who has made the moral choice to abort is prevented from doing so in her own community. She will have to either travel elsewhere or remain pregnant. A Supreme Court decision cannot force a group of people to provide an optional service if community values oppose the service.

Antiabortion forces worry about the social effect of the legalization of abortion and propose a version of the "wedge" argument described in Chapter 12 concerning euthanasia. It is thought by many that lifting the prohibition against the destruction of fetuses will inexorably lead to infanticide and other forms of socially approved killing. Indeed, they point to the rapidly heating debate over preserving the life of severely deformed and retarded neonates and fear that our cultural and religious reverence for life will be diminished and our ethical sensitivity become somehow blunted. No data exist to support the view that those who favor abortion also favor infanticide. Even a person who takes the most liberal position on abortion and who might favor infanticide in some extreme circumstances will acknowledge that the instances are not the same and the impact on society is vastly different. Killing an infant or allowing it to die, even if it could be morally defended, is a decision arrived at from a perspective totally different from that which approves of killing a fetus. The concept of personhood is then not simply theoretic.

Abortion and infanticide also cannot be equated in any social sense.

Unlike abortion, however, infanticide would involve the destruction of members of the species who had begun to play an explicit role within the social structure of the family and society, even though they had not yet assumed a full personal life. If nothing else, such destruction would erode the status of the individual within society by undermining the status of a positive active social role and relation.*

Because the fetus plays no role in society (the pregnant woman's social role may change, but the fetus itself is not a social being), a social and rational human is not being destroyed. One could argue that neither is an infant a rational human being, but it does play a social role, occupies a specific place in the family, and is an individual person with a definite identity. Even in cultures in which full person-hood is not accorded until late in childhood, the infant and young child play a social role and are qualitatively different from a fetus.

Another social issue of abortion concerns the permissibility of the state to enter the individual's private social sphere to regulate that individual's personal activi-ties. Increasing numbers of people subscribe to the belief that morality cannot be legislated, especially in view of new areas of civil concern such as race and sex discrimination, sexual behavior, and health practices such as smoking and lung can-cer that lead to increased risk for certain diseases. Examples of attempts to legislate sexual behavior can again be used. It is difficult to think of any reason why a state would want to interfere in the private sexual practices of adults and why it should be permitted to do so, but we find all kinds of repressive laws ranging from the prohibition of bestiality to forbidding fellatio and cunnilingus (these are mostly unenforceable laws, but occasionally a dramatic case comes to court), to discrimi-nating against homosexuals. With the exception of the gay rights movement, which is concerned more with civil discrimination than with sexual practice, no mass social movement exists to change laws concerning private sexual acts. The state has little interest in prosecuting sexual acts, however, and these laws are rarely en-forced. If instances of fellatio were prosecuted to the same extent as abortions prior to 1973, we would see a speedy liberalization of sex laws. When its own health or safety is not in jeopardy, society tends to legislate those acts it wants to legislate. Morality has little to do with obedience to laws concerning private behavior. The prohibition of alcohol was a perfect example; cigarette smoking is another, although it is less precise because the act of smoking is not forbidden by law. The law against cigarette advertising on radio and television and the health hazard warning on cig-arette packages caused a slight decrease in cigarette consumption for a short time, but almost immediately thereafter consumption surpassed existing levels. The pub-lic seems to think that one's lungs are part of one's private sphere and that their destruction by cigarette smoke should not be prohibited by law.

The same logic can be used concerning a woman's control over her own uterus. Laws regulating abortion and other private physical acts (sexual and nonsexual) can be seen as societal paternalism that abrogates individual autonomy and exercise of

---

*Engelhardt, H. Tristam, Jr.: The ontology of abortion, Ethics **84**:218, April 1974. Copyright © by The University of Chicago.

self-determination. Is abortion society's business? The state could be said to have a legitimate interest in abortion if public funds are used to finance the procedure. The Hyde amendment to prohibit the use of federal funds is being followed by similar actions in many states; the time may not be too far off when all abortions are privately financed, and the state will give up all right to interfere in abortion. This does not mean that states will withdraw from the issue, but their moral grounds for interference will be weakened if they have no financial stake in the matter.

ABORTION RESULTING IN LIVE BIRTH

Because some women delay abortion for a variety of reasons (indecision, fear, crowded clinic schedules, pregnancy test delays, and so on) and because physicians make errors in determining gestational age, some fetuses are born alive after saline instillation and prostaglandin abortions. This creates a host of ethical dilemmas. Veatch[7] presents the following case that illustrates the problem. A 24-year-old unmarried woman came to a hospital clinic in labor. The previous day she had had an abortion induced at another hospital. Between the time when she became pregnant and the time when the abortion was induced, many personal and bureaucratic delays occurred. The first hospital estimated the length of the pregnancy to be 22 weeks and replaced 1800 cc of amniotic fluid with an equal amount of saline solution. There is no indication why the woman had left the first hospital and chose to enter another when labor began; this is most unusual. When the infant was delivered, a heartbeat was discovered. In the next 2 hours no resuscitation attempts were made while the staff deliberated what to do. At the end of that time vital signs in the infant had ceased. While the discussions were going on, the woman showed no interest in the infant and no willingness to keep the child even though she knew it had been born alive. The physician had estimated that the baby weighed 1700 gm, but when it was finally weighed it was found to be 2000 gm. The policy at that hospital was to attempt to resuscitate any baby weighing over 500 gm.

The questions raised by this and similar cases compound the abortion dilemma. The first examining physician had made an error of about 10 weeks gestational age, but we have no way of knowing if it was an actual error or if he falsified his estimate because he wanted to justify what would have been a legally questionable procedure. A 32-week pregnancy is well into the third trimester. Let us assume that the physician was competent to make an accurate diagnosis and that his actions were quite deliberate. He injected the saline and then discharged the woman so that he would not be faced with a possibly live fetus. Could the physician in breaking the law have been morally justified by claiming that what he did was civil disobedience? If so, it would seem that he negated this claim by allowing the woman to leave the hospital and deliver at home or in other uncontrolled circumstances. It is unlikely that she left the first hospital by choice; she probably could have been persuaded to remain. This physician might be sued for malpractice though an unsophisticated woman is not likely to bring suit. But the fact that he could be held liable for his error should not be discounted.

What of the staff at the second hospital? They deliberately disregarded hospital policy by not resuscitating the infant, thus participating in passive euthanasia. The mother, although she demonstrated no interest in her infant, did not participate in the decision. Was the staff justified in letting the infant die?

Consider the likely consequences if the baby had been actively treated. It would have remained in a neonatal intensive care unit for several months while the cost of its care mounted to several hundred thousand dollars. If the mother chose to abdicate responsibility, as she gave every indication of doing, the baby would then become a ward of the state and a poor candidate for adoption because of its health history. Considering the technologic possibilities and its relatively high birth weight, it would have about an 80% chance of immediate survival but a 70% chance of permanent brain damage. It would be discharged to a state institution still needing extra care and special attention, which it might or might not receive depending on staffing and attitudes at the institution. The state would pay the financial bill, but the child would grow up with the emotional problem. Is this one child's life worth all that? To answer the question one must weight the physical existence of life against the amorphous concept of quality of life. More and more neonatologists and ethicists are beginning to question the morality of heroic efforts to save the life of every tiny premature infant and aborted fetus. They think that the cost to society is too great to be balanced by the quality of human life that emerges from these efforts. There are, however, many people who think that preservation of life is so strong an obligation that health professionals must use all means available to save life.

What responsibility did the mother have in this dilemma? She turned away from the infant, but should she have been compelled to participate in the decision? Any woman may choose to give up her baby for adoption, and this woman had clearly demonstrated by having an abortion that she wanted nothing to do with the baby. But until she stated her intention in writing, she was legally responsible for it, even if she seemed to feel no emotional attachment or moral obligation. It could have been assumed that if her opinion had been sought, she would have chosen not to resuscitate, but the knowledge that the infant was born alive could have changed her mind. Should people be permitted to walk away from responsibility that is legally and morally theirs? If a woman has delivered a full-term infant, takes it home, and then a month later simply turns her back and leaves it to die by starvation and dehydration, she is liable for child abuse and quite possibly murder. Is there a *moral* difference between turning one's back on a 2000 gm fetus that happened against all odds to be born alive and doing the same thing to a month-old healthy infant? Our emotional reactions to these situations are different: we visualize on one hand a scrawny, mewling thing hooked up to complex life-support systems and on the other hand a chubby baby just beginning to smile and relate to its environment. One baby has a reasonable chance for a satisfying life; the other has a greatly decreased chance and will live with almost no opportunity to overcome its tremendous handicap. Should these circumstances influence the moral decision? We are faced with the issue of the balance between societal cost and eventual societal benefit.

It could be argued that since an abortion was performed in the first place, the live fetus should be killed outright to carry the act to its intended conclusion, not only because it was the intention of the pregnant woman and the physician performing the abortion but also for a practical reason. It can be assumed that a fetus aborted during the second trimester has experienced grave damage either through contact with the saline or prostaglandin solution or by absorption of the general anesthesia given during hysterotomy. Is it then morally incumbent on the physician to complete the abortion to prevent development of a severely damaged or retarded infant?

In September, 1976, a law was passed in California that specified that a viable fetus born alive following an abortion was to be considered a ward of the state and that physicians were to perform all reasonable actions consistent with good medical care to preserve its life. "Extraordinary means" were excepted, and the live-born fetus was not given rights over its mother with respect to lifesaving treatment. A viable fetus was defined as one that is able to (1) increase in tissue mass, (2) increase in the number, complexity, and coordination of physiologic functions, and (3) develop into a self-sustaining organism independent of the connection with its mother.[8] The law leaves room for interpretation of the phrase "extraordinary means," and one wonders if the care of these infants will change as a result of the new law.

The increasing number of fetuses born alive will create an ambiguity in our concept of abortion. We are used to assuming that abortion automatically means fetal death, but as abortions are increasingly possible later in pregnancy, the concept needs to be broadened to include maternal-fetal separation with survival of the fetus. In "Abortion Surveillance 1974" the CDC projected, based on statistics from the state of New York, that approximately 196 fetuses each year will be born alive following abortion by hysterotomy or induction by saline or prostaglandin.[8] Of these, about six or seven will survive to grow to maturity. These figures can be expected to remain relatively constant if the use of prostaglandins for late abortion continues.

ETHICAL DILEMMAS

Most moral arguments about the permissibility of abortion revolve around the question of the personhood of the fetus. The polar extremes—that the fetus is a person from the moment of conception and therefore abortion is never permissible, and that the fetus is not a person until it is born and therefore abortion is always permissible—can be dismissed from the argument because they pose no moral dilemma. What causes most of the indecision is the problem of deciding when and if the fetus becomes a person, and the prospects for agreement are dim. It is true that the fetus takes on human characteristics remarkably early in its development, but human characteristics do not confer humanity. At what point does a seed become a plant? Let us agree that this question cannot be answered and instead suppose for the sake of argument that the fetus *is* a person and that every person has a right to life.

Thomson[9] asks us to imagine a scenario that may seem far-fetched but that, given the uniqueness of pregnancy, is an excellent analogy to abortion. You wake up in the morning and find yourself in bed with a famous violinist who is unconsious. He had been found to have a fatal kidney disease, and a thorough computer search of medical records had established that you alone have the blood type needed to help. During the night you were kidnapped, and the violinist's circulatory system was plugged into your own so his could be cleansed along with yours. The Society of Music Lovers has done this, and the hospital administrator is very apologetic, but he tells you that if you unplug yourself the violinist will surely die. He also says that the situation will last only 9 months; then the violinist will be cured and you can each go your own way.

Is it morally incumbent on you to accede to this situation? No doubt it would be very nice of you if you did, a great kindness. But do you *have* to accede to it? What if it were not nine months, but nine years? Or longer still? What if the director of the hospital says, "Tough luck, I agree, but you've now got to stay in bed, with the violinist plugged into you, for the rest of your life. Because remember this. All persons have a right to life, and violinists are persons. Granted you have a right to decide what happens in and to your body, but a person's right to life outweighs your right to decide what happens in and to your body. So you cannot ever be unplugged from him."*

Is the hospital director making an outrageous argument? Is it any more outrageous than telling a woman she must remain pregnant for 9 months and then remain "plugged in" to the responsibility for the child for at least 18 years if not for the rest of her life? The violinist may be seen as having an even greater claim to life than a fetus because he is already a developed human being and has proved his social worth. But you protest that you were kidnapped and had no part in the decision to plug in the violinist. The analogy in the case of rape does not change because the fetus is still a person, regardless of the circumstances under which it was conceived. It is not the fetus's fault that its mother was raped; the condition does not alter its personhood and consequent right to life. Those who would permit abortion only in the case of rape are distinguishing the personhood of one fetus from another; thus they destroy their own moral argument if they believe the fetus's right to life is absolute.

If we continue to assume that the fetus has a right to life, we need to ask what precisely this means. One might say that it is to be given the essentials to support life, but what if one of the essentials required is something he has no right to have (such as the essential need of the violinist of your circulatory system)? The Society of Music Lovers had no right to kidnap you, and the violinist has no right to hold you hostage. But if you cut yourself loose, he dies. Is his right to life greater than your need to keep your body for yourself? The right to life may be viewed as a positive right, that is, a right that confers corresponding obligations on others to see that the right is protected or provided. A somewhat weaker though still morally compelling view is that the fetus has the right not to be killed—a negative right—

*Thomson, Judith Jarvis: A defense of abortion, Philosophy and Public Affairs (Princeton University Press) 1(1):47-66, 1971.

that is, a right not to be interfered with. The right not to be killed is merely the converse of the right to life. The moral significance is slightly different, but the behavior of the pregnant woman would be the same.

Let us assume that the right of the fetus (or violinist) to live, or not be killed, is equal to the right of the woman not to be pregnant (or plugged in). Perhaps introducing the principle of justice will settle the argument. The violinist did you an injustice by using what he had no right to use, your circulatory system. If you unplug yourself and kill him in the process, has justice been served? You kill him, but the killing is a result of his injustice. Has his right to life then not been violated? Is this a circular argument or a rationalization? Perhaps it is, and it is not a perfect analogy to a fetus who had no responsibility for arriving where it is. A fetus cannot do or not do justice; it can only be the recipient of just or unjust acts. The point is that the fetus by its very existence makes demands and creates obligations. The *situation* can be seen as unjust, even if the fetus cannot.

Those who are opposed to abortion claim that if a woman voluntarily has intercourse and knows full well that intercourse can result in pregnancy, she is responsible for not destroying a pregnancy that occurs because she invited it in the first place. Thomson[9] draws two more analogies to the uninvited presence of the fetus. The room you are occupying is stuffy, so you open a window to air it. As a result of this a burglar climbs in. Are you now obligated to permit the burglar to remain and give him the right to use your house? It would be absurd to assent to this. Go a step further and recognize that burglars exist and are anxious to get into your house, so you have bars installed on the windows. But one of the bars is defective, and the burglar manages to squeeze through. It would seem that now you are even less responsible for making the burglar welcome. Thomson's second analogy involves "people seeds" that drift about in the air like pollen. If you open the window to your house the people seeds will blow in, take root in your carpet or upholstery, and grow into people. You need to open the windows, but you do not want people seeds sprouting all over the house, so you affix fine mesh screens to your windows to keep out the seeds. One of the screens, however, develops a tiny hole, and when you come home after a weekend away you discover a people seed well rooted and developing into a full-fledged person. Do you uproot it? Some would say that you must not because you could have lived without opening the windows or could have occupied a house with bare floors and no furniture. But breezes flowing through the house and attractive furnishings enhance the quality of your life, and you choose to live knowing that people seeds are everywhere. This might be analogous to having a hysterectomy prior to ever having intercourse or avoiding rape by walking around in a full suit of armor. It unjustly penalizes a woman for something that has not yet occurred.

If the arguments and analogies cited above are followed, abortion could be seen as morally impermissible. Let us imagine that you and the violinist have a long talk and the two of you agree that he can stay plugged in for the 9 months required for his own kidneys to heal. Things are progressing well, and laboratory studies show that he will indeed be cured in time. Seven months later you become bored lying in bed, the violinist's personality grates on your nerves, and you decide you can no longer stand the inconvenience and disruption to your life. Unplugging him at this point would be grossly indecent. You have instilled hope in him, and he has even begun to practice again. Your action would be monstrously immoral. Suppose the burglar that comes in through the open window turns out to be not such a bad fellow. You make up the guest room and tell him to help himself to whatever is in the refrigerator. He is just settling down to watch television after dinner, and *now* you call the police. That too would be morally unjust.

Suppose a woman who has three boys and who is 6 months pregnant decides that she does not want another boy. She obtains an amniocentesis by telling the physician that there is a history of Down's syndrome in her family and then incidentally asks about the sex of the fetus. If it is a male, would she be justified in demanding an abortion even though she is already 6 months pregnant though still in the second trimester? Most people would agree that this whim not to have another boy is not a morally acceptable reason for abortion, especially in view of the fact that it is not the *person* she wishes to abort but a specific *kind* of person. If the burglar had been unkempt and uncouth and smelled bad, would the police have been called earlier? This argument is summarized by Thomson:

While I am arguing for the permissibility of abortion in some cases, I am not arguing for the right to secure the death of the unborn child. It is easy to confuse these two things in that up to a certain point in the life of the fetus it is not able to survive outside the mother's body; hence removing it from her body guarantees its death. But they are importantly different. I have argued that you are not morally required to spend nine months in bed, sustaining the life of that violinist; but to say this is by no means to say that if, when you unplug yourself, there is a miracle and he survives, you then have the right to turn round and slit his throat. You may detach yourself even if this costs him his life; you have no right to be guaranteed his death, by some other means, if unplugging yourself does not kill him.*

Those who have fought hard for liberalized abortion laws have traditionally done so from the platform of the woman's right to control her own body taking precedence over the fetus's right to life. That argument, though pragmatic, does not come to grips with the moral dilemma. Whereas proabortionists use the language of rights, they seem to have overlooked the meaning behind that language. The right to control one's body is a *property* right or privacy right and should not be confused with a right to kill someone occupying one's property. If a trespasser happens to wander onto your property, you do not have a right to kill him even if his obvious intention is to harm you. You may kill him in self-defense, but that moral argument is different from killing him because he stepped across your property line. Slave owners were not allowed to kill slaves even though the latter were legally the property of their owners; the commandment against killing took precedence over property rights.

Thomson makes a strong argument that even if a fetus is a human being, this alone does not necessarily make it morally impermissible to kill it. Some antiabortionists maintain that because a fetus is an *innocent* human being, it is wrong to

---

*Thomson, Judith Jarvis: A defense of abortion, Philosophy and Public Affairs (Princeton University Press) 1(1):47-66, 1971.

kill it. However, there are situations in which it may not be morally wrong to take innocent human life (such as a noncombatant working in an enemy's munitions factory during wartime, euthanasia to end hopeless suffering, and the "crowded lifeboat" scenario in which one person is sacrificed to save many).

No matter what tack the moral arguments take, they always swing back to the one central overriding issue: is the fetus a human being to whom moral rights and obligations are due? Those who argue strongly for abortion often either ignore this questions or feel that the answer is so evident that it need not be examined. To argue for abortion and ignore the strongest plank in the platform is unwise. Fletcher's criteria for personhood (see Chapter 1) have been used to determine the fate of an individual at the end of life, that is, to determine whether he should be given continued artificial life support when he no longer has any characteristics of humanity. It is equally appropriate to apply the criteria to the beginning of life when personhood is equally in question in defining the fetus. None of Fletcher's criteria can be applied. It is impossible to know if the developing fetus will have minimal intelligence and it is ridiculous to consider giving an intelligence test to a fetus, but if it could be done the fetus would fail. The fetus has no self-awareness and no sense of time, futurity, or history because it is not a separate being. Self-awareness comes from learning to separate oneself from the environment; this the fetus cannot do. The fetus has no self-control because it is totally dependent on the body it inhabits. It cannot communicate, relate to others, or show concern for them. It has no control over its existence because it is subject to the control of its mother by nature of its existence. It shows no curiosity. It does demonstrate change, but the changes are all related to mere biologic growth and development, which is a condition of existence, not proof of personhood.

Biologically human beings are developmental: birth, life, health, and death are processes, not events, and are to be understood epigenetically, not episodically. All human existence is on a continuum, a matter of becoming. In this perspective, are we to regard potentials *als ob*, as if they were actual? I think not. The question arises prominently in abortion ethics.*

The fetus cannot balance rationality and feeling because it has capacity for neither, although because of early development of the central nervous system it may feel sensations such as heat, cold, or pain. But it cannot feel emotionally. It has an identity based solely on genetic structure, but it has no idiosyncracy that occurs as a result of personality development. Fletcher's criterion on which all others are based is neocortical functioning. By 8 weeks the fetus does have readable electrical brain activity (unlike the clinically "dead" individual who has an isoelectric EEG), but the functions of the cerebral cortex are not synthesized. The electrical activity does not imply the ability to coordinate it into useful function.

Using these criteria or any similar ones it can be said that a fetus is not a human being; therefore abortion is, though perhaps not always morally permissible, surely

---

*Fletcher, Joseph: Medicine and the nature of man. In Veatch, Robert M., et al., editors: The teaching of medical ethics: proceedings of a conference sponsored by the Institute of Society, Ethics, and the Life Sciences and Columbia University College of Physicians and Surgeons, New York, June 1-3, 1972, p. 55.

not impermissible. To say that the fetus is a potential human being, though a true statement, does not lend any greater force to the moral argument. Potentiality is not actuality. A fetus is not a human being, even though it has the greatest possible potential for becoming one. Becoming is not being.

The concept of personhood can be applied to membership in the moral community, that is, the state in which a person can claim rights and obligations and in turn owes them to others. It is not necessary to agree to *respect* these claims, although the moral community surely benefits from the respect of rights; what is necessary is the acknowledgment or recognition that rights and claims exist. It is commonly agreed that human beings are members of the moral community; all societies recognize this fact although they deal with it in different ways. In no way can a fetus be considered a member of the moral community, and therefore it is not owed rights or obligations.

Brody[10] takes an opposite position and argues that a fetus is a human being from the moment of conception for the following reasons. Because of its genetic code, the fetus is uniquely itself at the time of conception and will never be anyone else: that is, we are from the beginning what we are. Until conception the likelihood of any individual ovum and spermatozoan coming together is infinitesimal, but once they have done so, the likelihood that they will develop into an actual human being is great; therefore, once conjoining has taken place, it has a right to continue development. Because fetal development is gradual and one phase is never radically different from the preceding one, it is impossible to draw a precise line at the point at which the fetus becomes a full human being; therefore conception is the only possible point to establish humanness. Brody concedes that arguments can be made for determining personhood at other points on the developmental continuum, for instance, at the point where electrical activity in the brain begins (although this activity has been detected early in fetal life, it has not been proved that it does not exist from the moment of conception) because this is the same criterion by which someone is declared technically dead. A case can be made for declaring personhood at quickening, when the fetus is perceived as human by its mother and by other humans. The strongest case can be made for declaring personhood at viability, when the capacity to exist on its own is present.

The point to all these arguments about the personhood of a fetus is that a human being, practically speaking, is what other human beings decide it is. Individual people decide who is and who is not a human being, and states decide what to do with the consensus. For the time being in the United States the Supreme Court has decided not what constitutes a human being, for the Court avoided that question, but what we may legally do to act on our private convictions. The Court made no statement that it is morally permissable to abort a fetus; it simply prevented individual states from interfering with a woman's personal convictions. It is important to understand that difference.

SUMMARY

The debate about the morality of abortion has been going on as long as abortion has been practiced. Early Greeks and Romans argued about it, as have moral and religious philosophers in all cultures since. One can find Biblical injunctions to support or condemn abortion. The discussions about the morality of abortion involve two major issues: the rights of the pregnant woman in conflict with those of the fetus and the determination of the personhood of the fetus. Even in the unlikely event that we could settle these two issues, we still could not be certain that abortion is morally permissible.

The status of the fetus can be analyzed by two sets of criteria, the ontologic and the operational. The ontologic status refers to the meaning of a human person, of human life, and of rights and obligations owed to that human person or life. The operational status refers to measurable criteria to justify the statement that a person now exists where none existed previously. The latter is based on proof of a physical body, whereas the former could be said to be based on existence of a soul. Drawing a line distinguishing between the two has tantalized philosophers for ages and is crucial to discussing the morality of abortion. One method for drawing this line has been the concept of ensoulment, the time at which the soul is believed to enter the body. People believe it to be at almost any point on the continuum of fetal development; the question is open to endless debate.

The most common reason for a woman to choose abortion is that she does not want to be pregnant. There is also a variety of other reasons: the pregnancy may endanger her physical health or result in her death, there may be proof or strong suspicion that she is carrying a retarded or deformed child, or the fetus may have been conceived as a result of rape or incest.

The 1973 Supreme Court decision in *Roe v. Wade* drastically changed the legal status of abortion in the United States. The Court stated that a citizen's right to privacy includes a woman's right to control her body. States may no longer interfere with or prevent a woman from obtaining an abortion in the first two trimesters, although during the second trimester the state may regulate the conditions under which the abortion is performed. This restriction was included to protect the health and safety of the pregnant woman. *Roe v. Wade* contains ambiguous language and did nothing to solve the ethical debate about abortion, but it did change the reproductive patterns and attitudes of many American women.

A good deal of the abortion debate centers on attitudes toward sexuality; there is still a strong puritan streak in the way many people view sex. One hears the punitive attitude that pregnant women should be held accountable for their sexual pleasure by being denied abortion. Community acceptance influences the amount and kind of abortion services provided. Abortion cannot be prohibited by law, but no stipulation is made about health agencies providing access to abortion.

Antiabortionists use the wedge argument to predict that the legalization of abortion will lead to indiscriminate infanticide, but the two practices involve such different moral concepts and arguments that this is unlikely.

Abortions that result in live birth are part of the infanticide issue, although there are subtle moral differences between an abortus born alive and a full-term infant. More and more fetuses are being born alive (approximately 200 a year), creating yet another moral question of whether to work to save them or to let them die. California has passed a law making these infants wards of the state and ensuring that they are provided with aggressive medical treatment.

There are many ethical issues involved in abortion. The concept of the fetus as a person and the resulting rights and obligations owed if it is a person are the central issues in the ethical dilemma, which appears to have no universally agreeable solution.

REFERENCES

1. Carney, Frederick S.: Theological ethics. In Reich, Warren T., editor in chief: Encyclopedia of bioethics, New York, 1978, Macmillan Publishing Co., Inc.
2. Noonan, John T.: How to argue about abortion. In Beauchamp, Tom L., and Walters, Leroy: Contemporary issues in bioethics, Belmont, Calif., 1978, Wadsworth Publishing Co., Inc.
3. Engelhardt, H. Tristam, Jr.: The ontology of abortion, Ethics 84:218, April 1974.
4. Beauchamp, Tom L., and Walters, Leroy: Contemporary issues in bioethics, Belmont, Calif., 1978, Wadsworth Publishing Co., Inc.
5. Majority opinion in *Roe v. Wade* (delivered by Mr. Justice Blackmun), United States Supreme Court, 410, United States Reports 113, decided January 22, 1973.
6. The fanatical abortion fight, Time 114(2):26-27, July 9, 1979.
7. Veatch, Robert M.: Case studies in medical ethics, Cambridge, Mass., 1977, Harvard University Press.
8. Bok, Sissela, Nathanson, Bernard N., Walters, LeRoy, and Nathan, David C.: The unwanted child: caring for the fetus born alive after an abortion, Hastings Center Report 6(5):10, October 1976.
9. Thomson, Judith Jarvis: A defense of abortion, Philosophy and Public Affairs (Princeton University Press) 1(1):47-66, 1971.
10. Brody, Baruch: On the humanity of the foetus. In Perkins, Robert L., editor: Abortion: pro and con, Cambridge, Mass., 1974, Schenkman Publishing Co., Inc.

BIBLIOGRAPHY

Annas, George J.: Abortion and the Supreme Court: round two, Hastings Center Report 6(5):15-17, October 1976.

Augenstein, Leroy: Come, let us play God, New York, 1969, Harper & Row, Publishers, Inc.

Beauchamp, Tom L., and Walters, LeRoy: Contemporary issues in bioethics, Belmont, Calif., Wadsworth Publishing Co., Inc.

Bok, Sissela, Nathanson, Bernard N., Walters, LeRoy, and Nathan, David C.: The unwanted child: caring for the fetus born alive after an abortion, Hastings Center Report 6(5):10-15, October 1976.

Brody, Baruch: On the humanity of the foetus. In Perkins, Robert L., editor: Abortion pro and con, Cambridge, Mass., 1974, Schenkman Publishing Co., Inc.

Carney, Frederick S.: Theological ethics. In Reich, Warren T., editor in chief: Encyclopedia of bioethics, New York, 1978, Macmillan Publishing Co., Inc.

Davis, Anne J., and Aroskar, Mila A.: Ethical dilemmas and nursing practice, New York, 1978, Appleton-Century-Crofts,

Ely, John Hart: The wages of crying wolf: a comment on *Roe v. Wade*, The Yale Law Journal 82:923, April 1973.

Englehardt, H. Tristam, Jr.: The ontology of abortion, Ethics 84:217-234, April 1974.

Fletcher, Joseph: Medicine and the nature of man. In Veatch, Robert M., et al., editors: The teaching of medical ethics: proceedings of a conference sponsored by the Institute of Society, Ethics and the Life Sciences and Columbia University College of Physicians and Surgeons, New York, June 1-3, 1972.

Majority opinion in *Roe v. Wade* (delivered by Mr. Justice Blackmun), United States Supreme Court, 410, United States Reports 113, decided January 22, 1973.

Moore, Emily C., Edgar, Harold, Lebacqz, Karen A., and Callahan, Daniel: Abortion: the new ruling, Hastings Center Report 3(2):4-7, April 1973.

Nelson, James B.: Human medicine: ethical perspectives on new medical issues, Minneapolis, 1973, Augsburg Publishing House.

Noonan, John T.: How to argue about abortion. In Beauchamp, Tom L., and Walters, Leroy: Contemporary issues in bioethics, Belmont, Calif., 1978, Wadsworth Publishing Co., Inc.

Potter, Ralph B.: The abortion debate. In Cutler, Donald R.: Updating life and death: essays in ethics and medicine, Boston, 1968, Beacon Press.

Ramsey, Paul: Ethics at the edges of life, New Haven, Conn., 1978, Yale University Press.

Smith, Harmon L.: Ethics and the new medicine, Nashville, 1970, Abingdon Press.

The fanatical abortion fight, Time 114(2):26-27, July 9, 1979.

Thomson, Judith Jarvis: A defense of abortion, Philos-ophy and Public Affairs (Princeton University Press) 1(1):47-66, 1971.

Veatch, Robert M.: Case studies in medical ethics, Cambridge, Mass., 1977 Harvard University Press.

Warren, Mary Anne: On the moral and legal status of abortion, The Monist 57(1), January 1973.

8

Behavior control

DETERMINING ACCEPTABLE BEHAVIOR

Acceptable behavior is often what other people define it to be. Problems arise when different groups of people define acceptable behavior in different and sometimes conflicting ways. Loud music played on the sidewalk late at night would be tolerated differently in different neighborhoods. A public display of strong emotion is viewed differently depending on the culture in which it takes place. We usually wish to change or control a person's behavior because we are convinced that the person is out of sync with the rest of society and that he should conform at least outwardly to the behavior of others. But increasingly people are asking the question of *why* certain types of behavior that society has labeled "sick," "deviant," or "crazy" should be changed. Who will ultimately benefit from the change—the person, those who associate with him, or society in general? This chapter will explore some of the methods by which behavior is changed and the ethical issues involved in doing so.

Mental illness and deviant behavior are defined in a number of ways, and the concepts can be variously used. In 1843 Daniel M'Naughten, intending to kill Sir Robert Peel, shot and killed Peel's private secretary instead. Evidence was introduced at the trial showing that M'Naughten suffered from insane delusions of persecution by enemies that included Sir Robert, and he was acquitted on grounds of insanity. From this decision the famous M'Naughten rule in law was derived. M'Naughten was not, however, set free as usually happens when a person is acquitted of a crime. He was sentenced to life imprisonment in an insane asylum and died in one 22 years later. He was acquitted of the crime but convicted for the illness. According to Anglo-American law an act is considered criminal only if it is committed with criminal intent; therefore a way must be found to distinguish between one intent leading to an illegal act and another. The M'Naughten rule maintains that a person cannot be found guilty if at the time of committing the act he was laboring under such delusions that he either did not know what he was doing or did not know that what he was doing was wrong. In 1954 in the United States the M'Naughten rule was replaced by the Durham rule, which states that a person cannot be held responsible for a criminal act if the act was a result of mental disease or defect.[1] The application of Durham can be broader than that of M'Naughten. Various courts and juries have interpreted the definitions of insanity and mental

235

illness in different ways at particular times, making the legal definition of insanity ambiguous. If a defendant is found not guilty of a crime by reason of insanity, he is sometimes committed to a mental hospital for an indeterminate time rather than imprisoned for a specific sentence, and in many instances this commitment has turned out to be a harsher punishment than an ordinary conviction. In these instances it might be said that the designation of unacceptable behavior was used as a punishment.

Mental illness or deviant behavior can be seen as something that society does not approve of or cannot accomodate. This kind of illness usually involves a social role occupied by a person either voluntarily or involuntarily. Evidence is mounting, however, that certain types of mental illness have a biologic or chemical basis, and these types are no longer being classified as social or behavioral disease.

Szasz[2] believes that mental illness is a designation made by some members of society (psychiatrists) about other members of society because the former do not understand the latter. He believes that unacceptable behavior may be a defect in communication: "sometimes they talk differently than others do. Sometimes they say things that offend others. In short, they speak just as you do and I—though perhaps in accents and metaphors that we do not understand or, if we understand them, that we do not like."[2, p. 89] Szasz maintains that some people are labeled sick simply because they are misunderstood or disliked by other people. This labeling covers behavior ranging from the bizarre to the political (expressing an opinion counter to the conventional thinking of the day). Many political reactionaries or highly original thinkers have been deemed crazy by one segment of society or another. Szasz sees much of what is considered unacceptable behavior as a matter of language, which can be used to deprive people of humanity in the same way that it can be used to deprive them of liberty. People who stood on street corners and shouted iconoclastic speeches once were called heretics and burned at the stake; now they are called mentally ill and urged (sometimes forcibly) to seek psychiatric treatment. The gruntings and squealings of inmates in early lunatic asylums were likened to the noises made by caged wild animals, and they were treated as such. Now animal behaviorists are studying the squeaking and whistling of porpoises and the grunting and gesticulating of apes and are likening it to human language. The thought processes of the mentally ill, which may seem incomprehensible to us are believed to emanate from a sick mind. But how do we know this? Szasz believes that the switch from calling unacceptable behavior criminal or heretical to labeling it illness is no improvement; a service has not been done for those thus designated. He sees them as victims of a paternalistic system that needs to label them to differentiate them from the rest of society so that they can be isolated for treatment or punishment.

Szasz is not alone in thinking that there is no such thing as mental illness but only wide variations in human behavior. Certain specific organic diseases of the brain or chemical imbalances should be classed as organic or chemical disease rather than mental illness. Diseases of the brain are reflected behaviorally, whereas diseases of other organs are reflected physically. Diseases of the *mind* do not exist, according to Szasz, but only differences in interpreting communication and function. Therefore there is no such thing as behavior that is so unacceptable that society has the right to change it, except in those cases in which physical harm is done to others, and these cases involve only a small percentage of people who are labeled mentally ill.

Unacceptable behavior is often considered that which is in disharmony with the rest of society or that which the majority does not understand or approve. For example, each year at the end of June, homosexuals in New York, San Francisco, and other large cities take to the streets in a demonstration of solidarity and gay pride. All kinds of people march, including those who are quite average looking, those who cross-dress, and those who make flagrant display of their homosexuality. One person watching the parade might be angry saying that he had no objection to private homosexual acts but, "Why do these people have to flaunt it in everyone's face?" Szasz or others might have responded that homosexuals have as much right as other groups to parade down a street in costume. They were behaving no differently from drum majorettes or a platoon of soldiers. Soldiers may seek applause for their military role, which happens to be socially acceptable, and homosexuals are asking for civil rights even if their behavior may be socially unacceptable. The difference in these two groups is the social acceptability of their behavior. In another culture militarism may be regarded as a ludicrous waste of time whereas a demonstration of sexual freedom might be regarded as a joyous celebration.

The judgment of mental illness or deviant behavior is based on established social, ethical, and behavioral norms. If there are no norms of behavior, then there is no deviance. "Difficulties in human relations can be analyzed, interpreted, and given meaning only within specific social and ethical contexts. Accordingly, the psychiatrist's socio-ethical orientations will influence his ideas on what is wrong with the patient, on what deserves comment or interpretation, in what direction change might be desirable."[3,p.15] Thus we see that the determination of what is and is not acceptable behavior can result from personal opinion and prejudice. Psychiatrists frequently formulate public policy on the basis of personal prejudice. It is one thing to call someone crazy in private conversation if he says something disagreeable or incomprehensible, but it is another to publicly label that person mentally ill. Galileo proclaimed that the earth was not the center of the universe but with the other planets revolved around the sun. The Catholic Church was so distraught that it excommunicated him and tried to force him to recant. In another time such an iconoclast would have been burned or stoned. In our time a person with such publicly unconventional views and with such passion of belief might be consigned to the psychiatrist's couch.

Unacceptable behavior, or deviation from the norm, can be viewed in terms of a revocation of liberty. Mill[4] believed that society has only an indirect interest in the portion of a person's life that affects only himself or others with their free and voluntary consent. Human liberty involves the inward domain of consciousness, thought, feeling, opinion, and sentiments on all subjects. Publishing or publicly speaking these personal opinions may affect others, but the importance of the liberty of expression is as important as the liberty of thought itself and therefore cannot be separated from it. Liberty also involves a freedom of preference to pursue one's life as befits one's character. No impediment should be instituted by others unless it is to prevent harm to others. There also follows the liberty to join with others for any purpose that does not involve harm to others.

No society in which these liberties are not, on the whole, respected, is free, whatever may be its form of government; and none is completely free in which they do not exist absolute and unqualified. The only freedom which deserves the name, is that of pursuing our own good in our own way, as long as we do not attempt to deprive others of theirs, or impede their efforts to obtain it. Each is the proper guardian of his own health, whether bodily, *or* mental and spiritual. Mankind are greater gainers by suffering each other to live as seems good to themselves, than by compelling each to live as seems good to the rest.*

Confinement to a mental institution has been said to be one of the greatest deprivations of liberty ever devised by human beings. It is far worse than being *only* imprisoned. In a mental hospital one is considered both sick and evil, particularly in those institutions for the "criminally insane," a term used to describe people who commit unlawful acts but who are judged not to have known what they were doing or what the consequences of the act were. It is a legal rather than behavioral term.

More than 120 years ago Mill wrote that since ancient times society has contrived to compel people to conform to existing social standards. He believed that the state assumed an interest in all the mental and physical energies of its citizens, an interest that might have been permissible when people lived in small republics and were subject to constant threat of attack by powerful enemies. In modern times temporal and spiritual authority were separated as communities grew, and thus public law controlling private life could no longer be justified. To do so is to behave in a despotic manner "surpassing anything contemplated in the political ideal of the most rigid disciplinarian among the ancient philosophers."[4,p.139] Mill believed that this encroachment on the liberty of others tends to increase in power because it is supported by some of the best and some of the worst characteristics of human nature, a spirit of paternalism that combines extremes of beneficence and nonmaleficence. Mill felt that this "mischief" would increase unless a "strong barrier of moral conviction" could be raised to prevent it. His prediction was correct.

Szasz believes that health values have replaced moral values and thus it becomes easy and not morally incorrect to deprive a person of liberty when moral values play no part in making the decision. Another way of subverting liberty is to confuse moral values with health values by applying moral value judgments to health behavior. A broken leg is seen as a morally neutral behavior, but exposing one's genitals in public is regarded as a morally wrong health behavior. We do not like it and are frightened by it; therefore we label it sick. The sight of genitals in an appropriate semipublic place (for example, a locker room) is neutral, however, and in private it is often positive and exciting. The *place* the genitals are uncovered is the focus of the judgment, not the fact that they are uncovered.

---

*Mill, John Stuart: On liberty (1859). In Utilitarianism, New York, 1962, The New American Library, Inc., p. 138.

The interpretation of behavior and the place in which behavior occurs can change its moral content and therefore its societal label of sickness or health. For example, some soldiers returning from Vietnam had difficulty controlling reflexes adapted to the least suspicion of threat. Many soldiers had spent months or years fighting in jungles where the snap of a twig could prefigure death. They learned to react instantly, often by shooting. Society trained and encouraged them to behave in this way and provided positive reinforcement for doing so. It was considered healthy and morally correct behavior. But if a soldier came home, had a few drinks, and reacted in the same way to what he perceived as a threat, his behavior was judged sick and immoral. Perhaps he should have known where he was, and perhaps a healthy mind should recognize the difference between a jungle and home, but society had devoted time, money, and energy into turning him into an efficient killer and should not have been surprised if the behavior continued longer than anticipated.

Liberty can be subverted when the psychiatrist steps from his private office, where people voluntarily come to be treated, into the public arena, where he in concert with his colleagues establishes norms for acceptable social behavior. Although this is done under the guise of protecting and maintaining general mental health, it comes close to violating morality by controlling the freedom of personal behavior. Liberty is a right most dearly cherished by Americans, second only to life itself; yet it is amazing how willingly we give up the right to freedom of personal behavior when we would not give up other rights. If we found government troops standing in a church or synagogue making certain we prayed in a healthy and socially acceptable way, government would hear about our displeasure in no uncertain terms. Yet when personal behavior is judged not to be within acceptable norms that were arbitrarily established in the first place and are subject to changes in social climate, many people begin to worry and seek help to change their behavior so that they have the approval of people who mean nothing to them. It is a frightening arrangement.

Skinner[5] disagrees and thinks we need to make "vast changes" in human behavior. He points to the breakdown of the educational system, the revolt of the young, and the deterioration of social systems as proof of this needed change. He calls for a "technology of behavior" as powerful and precise as physical and biologic technology. People have an understanding of the physical world but according to Skinner have almost no understanding of themselves. He advocates applying the experimental tools of the physical sciences to study human behavior.

In Skinner's novel *Walden Two*, one of the characters uses cultural and behavioral engineering to achieve a utopia. In the novel a psychologist and philosopher visit Walden Two and find that Frazier, its social and behavior architect, is utterly convinced that his methods to achieve utopia are not only workable but entirely moral.

"It's a little late to be proving that a behavioral technology is well advanced. How can you deny it? Many of its methods and techniques are really as old as the hills. Look at their frightful misuse in the hands of the Nazis! And what about the techniques of the psychological clinic? What about education? Or religion? Or practical politics? Or advertising and salesmanship? Bring them all together and you have a sort of rule-of-thumb technology of vast power. No, Mr. Castle, the science is there for the asking. But its techniques and methods are in the wrong hands—they are used for personal aggrandizement in a competitive world or, in the case of the psychologist and educator, for futile purposes. My question is, have you the courage to take up and wield the science of behavior for the good of mankind?"*

A bit later in the conversation Castle, the philosopher, asks Frazier about the freedom and dignity of the individual in the utopian Walden Two. Frazier replies that by the technique of positive reinforcement a social structure will be built in which everyone's needs will be satisfied and everyone will *want* to observe the Walden Two Code. The feeling of freedom is increased "through the psychological management of our adult membership."[6,p.248] Castle remains unconvinced that freedom and liberty can survive this kind of strong behavioral engineering, which begins at birth, and maintains that the capacity for evil is too seductive.

The book was written in the summer of 1945 when the world had just had its closest escape from the death of liberty; yet Skinner believed even then that total liberty was not the correct path to personal happiness and societal peace. He and Szasz can be seen as holding opposite views about the role of social scientists and psychiatrists in shaping public policy about what behavior is considered acceptable and what might be done to achieve it.

HOW BEHAVIOR IS CHANGED

Behavior can be changed, or attempts made to change it, by a variety of methods. Some are used commonly and are almost as routine as eating, some are used only in the most drastic circumstances, and some are still experimental.

Chemical and pharmacologic methods are among the most common; tranquilizers are one of the largest-selling drug classifications in the United States. Chemical interference with behavior ranges from massive doses of phenothiazines used in hospitals to subdue violent or aggressive behavior (and potentially violent or aggressive behavior) to tranquilizers taken by people daily to function in a way they feel is appropriate. Tranquilizers affect both the central and autonomic nervous systems and parts of the brain itself, notably the limbic system, amygdala, and reticular formation. The mechanism by which tranquilizers work is not fully understood, but their use despite this is not necessarily objectionable. The full pharmacologic effect of aspirin, many antibiotics, and other common drugs is not known either; this does not decrease their efficacy or mean they should not be used. Tranquilizers are, however, among the most overused, misused, and abused drugs in the pharmacopoeia.

Other chemicals change behavior as well. Everyone is familiar with the effects of alcohol, and substances that alter the mind's ability to perceive and interpret reality are in common use. Marijuana is used most frequently, but hashish, LSD,

---

*Skinner, B. F.: Walden two, New York, 1976, The Macmillan Co., p. 241. Copyright © 1948 and 1976, The Macmillan Company.

peyote, mescaline, and dozens of others used alone or in combination, are swallowed, snorted, smoked, or injected by thousands of Americans every day. Some, like marijuana, appear relatively harmless when used in moderation. Others, however, are dangerous and should be used only in the most carefully controlled circumstances. "Hard" drugs such as heroin, other narcotics, and amphetamines change behavior also, almost always for the worse. The reasons people choose to take these drugs are so sociologically and psychologically complex and different from those involved in deliberate behavior control that they can not be discussed here.

Electricity also is a potent force for changing or controlling behavior. Electroshock therapy was once used commonly in mental hospitals because it was found to change behavior, usually by subduing destructive or depressive characteristics, but these changes were frequently only temporary. The treatment itself was cruel and painful. Major tranquilizers were found to be more efficient. Therefore the use of electroshock therapy has decreased in recent years but has not disappeared altogether.

Electricity can be used in a way more sophisticated than simply jolting the entire brain. Electrodes can be implanted into those parts of the brain that are thought to control specific kinds of behavior; by charging these electrodes for varying periods of time the function of brain cells coming in contact with the electricity can be altered, and behavior is modified. The implications of this technique are only just being discovered, but what is already known is awe-inspiring because of the potential for political and social control of individual and group behavior.

Psychosurgery, another method of behavior control, has been in existence for many years. Frontal lobotomies have been used since the 1930s, although their use has decreased. Psychosurgery now is done more delicately and intricately than simply removing an entire lobe of the brain. Those portions of the brain that are known to control certain kinds of behavior can be removed or altered so that particular behavior is changed or reversed. Psychosurgery is now used almost exclusively to control violently aggressive behavior, such as psychomotor (temporal lobe) epilepsy.

Psychotherapy is a generic term used to describe almost any kind of verbal interaction between a therapist and a client. The variations in kinds of therapy are endless and run the gamut from classic Freudian analysis to primal scream therapy, from rebirthing in hot tubs to behavior modification. Therapy can be done individually or in groups and may take years or weeks, and the results range from a complete change in personality structure to no change at all. Therapists are as varied as therapies, from physicians who have had several years of postmedical training and have been analyzed themselves to lay therapists who simply hang out a sign and attempt to help people. Another widespread form of psychotherapy is the do-it-yourself variety, that is, reading books written expressly for the lay person that give all kinds of good, bad, or indifferent advice about how to cope successfully with the exigencies of daily life. Some of the books are written by knowledgeable psychologists; most are filled with commonsense advice that could be gained by talking with an intelligent and sensitive friend.

Psychosurgery

Psychosurgery is interesting, dramatic, and potentially dangerous. For these reasons it will be used as an example to illustrate the moral and ethical dilemmas involved in all behavior control. The first prefrontal lobotomy was performed in 1935 in Lisbon, Portugal, on a person whose behavior was considered refractory and not amenable to other forms of treatment. Dr. Egas Moniz, who pioneered this surgical research on humans, received the Nobel Prize in Physiology and Medicine in 1949 "for his discovery of the therapeutic value of prefrontal lobotomy in certain psychoses."[7,p.159] In 1936 the first lobotomy was done in the United States, and it is estimated that about 40,000 such operations were performed until its popularity declined in the late 1950s when psychotropic drugs were developed.[7] It was also found that prefrontal lobotomy had more deleterious effects than had been anticipated, such as personality deterioration, extremely passive behavior, lack of foresight and ability to plan, and a general blunting of the emotions.

Psychosurgery is still being performed, although not as commonly as in the past. Prefrontal lobotomy was usually performed on people who were considered beyond the reach of other forms of treatment. They had usually been institutionalized for years, and the surgery was considered a last-ditch effort. It rarely returned anyone to effective independent functioning.

Today's psychosurgery is reserved for those who have a reasonably good prognosis, although it is not yet possible to predict ultimate long-term effects. Psychosurgery is still in its infancy, but some segments of the public believe that total mind control is just around the corner. That corner is at the end of a very long block; between now and then people would have to become willing to consent to surgery, to voluntarily relinquish liberty. Popular novels such as Daniel Keyes's *Flowers for Algernon* and Michael Crichton's *The Terminal Man* are science fiction. Before that fiction could become fact, people would have to subject themselves to a neurosurgeon's suggestion that their behavior be drastically changed. Psychosurgery is far from an exact science, and the outcome of each operation is by no means predictable. The potential danger of psychosurgery involves individuals rather than a whole society, for any government that could coerce a significant portion of a society to submit to involuntary psychosurgery would already be dealing with highly malleable people, mental and emotional slaves, and would not need to waste resources on surgery. The problem with psychosurgery lies in the abrogation of the liberty of individuals and in the protection of their personhood while significant aspects of their behavior are changed.

Is a person's identity altered after surgery—is he indeed the same person? William Scoville, president of the International Society of Psychiatric Surgery in 1973, believes that the ethical question of psychosurgery is no different from surgery on any other part of the body.

If surgery benefits overall function it is justified. If overall function is made worse by the operation than by the disease, then surgery is not justified. Certainly all surgical lesions of the brain are destructive of some function; but continuing mental disease may be more destructive of function. Surgical lesions can cut out pathological thought processes or "sick circuits" so that there may result an impressive benefit in overall brain function, thus resulting in a happier and more productive social being.*

This is a rather black and white view of psychosurgery; in actuality the issues are more complex. Operating on the brain with the intent of altering the mind, that is, that part of the brain that controls thought and emotion, is not the same as operating on any other part of the body. Our personhood and very being reside in the brain as they do not in other body parts, and therefore surgically interfering with it involves ethical dilemmas entirely different from those involved with any other organ or body part. Scoville makes the assumptions that the brain is operated on because it is diseased in some way and that the cause of certain types of behavior can be directly traced to specific spots in the brain. Except in cases of detectable tumors this is not necessarily true. Socially unacceptable behavior, even that which is murderously violent, is caused by so great a variety of internal and external circumstances that thinking psychosurgery can benefit overall brain function is dangerously simplistic.

Another problem with Scoville's statement is the paternalism of his belief that psychosurgery can produce a happier and more productive social being. Happiness is entirely subjective, fleeting, and amorphous. Social productivity is also subjectively determined, although admittedly it is not as internal as happiness. It is true that persons who have undergone psychosurgery have expressed their gratitude to Dr. Scoville and others; they may indeed be much happier and able to hold a job now though they could not before, and they may even have developed satisfying human relationships. But even if these kinds of results occur more often than not after psychosurgery, the goals of happiness and social productivity are alone not sufficient to warrant surgery. These goals are too ephemeral and intangible to justify subjecting a person to considerable risk without the person's fully informed consent, which may be impossible to obtain under the circumstances.

One also needs to control carefully the population on whom psychosurgery is performed. What characteristics of behavior would make a person a candidate for surgery—how aggressive is too aggressive? If happiness and social productivity are goals, could anyone who feels unhappy or lazy be a candidate? How can one determine that antisocial behavior is the result of brain disease rather than the influence of a corrupt society?

The National Commission for the Protection of Human Subjects of Behavioral and Biomedical Research (hereinafter referred to as the Commission) studied the problems of psychosurgery and made a report to Congress in March, 1977. The Commission stated that psychosurgery is an experimental procedure and that safeguards should be established to ensure that it is performed only when it is medically indicated and when the subject has given informed consent. The Commission also recommended that because of its nature the surgery be done only in hospitals that have an institutional review board (see Chapter 9 for a discussion of IRBs) and

---

*Scoville, William Beecher: Only as a last resort, Hastings Center Report 3(1):3, Feburary 1973. Reprinted with permission of the Hastings Center, © Institute of Society, Ethics and the Life Sciences, 360 Broadway, Hastings-on-Hudson, N.Y. 10706.

only if the IRB has determined that (1) the surgeon is competent to perform the procedure, (2) the patient has been sufficiently assessed to determine that the procedure is appropriate, and (3) adequate preoperative and postoperative evaluations will be performed.[8] If there is any reason to question the person's consent (considering the nature of the surgery, this is highly likely), further safeguards should be required, such as a court hearing for a prisoner or an involuntarily committed mental patient. The Commission dealt only with safety and efficacy of surgery, not with the conditions under which it might be performed or questions involving the reasons for the surgery or who will receive it. Annas feels that the issue of safety and efficacy should be secondary to that of the uses to which the surgery might be put:

> An "approved" procedure is likely to take on a technological imperative of its own, with unpredictable results. I would submit that psychosurgery that "works" poses a greater danger to society than psychosurgery that doesn't, and that this issue demands attention to such things as deviance and violence *before* "safety and efficacy" are demonstrated.*

The Commission reviewed four different psychosurgical procedures on 61 adults conducted by researchers at Boston University and the Massachusetts Institute of Technology and found that there is "tentative evidence" that some forms of psychosurgery can be a significant treatment of certain disorders. The Commission did not specify which types of surgery, the degree of success, and which disorders would be beneficially treated. The vagueness of the report makes one suspicious about the surgical success rate. Several variables might have skewed the report: (1) psychosurgery might have included operations to relieve emotional reactions to pain, (2) the surgeons' attitudes might have affected the clients' attitudes, (3) only surgeons who volunteered their cases for study were included—and surgeons usually do not volunteer failures for inclusion in a report, and (4) the sample size was limited. Thus it is difficult to draw any positive conclusions about psychosurgery from the Commission's report.

In addition the Commission's recommendations about privacy, confidentiality, and consent are ambiguous. The client may have a face-to-face meeting with the IRB, but it is not required because his privacy must be respected. Therefore the IRB, if it does not meet the client, might simply rubber stamp the surgeon's recommendations. Adult prisoners and mental patients have an absolute right to veto psychosurgery, although children may be subjected to it by proxy consent. There is, however, no evidence that psychosurgery is beneficial with children. One could also wonder about the quality of the consent given by adult clients. Not all candidates for psychosurgery are psychopathic or psychotic, but some are; therefore informed consent might be difficult to obtain.

A typical condition for which psychosurgery is performed is focal epilepsy of the temporal lobe with foci occurring in the limbic system. Episodes of violence

---

*Annas, George J.: Psychosurgery: procedural safeguards, Hastings Center Report 7(2):11, April 1977. Reprinted with permission of The Hastings Center, © Institute of Society, Ethics and the Life Sciences, 360 Broadway, Hastings-on-Hudson, N.Y. 10706

are occasionally related to this form of epilepsy, along with a variety of other symptoms. If drugs are not effective in controlling the symptoms (abnormal aggression and rage), surgery with removal of the anterior portion of the temporal lobe, including the amygdala and hippocampus, may be performed.[9] Critics of the procedure maintain that it is difficult or impossible to accurately locate diseased portions of the brain in temporal lobe epilepsy and that the implantation of electrodes is equally effective in controlling seizures without requiring destruction of brain tissue.

Mark[9] reports several cases of individuals who either had brain tumors or sustained traumatic head injuries that were visible in x-ray views. Surgery in these cases drastically improved the violently aggressive behavior and in most cases returned the client to normal. It is difficult to draw a moral line between psychosurgery for someone who has come into an emergency room with a head injury causing such violent behavior that he tries to kill the nurse and psychosurgery for someone who has become progressively more violent over the years and finally ends up stabbing a stranger. If both conditions are distressing to the clients and their families, and if both involve equally bizarre behavior, but if only one condition can be detected on an x-ray film or CAT scan, what is the moral difference between the two operations? Chorover[10] believes that there is no conclusive proof of the merits of psychosurgery and that the continued performance of psychosurgery in the absence of medical justification is questionable. He sees psychosurgery as an ominous means to control deviant behavior, including abnormal agression and violence directed toward the self and others. Dr. M. Hunter Brown at the 1970 International Conference of Psychosurgery recommended initiation of a pilot program to "rehabilitate" by surgical means those intelligent young prisoners who could not control violent outbursts.[10] It has been suggested, however, that this surgery was used only on prisoners who viewed their punishment in socioeconomic or racial terms. In 1972 a group of neurosurgeons in Germany destroyed a portion of the hypothalamus of 22 males, 20 of whom were sexual deviants.[10] Fifteen of the 22 were reported to have "good" results, that is, sexual behavior that was in harmony with current societal norms. Psychosurgery on hyperactive children, particularly those who are mentally retarded and engage in self-destructive behavior, has been performed in the United States and several other countries.[10] The purpose of the surgery has been to make the children more docile, and "good" results are generally reported. Because psychosurgery is so controversial and its merit so hotly debated, Chorover[10] recommends that the medical profession and state and federal regulatory agencies take the following steps:

1. Psychosurgery should be explicitly designated as an experimental rather than a therapeutic procedure.
2. Psychosurgery should not be performed on children, prisoners, the mentally retarded, or anyone involuntarily committed to a mental hospital.
3. A registry should be established to assess psychosurgical practices and to publish the results of postmortem examinations of brain tissue.
4. A temporary moratorium should be called on all psychosurgery until the risks and benefits can be more adequately weighed.

5. Basic research on brain mechanisms and behavior should be increased.
6. Target behaviors for psychosurgery should be defined more clearly and specifically than the current vague designations such as "aggressive," "hostile," "dangerous," and so on.

One of the most famous court cases involving psychosurgery was *Kaimowitz v. Department of Mental Health,*[11] better known as the case of John Doe. In 1972 John Doe, then 36 years old and an inmate of Ionia State Hospital in Michigan, was asked by the Department of Mental Health to participate in an experiment comparing methods of reducing aggression in the chronically violent.[12] One group was to receive the drug cyproterone acetate, which would make the recipient impotent as well as docile, and the other group was to undergo psychosurgery. John Doe, who had been admitted to the hospital at age 18 as a sexual psychopath after raping and murdering a student nurse, consented to the surgery, and his parents agreed. However, the research program was stopped because Michigan Legal Services attorney Gabe Kaimowitz brought suit to block the experiment. John Doe resented the intrusion and requested that the surgery proceed. The state withdrew the funds for the experiment pending the outcome of the suit, and during the hearings John Doe reversed his decision to have surgery.

The court issued the following rulings: (1) people involuntarily committed to state institutions are incapable of giving informed knowledgeable consent for experimental psychosurgery that will permanently destroy brain tissue, (2) the First Amendment right to freedom of speech and expression of thought would presumably be denied these individuals by the surgery, and (3) the constitutional right to privacy would be frustrated by an unwarranted intrusion into a person's brain.

The competency of committed mental patients in consenting to surgery is subject to many variables. John Doe had been hospitalized for 18 years and was dependent on hospital personnel to make almost all his decisions, including going for a walk on hospital grounds. In institutions where vigorous psychotherapy is offered and where clients are encouraged to think and act independently, informed consent might be possible. Whether the consent is truly voluntary, however, would be difficult to ascertain considering the inequality of physicians and clients in the hospital atmosphere and the coercive nature of the institutional setting.

As a result of *Kaimowitz* virtually all experimental psychosurgery in mental hospitals has been halted; the tone of the decision makes it seem that the court would have liked to ban psychosurgery altogether. Because knowledge gained from animal studies cannot be transferred to humans in toto, it may not be possible for anyone to give knowledgeable informed consent for psychosurgery. All people who agree to have their minds operated on are taking a chance because the results can never be precisely predicted.

There is an interesting postscript to the John Doe case.[8] In March, 1973, he was released from the hospital and worked for a few months as a silk-screener in Detroit. Shortly afterwards he was arrested for shoplifting a woman's girdle. When he was booked and searched he was found to be wearing 19 pairs of women's underpants and 10 slips. He pleaded guilty and was sentenced to prison. While he was in custody he finally confessed to the crimes for which he had been sent to the state mental hospital 21 years before (rape and murder) rather than being brought to trial. He was tried in 1976 and pleaded innocent by reason of insanity. The jury convicted him, and he is now serving a life sentence.

There are advantages and disadvantages to psychosurgery. Some people think that medical intervention should be undertaken to improve behavior whenever possible. They point to the fact that normal people, that is, those who are not violently aggressive, take tranquilizers in record numbers in an effort to improve their behavior and functioning and to increase their happiness. Physicians prescribe these drugs sometimes for questionable medical reasons and sometimes merely because the client requests them. Tranquilizers have been found to control anxiety and some forms of depression, but they have no measurable effect on neurotic behavior. Nevertheless, they are still prescribed. Therefore, the argument goes, when a person's behavior is seriously psychotic and dangerous to himself and society and when the only alternative is to place him in chemical restraints and lock him up forever, psychosurgery even on an experimental basis is justified. This argument would be perfectly reasonable only if there was no doubt that life in the back ward of a state hospital was the only alternative to psychosurgery and if the surgery had a better than even chance of success. However, doubt does exist. Another problem with the argument is that it is not always possible to prove that unacceptable or violent behavior has a physical cause. Even if the person has not responded to years of other forms of therapy, it cannot be assured that surgery will provide a benefit. On the other hand, it could be argued that every technique available should be employed to relieve the person's mental suffering; if nothing thus far has worked, then psychosurgery should be tried. Some think that if the person is left with a decreased ability to think, he is still better off than when living in a state of unpredictable violence. Because psychosurgery is irreversible, critics feel it should be used only with extreme caution or not at all.

Proponents point out the irreversibility of *all* surgery and some of the permanent side effects of psychotherapeutic drugs, especially large doses of major tranquilizers. Even some of the temporary side effects of these drugs may be extremely severe including sudden unexplained death. An intractably violent person might be made overly docile by psychosurgery, but the long-term use of drugs causes equal if not greater passivity. These have been aptly dubbed "chemical straight jackets." And some people who are tortured by the effects of their violent outbursts and are filled with remorse voluntarily request psychosurgery. Should they be denied the opportunity to be relieved of their suffering?

ETHICS OF CHANGING BEHAVIOR

The primary ethical issue in behavior control concerns behavior itself and the desirability and acceptability of certain kinds of behavior. It is tempting to gloss over the question of what behavior is normal and suggest that it be left to experts in psychology to define. The problem, however, involves questions of who the psychologic experts are and who gives them the right to establish the parameters of normal behavior. An expert in the field of psychology ostensibly has had a significant amount of education and training concerning human behavior and can differentiate the normal from the abnormal. How much and what kind of training is sufficient, and who is qualified to provide it? Who teaches the experts? What is the difference between very crazy and slightly crazy or intermittently crazy? We could go round and round with these kinds of questions and still never face the ethical issues.

One must then somehow agree that certain types of behavior are unacceptable to the individual and to others. For example, some compulsive behavior is intolerable to a person because his functioning is decreased. If after leaving for work one has to return home exactly 11 times to check that the gas stove is turned off, or if one refuses to enter a room in which there are more than three people, the behavior does not disturb society but is highly unacceptable to the person who seeks to change it. On the other hand, a peeping Tom is distressing to the people into whose windows he peers, but he may feel no need to change his behavior because he finds it pleasurable, gratifying, and exciting. However, the neighbors want his behavior changed.

We will assume also that some people know more about behavior and behavior control than others. It must be acknowledged that everyone does not have an equal amount of expertise in this area. It can also be acknowledged that a diploma or certificate does not automatically confer sensitivity and humanity or the ability to make correct decisions about what is acceptable behavior and what procedures if any should be undertaken to change it.

If the aim of any kind of psychotherapy (including all forms of treatment, such as verbal, chemical, electrical, and surgical therapy and all variations thereof) is to change behavior, at issue is the problem of *whose* goals therapy is directed toward achieving—the clients, therapist's, or society's. The person with a compulsion to turn off the gas might seek treatment only for relief of this symptom, but the therapist may interpret it as a manifestation of a deeper and more serious illness and create an entirely different goal for the client. The same person may want to talk about his fear of entering crowded rooms whereas the therapist believes that drastic behavior modification involving implanted electrodes would solve the problem. A homosexual seeking therapy not because he *is* a homosexual but because he needs help living a gay life in a straight world exemplifies this problem of conflicting goals. In his view the problem is as much society's inability to accept his minority behavior as his difficulty in trying to fit in with the majority. The therapist, however, may not share his point of view and may attempt to convince the homosexual that he is exhibiting sick behavior and establish a goal of enjoyable intercourse with a woman. The therapist believes that he is acting in the client's best interest when he imposes his own and society's goals on the client. Because the client does not share these goals and does not view his homosexuality as a problem, the therapist has acted unethically. The problem of goals can be stated in terms of values: when the values of the therapist and those of the client differ, an ethical dilemma arises. The dilemma is compounded when the client has wholly or partly lost his ability to reason and the therapist does not know if the client means what he says and says what he means. One can never be certain if the established goals are those of the client, because it cannot be known if the client knows what he wants. Therapy runs the risk of being coercive even when the client's presence in therapy is voluntary.

To control or change someone's behavior or even suggest that behavior should be changed is to exert power over a person or group of people (usually a family). Psychologic "experts" are increasingly exerting power and influence over private behavior and public consciousness and establishing behavioral norms that usually embrace those human characteristics that appear least unusual to the greatest number of people. Individuals are often asked to take psychologic tests before being considered for certain jobs. Hospital nurses who ask too many questions and who challenge the established routine are frequently branded troublemakers and iconoclasts and may find themselves socially ostracized by the rest of the staff. In many corporations a certain standard of dress is required and expected, and deviation from the standard is not easily condoned regardless of the excellence of the person's work.

This kind of influence on mass behavior is frightening. The moral problem comes in achieving balance between personal behavioral liberty and social order. Every human being has personal and public behavior. We may hold in towering anger and frustration all day at work and when we get home burst into tears or smash crockery. This behavior is accepted because there is no one there to see it or because the only witnesses have been admitted to the sphere of our intimate selves. The problem for some lies in differentiating the times and places for exhibiting certain kinds of behavior; more and more we are limited to certain circumstances for certain behaviors. Those who set limits on behavior are generally seen as the establishment, that is, the controllers of societal goods and benefits.

It is difficult to develop an absolute ethic for the management of behavior control, the technology of which is still not sufficiently developed for us to know how far one can go in experimenting with or controlling behavior. An absolute ethic may be too rigid to be useful in studying behavior or in trying to change or control behavior that is so asocial or antisocial that almost everyone agrees to its unacceptability. A practical or temporary ethic, however, could be seen as too expedient or flexible to be called an ethic. A set of values or ethics that changes with society's moods or mores might as well not exist if moral principles cannot be extracted from it and applied to behavior control technology and experimentation. Viewing the abstract and the concrete in their proper relationship is difficult, and developing an ethic for behavior control that separates the two is even more so.

Behavior therapy research is increasing, as is the therapy based on this research. Some therapy is voluntary, but much is coerced, particularly that performed in institutions. The moral dilemma of behavior therapy arises in determining why behavior should be changed if the client does not agree. It is facile to say that a man who has been committed to a state mental hospital and who has not spoken since the day of admission should be made to speak. Speech might hasten his return to the outside world, but it cannot be assumed that he wants to return or that he has any reason to speak. He may have decided that he has nothing further to say and wants to spend a period of time, even the rest of his life, communing only in his mind. Is this necessarily sick? Almost all of us have ignored a ringing telephone simply because we did not want to be bothered with speaking to anyone at the time—this behavior is considered perfectly acceptable up to a point. But we might consider someone who never answered the telephone bizarre or even sick, simply because we do not understand or agree with this behavior. The man who has decided to stop speaking has carried this behavior to an extreme, but to automatically label it sick is to enter dangerous ethical waters, especially if his reasons are not known. In institutions people often refuse to eat, and if this behavior lasts long enough, death by starvation will result. Perhaps the person is indeed intent on committing suicide but the thought of suicide by direct action is too frightening to him. Or perhaps the food is inedible. Is it ethical to coerce a person into eating by using behavior modification or by actual force feeding?

When behavior that is harmful to no one else is at issue, so is personal liberty. If a person not in an institution chooses not to eat, nothing is done to him until he becomes too weak to function. If an institutionalized person chooses not to eat, the fact that he has already lost most of his liberty by being where he is does not make it morally permissible to deprive him further of liberty and choice by forcing him to eat. If an institutionalized person is deprived of liberty, the ethical tone is then set for further abuses. An institution has no more right to deprive a person of liberty unjustifiably than an individual or even a court.

The ethics of aversive therapy are even more questionable. Applying an electric shock to the testes of a child molester while showing him pictures of nude children would be considered cruel and unusual punishment if it were carried out in any set of circumstances other than a therapeutic one. But does the therapeutic environment neutralize the fact that harm is done by inflicting pain? When if ever does infliction of pain become morally acceptable? The ethics of using evil means to achieve good ends will be discussed in relation to human experimentation. It is difficult to justify aversive therapy morally when painful, dangerous, or highly unpleasant stimuli are used to achieve a therapeutic goal.

In language and law, cure and control are like two banks of a river clearly separated by a body of water—that is, they are clearly separated by a willingness to distinguish between the interests of two parties in conflict with each other. The word *therapy*—as in psychiatric therapy or behavior therapy—is a bridge over the water: it unites the two parties in a fake cooperation and enables one or the other or both of them to declare the nonexistence of any difference between cure and control, contract and coercion, freedom and slavery.*

Behavior therapy, whether free or coerced, aversive or positive, takes place because a particular behavior is deemed unacceptable by the client or someone in society. If the client himself wants to change his behavior for rational reasons and cannot do it alone, certain kinds of behavior therapy are probably quite effective and ethical, for example, anti-smoking clinics that are based on rewards for a certain number of cigarettes not smoked. Rewards are delineated by the client himself, and no punishment is exacted by the therapist. Negative reinforcement comes from the client's sense of failure.

If unacceptable behavior is determined by society (except that which causes

---

*Szasz, Thomas: The theology of medicine, Baton Rouge, 1977, Louisiana State University Press, p. 58.

physical harm to another), it is difficult to justify forcing a person to change his behavior unless he himself specifically requests help. Shoplifting, for example, is a behavior that is becoming more common, and society frowns on it for a number of reasons. Some people shoplift because they are true kleptomaniacs; that is, they are unable not to steal. Some people do it because they are hungry or too poor to buy what they need, and others shoplift because it provides excitement. Possibly except for the person who steals because he cannot afford to buy food, shoplifting can be classed as unacceptable or undesirable behavior. Should the behavior be *changed* because it is deviant or unacceptable, or should it be punished? Should the shoplifter be put in jail for breaking the law or in therapy for engaging in antisocial behavior?

The following example involves a different case but concerns the same issue. A man who seems otherwise perfectly respectable and functional steals small items of gourmet food. He can afford to buy them and does not live the kind of life in which imported brandied chestnuts are essential. In an interview with a psychiatrist he demonstrates no compulsion to steal. On the surface his reasons seems logical: he likes the idea of serving exotic foods to guests but does not like "paying all that import duty so the government can waste more money at my expense." He seems to be stealing for political reasons and exhibits no remorse or guilt. He is quite good at shoplifting, but recently he has been getting caught frequently because the shopkeepers in his neighborhood keep a sharp eye on him. Usually he receives a fine and suspended sentence because he always pays for the merchandise as soon as he is caught. This time, however, he is sentenced to 30 days in prison, and the judge recommends that he be evaluated by the prison psychiatrist. Now the psychiatrist faces a problem. The man has said that he will stop stealing in his own neighborhood because being in prison has dampened his enthusiasm for shoplifting, but he shows no indication of wanting to change his behavior. He understands the consequences of stealing and will probably simply perfect his technique to decrease his chances of being caught. Should the psychiatrist use coercive means to try to get this man to accept behavior therapy, or would that restrict his liberty? His habitual shoplifting is an activity that will eventually lead to a restriction of his liberty because sooner or later he will be caught again and will receive a longer prison sentence. Would it be ethical to try to prevent this ultimate limitation of liberty by using coercive tactics now if the psychiatrist thinks the man might ultimately benefit?

Beauchamp and Childress[13] present a case that demonstrates the issue involved in restricting a person's liberty now so that he might benefit in the future. A 65-year-old retired army officer who had had several abdominal operations was admitted to a psychiatric ward because of severe chronic pain, weight loss, and social withdrawal. He gave himself six injections a day of pentazocine (Talwin) but still could not control the pain, even when he assumed awkward and embarrassing postures. His goal for therapy was to "get more out of life in spite of my pain." He was finding it increasingly difficult to give himself injections because of tissue breakdown. The hospital staff ignored his pain behavior to avoid reinforcing it, and positive reinforcement was limited to relaxation techniques, cognitive relabeling, and the like. The client when he voluntarily admitted himself knew of the hospital's expectation of a downward adjustment of medication. However, he refused to allow modification of his Talwin dosage, claiming that the amount he took was essential to control his pain. The staff discussed the problem at length and decided to decrease the dose of Talwin without informing the client by gradually diluting it with saline. Three weeks later the staff told him what they had done. At first he was angry but then asked that even the saline be discontinued and only the self-control techniques used. He was discharged after another 3 weeks, still experiencing some pain but able to control it sufficiently to resume social activities and part-time teaching. The therapists had felt ethically obligated to treat this man with a means that had a high probability of success even though it meant temporarily depriving him of a certain amount of liberty (informed consent and knowledge of the treatment he was receiving). Complete openness would not have been in his best interest.

If autonomy is a primary principle of informed consent and if behavior control without informed consent is unethical except in highly unusual circumstances such as those involving violence, how does autonomy relate to behavior control? Various forms of therapy simply by their existence decrease autonomy. For example, if a person's mind is altered by drugs, surgery, or electricity, a good deal of his autonomy has been removed. Anyone who has seen the behavior of a person who is taking 700 to 800 mg of Thorazine or Mellaril a day has observed the decrease in ability to think logically. Autonomy has been totally or partially destroyed. Is it ever ethical to alter a person's capacity to think? One can argue that no one has complete autonomy, that we all operate within a set of restraints and constraints applied either by societal judgment and mores or by our own value system. None of us is free to act completely as we wish. Therefore chemically or electrically reducing autonomy in a person who has demonstrated that he cannot or will not live within a set of reasonable constraints is morally justified, just as it is justified to deprive someone of liberty when he has been convicted of a crime. The argument rests on choice. If a person chooses to behave in a certain way, can he then be forced to pay for the incorrect choice by having to give up his autonomy? This argument

leads to a paradox in the relationship between autonomy and moral goodness. Autonomy, on this view, demands that the agent choose his moral principles independent of external constraints. But for many moral philosophers the principles of morality are such that their correctness or truth is independent of whether they are chosen or not. So we have a conflict between being subject to the constraints of a correct set of principles and the notion of choosing whatever the self decides upon.*

The conflict can be resolved somewhat by stating that the self does not have total autonomy and that selected beliefs, desires, and consequent behaviors occur as the result of being manipulated by society—that there is no such thing as com-

---

*Dworkin, Gerald: Autonomy and behavior control, Hastings Center Report 6(1):24, February 1976. Reprinted with permission of The Hastings Center, © Institute of Society, Ethics and Life Sciences, 360 Broadway, Hastings-on-Hudson, N.Y. 10706.

pletely free choice. This does not solve the ethical dilemma but may partly explain its origins.

Autonomy is a characteristic of independence, and if one's autonomy is interrupted by behavior therapy, he becomes less independent, further decreasing his autonomy. The ostensible goal of most forms of therapy is to increase the client's independence and ability to function in society. Again there is a means-ends dilemma as well as a practical question. What purpose is served by committing a person to an institution, giving him so much Thorazine that he cannot think straight, and calling that therapy? His chance of functioning autonomously will surely be decreased. Autonomy is removed, dependence is fostered, and the therapeutic goal will never be reached. Some then rationalize the situation: "We have to protect people; we can't just let them wander around out there; they might get hurt." If this is the goal, why not label the situation protective custody rather than therapy?

If another purpose is to protect society from the bizarre or unacceptable activity of others by changing the behavior of those others, then calling it therapy in this case is also misleading. This does not mean that the act of changing or controlling behavior is necessarily immoral, although a different justification has to be made; it does mean, however, that it should not be labeled therapy unless it can be said that the person whose behavior is being changed will benefit the most and that the behavior is being changed because the client wishes it to be.

Dworkin[14] has proposed guidelines for preservation of autonomy in the process of behavior control:

1. We should favor those methods of influencing behavior that support the self-respect and dignity of those who are being influenced. A guideline at this level of abstraction does not provide much help in selecting specific techniques, but "it is important to be clear about the distinction between expressing and supporting self-respect, and being causally connected with producing a state of affairs which might be called increased self-respect or dignity."[14,p.27] Dworkin uses psychosurgery as an example: because after therapy the client may be able to function, it could be said that his dignity is increased or fostered. But the methods used might not be expressive of the dignity of the client if he is treated as an object rather than a subject.

2. Methods of influence that destroy or decrease an individual's ability to think rationally in his own interests should not be used. Dworkin does not specify which methods should not be used, but we can assume that large doses of tranquilizers or central nervous system depressants and electroshock therapy as well as other forms of behavior control can be included in this category. Institutionalization, which fosters dependence, might also be included though Dworkin does not comment on this.

3. Methods of influence that fundamentally affect the personal identity of the individual should not be used. If the method of treatment (such as psychosurgery, electricity, and certain chemicals) raises questions about whether the person is the same after treatment, it should not be used. Change is acceptable, but it must be within a framework of personal continuity.

4. Methods of influence that deceive or keep relevant facts from the individual should not be used.
5. Methods that are physically intrusive (such as drugs, psychosurgery, and electricity) are less preferable than methods that are not. Each person needs a realm of physical integrity that cannot be violated, an assurance of a measure of dignity and privacy.
6. The person should be able to resist the method of influence if he so chooses. Changes in behavior that are reversible are preferable to those that are not. The duration of the effect also makes a difference in the amount of autonomy a person retains. A shorter effect is preferable to a longer one.
7. Methods that work through the cognitive and affective structure of a person are preferable to those that short-circuit his beliefs and desires and cause him to be passively receptive to the will of others.

In recent years paternalistic justification for behavior control has increased, notably in the area of involuntary commitment to mental hospitals for behavior that may or may not be dangerous to the self and others. Behavior control may be forced on a person after legal commitment has taken place. Eugenic sterilization, notably for the retarded and recidivist criminals, is another form of paternalistic control of behavior. Psychosurgery is highly paternalistic, as are many forms of behavior control such as giving drugs to hyperkinetic children and aversion techniques for socially unacceptable behavior. Beauchamp[15] lists the following ways in which paternalism in behavior control has been justified by others in the past:

1. The person was thought to need protection from himself.
2. The person either did not know what his own best interests were or was not sufficiently motivated to achieve them.
3. It was believed that a wider range of freedom could be achieved or an unreasonable risk prevented.
4. The person was not able to prevent evil from occurring to himself or others.

Beauchamp believes that these paternalistic decisions should be made only in the most extreme instances of involuntary behavior, most of which result from an ignorance of consequences, such as drunkenness, retardation, mob-incited violence, and the like. A person in such a situation should be protected from his own actions only up to a certain point. After being "informed of the dangers of his actions, if and when a context can be provided where voluntary choice is meaningfully possible, he cannot justifiably be further restrained."[15] Coercion or paternalism is justified only when the person's ignorance cannot be overcome because of some innate and immutable condition such as severe retardation. The paternalistic action, however, should be directed at nonexploitation.

LEGAL AND POLITICAL IMPLICATIONS

Most instances of legally authorized behavior control have involved prisoners and involuntarily committed mental patients. Courts have frequently been swayed by researchers who deliberately or inadvertently confused punishment or control with therapy. Informed consent from people who are incarcerated is often not obtained because it is assumed that the mere fact of loss of liberty implies loss of competence. Legislation is now, however, beginning to protect such individuals. In 1974 the California legislature passed a bill to control the use of organic therapies in California prisons.[16] Organic therapy included psychotropic drugs and provided the following protection:

1. Integrity of thought and mentation is believed to be a fundamental constitutional right.
2. Informed consent is a necessary condition for all therapy (except electroshock in certain emergencies) regardless of the mental capacity of the person. Simple refusal is final.
3. Psychosurgery, electrical stimulation of the brain (ESB), and certain other therapies require judicial authorization in all instances.
4. If the person lacks capacity for consent, therapy cannot be performed; stringent procedures are established for circumstances under which this rule can be overridden.

The goal of the bill was to provide a buffer against the power of the state without making it impossible to help a prisoner regain the ability to function freely. Shapiro correctly points out the "catch-22" of this stance: if a therapy works, it is forbidden, but any therapy that does not work may be used. Prisoners may be protected from harm, but they are also "protected" from any help they might have received. The catch can be stated another way: if a treatment is potent or effective enough to provide real help, then it is also potent and effective enough to do real harm and as a result may be banned from use.

The political implications of this and similar statutes are enormous. If a person's thought and mentation are protected by the Constitution, then it should be impossible for any court to grant permission for therapy that might jeopardize that mentation. Theoretically, then, any form of behavior control would be unconstitutional. But to help people regain lost mental function it is sometimes necessary to interfere with their capacity to function; therefore the process of regaining mental control may involve further diminishing that control. The risk is great, and the problem lies in deciding whether possible benefits are worth the risk.

If a person or group espouses ideas that are politically radical or thought to be dangerous, it is now too easy to consider their thought processes disturbed mentation and seek a cure for what is not an illness. Under what circumstances can the state intrude on the mental processes of a citizen? The criteria usually involve concepts seen as abnormal or unnatural or thought to present some physical danger to others. The problem as always is to determine the parameters of normalcy and decide if the threat or potential for danger is real. The safest course of action is to assume that any form of mentation is valuable to the person himself and should be legally protected unless there is *clear and present* danger to others.

There will always be conflicts between those who would guard civil liberty and those who wish to impose psychiatric therapy. To a great extent the conflict involves different views of the nature of crime. A psychopathologic orientation maintains that most criminal acts occur as a result of a disturbance in mentation; therefore criminal behavior can be "cured" by behavior control. In light of the dismal failure of the American penal system, this view has many adherents. It is a mistake to assume, however, that because prisons do not reform criminals, behavior control will prove more successful. Libertarians frequently view crime not so much as a result of mental illness but as an undesirable manifestation of free will; they see no reason to tamper with a person's mind simply because he has committed a crime, regardless of how senseless or brutal it was. Even if a person is found not guilty because he obviously was not able to comprehend the consequences of or reasons for his criminal act, there is not necessarily a rationale for forced behavior control. Even a mass murderer who suffers from the most bizarre delusions should not be treated unless he wants to be treated. Punishment is not the same as therapy.

Mental illness or mental incapacity has been used as an excuse for immoral or criminal behavior, but physical illness never is. One never hears that a person shot another because he was crazed by the pain of a leg broken in several places. A physical disability may be as great a burden as a mental one, but dishonesty and violence are not excused because of it. A similar comparision can be made with sociocultural factors that lead to crime. If a poor person in a crowded slum shoots his neighbor on a hot night, his attorney may plead that he was unable to cope with the squalor of his living conditions and was thus driven to a violent act. If a millionaire shoots his neighbor, the defense is not likely to plead that the pressure of living with all that money drove him to uncontrollable violence. This does not mean to imply that no criminal behavior has psychiatric overtones; it does mean to imply that the distinction between morality and illness is not finely drawn. Therefore the consequences of behavior cannot be clearly indicated. Criminal acts are frequently justified by mislabeling the behavior as that resulting from mental illness. By being unable to differentiate between evil and illness in many instances, American society may subtly not discourage crime or give it negative reinforcement.

Dershowitz[17] presents two cases that clearly demonstrate the dilemma of using psychiatric judgment to control behavior or impinge on personal liberty. In the first instance an American of Korean origin, Bong Yol Yang, appeared at the gate of the White House asking to see the President. He wanted to tell the President about the people who were following him and "revealing his subconscious thoughts." He also wanted to offer his talents as an artist to the government. The gate officer at the White House had him committed to a mental hospital. Yang demanded a jury trial, and there a psychiatrist testified that he was a paranoid schizophrenic. The psychiatrist admitted that there was no evidence that Yang had ever attacked anyone but said there was a possibility that he would. The jury with permission of the judge committed him to an indeterminate term in a mental hospital. Yang's only "crime" was wanting to discuss his private thoughts with the President.

The other case involved Dallas Williams, 39 years old, who had spent half his life in jail for seven convictions of assault with a deadly weapon and one conviction of manslaughter. Just before his scheduled release the government petitioned for civil commitment, and two psychiatrists testified that he was likely to repeat his homicidal pattern. The judge denied the government's petition and maintained that one cannot be confined before a crime is committed, no matter how likely it is that the crime will occur. Two months after Williams was released he shot and killed two men in an unprovoked attack.

Could Yang be considered mentally ill because he thought people were following him? If he had not shown up at the White House, he might not have found himself in his present situation; he could have continued his life as usual, perhaps being thought a bit weird by his associates, but he would have remained undisturbed. His naiveté in thinking he could see the President put him behind locked doors. On other other hand, should Williams have been released? If society chooses not to put up with people who are unable to control their violent impulses, provision must be made to remove them in some way, such as life imprisonment without parole or execution if a certain number of offenses have been committed. If society does not mind having violent people in its midst or is willing to risk further abuses by permitting such people to be at liberty, then why should society often delude itself by labeling someone sick instead of evil?

Every society has people who cause some kind of trouble, ranging from offensive behavior to outright violence. Dershowitz[17] says that several questions need to be asked when a determination is made about what to do with such people. What sorts of harm warrant involuntary confinement, or what kinds of behavior is society willing to tolerate? How likely is it that harm will occur, and should this include self-harm? If harm to oneself is sufficient to deprive a person of liberty, must that person be capable of weighing the risks of incarceration against the urge to harm himself? Must he be able to ask, "Do I want to cut off my hand badly enough to risk being locked up for a long time, possibly forever?" If he is not rational enough to pose this kind of question, should he be considered mentally ill? If a person is involuntarily confined, how much time is required to decrease likelihood of his causing trouble, and how does one know when the danger has passed? The questions are complex, but the answers, if answers are possible, will reveal the political and legal tone of the society that answers them. "Whether or not it is constitutional for the state to use mental hospitals to deprive citizens of their liberty is for the authorized interpreters of the Consitution to judge. Until now, the courts have found such detention consitutional. We might recall that earlier courts had found slavery constitutional."[1,p.205]

The decision to involuntarily incarcerate a mentally ill person and force him to change his behavior is essentially a political one. Politics itself is a form of behavior manipulation. Most people are familiar with the phrase "office politics," that is, acceptable modes of behavior at work, a more or less benign form of behavior control. However, a societal decision to deprive a person of liberty is a continuation of that benign activity to a form that can become malevolent. As society becomes more complex, individual regulation tends to increase and political controls become more intense. The line between liberty and coercion is blurred, and the range of behavior that is deemed acceptable narrows. In most states, for example, a paroled prisoner is not permitted to associate with known criminals, presumably to prevent him from being tempted back into a life of crime. Thus even after a prisoner is physically released, his behavior is still to some degree controlled. This is a political decision that could be extended to us all. The FBI has in the past kept dossiers on political activists and people with whom they associate. Democracy is partially based on the idea that an individual is responsible for his own behavior; if society chooses to control that behavior wholly or partly, what happens to the concept of democracy?

Veatch[18] presents a case that clearly illustrates the political and legal implications of forced treatment for unacceptable behavior. A man in his late 30s had been convicted of a series of alcohol-related petty offenses. He was found holding a hammer and standing over the dead body of a friend and was charged with murder. Conviction would have been difficult because all the evidence was circumstantial except for the testimony of his wife, which was not admissible in court. He had a long history of alcoholism and was therefore sent to a state mental hospital for diagnostic evaluation. After 9 years there, during which time he underwent group and individual psychotherapy, he showed no change, and he was denied parole each year. The staff felt that therapy should be continued indefinitely because if he were released, his alcohol-related violence would eventually be manifested. One staff member proposed psychosurgery so that the man could drink without the danger of violent episodes. Another proposed the use of disulfiram, a drug that causes a person who has ingested alcohol to feel dizzy and nauseated and eventually to fall unconscious. The staff refused to perform surgery, and the client refused the drug. Another staff member argued that even though the man was an alcoholic, he should not be considered mentally ill because he could stop drinking if he wanted to; therefore he should be returned to prison to serve his sentence. Yet another staff member favored behavior modification therapy with rewards to the man for not drinking.

The dilemma concerns how this man is viewed and what action should be taken as a result of that view. If the man is considered sick, should his treatment be temporary, thus assuring this return to alcoholism when treatment is discontinued? Should it be permanent, as is psychosurgery, thus depriving him of liberty forever? Should he be coerced into behavior modification even though he likes to drink and wants to continue? Or should his alcoholism be legally ignored and he be made to stand trial and let the jury decide if he did commit the murder and if so whether his drinking was relevant to the crime? Should the man be offered paternalistic continued treatment that necessitates involuntary commitment, or should he be offered his constitutional right to a trial by jury even though he might be convicted of murder and sentenced to death, life imprisonment, or a longer sentence than he would have had in the mental hospital? The decision is not a medical one even though the man is confined to a hospital. It is a political decision with strong legal overtones.

SOCIAL IMPLICATIONS

The aspect of behavior control that arouses more public interest and controversy than any other concerns the study of violently aggressive behavior. No one escapes being affected by such behavior, and there is no way to prevent completely the possibility of violent attack. In February, 1978, the UCLA Center for the Study and Reduction of Violence held a conference sponsored by the Hastings Center.

The three purposes were (1) to survey present and study future capacities to understand and control violent and antisocial behavior, (2) to examine specific cases to try to determine the dynamics of behavior, and (3) to ask under what conditions further scientific research should take place and to bring into account social and ethical problems and past pitfalls.[19]

The UCLA violence center met with much public opposition and the project had to be abandoned, but the problem of what to do about violence remains. It is a form of unacceptable behavior that is steadily increasing and about which the public is becoming particularly vociferous. "Law and order" public rhetoric and police behavior can do no good unless the causes of increased violence can be determined. We must know why a man was driven to murder 36 women, why a young man in a completely unprovoked attack suddenly pushed a 17-year-old girl into the path of an oncoming subway train, and why 17 or 18 Mom and Pop grocery store robberies in San Francisco ended in murder though in each the robbery had already been successfully accomplished. Violence is one of the major social problems of our time, and the chance that any individual will be attacked is increasing.

One of the many interesting results of increasing violence, possibly because we are so appalled by its existence and our inability to control it, is blaming the victim for the crime. A woman who is raped is frequently thought to have brought it on herself if she wears a certain kind of clothing or walks alone at night. If a man is mugged on the street, the police ask what he was doing in the neighborhood, as if the crime resulted from his presence rather than the criminal's intent. If a friend's car is broken into, we feel he was asking for it by leaving a camera on the front seat.

Society seems to be asking how it brought this state of affairs onto itself. We do not know how to begin looking for causes of violence in either societal structure or individuals' minds, which are inextricably intertwined. One of the public's positions that contributed to the demise of the UCLA violence center is that studying violent individuals will shift attention away from the class struggle and maldistribution of power, which many believe to be the real source of violence in the United States and other countries. Proponents of this view think that if society is reformed, violence will disappear. Louis Jolyon West, who has studied violence for 20 years and was one of the conference participants, believes that individuals who engage in violent behavior are generally not able to fit into a societal group and have been alienated from their own groups. He found that most people who commit acts of violence direct them toward people who are most like themselves: blacks murder blacks and whites murder whites. The two causal views of violence conflict: if the powerless commit violent acts because of their rage at the powerful, why do so many people kill others in their own social groups? Has the class system become so entrenched that we will not leave our own social group even to commit violence? One of the purposes of the UCLA violence center was to predict the kinds of people who would likely engage in violent acts, for example, potential child abusers or rapists. The theory was to engage them in therapy before they acted or to provide therapy to dissuade them from continuing their violence.

The opposition to the center reached a rather hysterical pitch with accusations of forced psychosurgery and drug treatment that turned people into zombies. The rational opposition to the center was based on the fact that its goals and purposes seemed vague and inconsistent. The target client population would likely have been society's disenfranchised, on whom so much experimenting has already been done, and there did not appear to be sufficient ethical controls built into the operation of the center.

Public pressure succeeded in blocking the UCLA center, which may or may not have been a wise choice, and we are still left with the problem of knowing little about the causes of violence, although we are well aware of its intensely negative effects. Society must answer the basic questions whether it *wants* to know what causes violence, and if answers can be determined, whether preventive action should be taken. Are there some things we are better off not knowing, such as the intricate workings of the human mind? If so, will we agree to pay the price that seems to be increasing with each passing year? Is the study of human behavior so dangerous in itself that it is better not to do it because adequate safeguards cannot be instituted?

Let us assume for the moment that violence in society has reached the point at which it is no longer tolerable and that federal funding for behavioral research has become readily available. Further assume that the research proves that certain groups of people are naturally more prone to violence than others and that particular environmental circumstances aggravate that natural proclivity. Will society be willing to subject these groups to genetic engineering in an effort to decrease the tendency to violence, to assure that their environments are the most favorable in view of what could happen if they are not, and to provide ongoing research and therapy at the taxpayer's expense in an effort to decrease the frequency of violent acts? How far into behavior control are we as a society willing to go to assure reasonable safety on the streets? The technology to turn all violent criminals into more or less docile people presently exists. This could be done relatively easily, although at great expense, by means of surgery or ESB. Each new act of violence, no matter how minor, could be dealt with in this way, and we would all breathe easier when we took the subway home late at night. The other extreme is to prevent anything from being done by imposing such stringent safeguards on research that new knowledge becomes impossible to obtain. If an effective compromise is to be reached, decisions must be made about what kinds of behavioral research will be permissible and the uses to which the results can be put.

In her book, *Woman on the Edge of Time*, Marge Piercy paints a vivid picture of life 200 years from now. There are no prisons, and acts of violence occur only rarely. When a person commits a violent crime, he atones by making reparations to the person or family he has hurt. He is marked for life by a tatoo on his hand. If he commits a second violent offense, he is executed. This society has decided that it will not tolerate violence and that those who choose violence will not be permitted to live. It is not concerned with the cause of violence but only with the acts themselves. Not only could truly malevolent people be executed, but also the violent retarded and those who do not understand the consequences of their behavior. The society would be calm and safe, but it would not be just.

In *Walden Two* B. F. Skinner depicts a utopia in which violence is unheard of not only because the society meets all the needs of individuals but also because behavioral engineering teaches people from infancy onward how to cope effectively with frustration.

The structure of American society today appears to foster violence, and one frequently wonders if this is the way we *want* to live. Have we chosen a violent life for ourselves, or have we become too passive to prevent it? How can present violent patterns of behavior be altered? Hoagland[20] believes that major forms of behavior control, such as psychosurgery or drugs, are one effective answer. He reports a study at Massachusetts General Hospital involving 200 people who suffered episodic losses of control. Sixty percent had been arrested for violent crimes; eight were murderers. Many had used an automobile to assault others. Twenty-five percent were found to have EEG disturbances characteristic of temporal lobe epilepsy. Hoagland is in favor of using ESB to treat these people and others whose violence can be traced to brain lesions.

Male sex hormones and genetic factors play a large role in violence. An extra Y chromosome is sometimes found in males who commit violent crimes, and it is well known that the castration of male animals decreases aggressive tendencies. Should all males be karyotyped at birth, or should we castrate every man who commits a violent act and turn him into a docile eunuch? Again, we might be safer, but would we be fair? If 25% of all violent crime could be prevented by destroying a part of the temporal lobe, would society be justified in doing so? An argument could be made that when a judge sentences a man to life imprisonment for murder, he does not seek informed consent from the man about to be imprisoned. Society has given the judge authority to deprive a person of liberty for certain acts. Why then is informed consent necessary to perform psychosurgery or ESB on a person who has committed a violent act? He too is being deprived of liberty, but he may end up freer than the prisoner and eventually more able to exist amiably in society. One wonders why society is permitted or permits itself to inflict some kinds of punishment but not others. It cannot be said that in all cases psychosurgery is worse than life imprisonment or that 5 years of using tranquilizers is worse than 20 years in a mental hospital without them. The point is that we do not know which punishments are worse than others, but society proceeds on the premise that it can distinguish between them. Further behavioral research may provide answers.

Behavior control is also related to social class. A certain behavior, for example, talking out loud with an imaginary person, may be considered merely eccentric in the upper class and crazy in the lower class. What is done about the behavior varies even more from class to class. The upper classes may do nothing, or if treatment is sought it is private, expensive, and discreet. If the behavior is so unacceptable that the person requires confinement or restraint, he is likely kept at home or placed in an institution with others of his class, and a great effort is made to treat him. The poor person's illness is treated publicly, as cheaply as possible, and with little thought given to his dignity. He is placed in a state mental hospital. This difference in reactions to unacceptable behavior is not surprising; it simply reflects the larger health care system and society in general. The situation will not change unless the entire structure of society changes.

Szasz[3] uses the caste system of the military as an analogy. An officer can order an enlisted man evaluated for psychiatric treatment (the fact that he requests it indicates that he has already made a negative judgment), but the enlisted man cannot order an officer to be examined no matter how bizarre his behavior is. In considering the issue of social class we can simply shrug our shoulders and say, "Life isn't fair," which may be the truth, or we can examine why certain behaviors are viewed and dealt with differently according to social class. That examination itself is likely to reveal some of the causes of unacceptable behavior.

The social control of unacceptable behavior involves several problems that can be summarized as follows:

1. Any treatment of criminal violence can be viewed as a political act and therefore should be dealt with only as permitted by society.
2. The causes of unacceptable or violent behavior remain unknown for the most part; therefore treatment is mostly guesswork and is in large measure ineffective.
3. Society maintains that it is uncomfortable with the present degree of violence but has established such strict sanctions against researching the causes of violence that it prohibits itself from changing present patterns; therefore perpetual conflict continues.
4. Accusations of racism, sexism, chauvinism, and elitism follow most suggestions that certain groups of people tend to engage in certain violent acts; again research is prohibited and the conflict continues.
5. The direction of most behavioral research is unknown and therefore frightening, and continued violence is also frightening. Society appears not to know which it fears most.
6. Moral problems in dealing with unacceptable behavior are so complex that it seems easier in many instances to ignore the problem of violence and retreat as far as possible from its center, thus creating an even wider social class chasm.

The conflict between personal liberty and social control remains at the heart of the issue, and unless some reasonable compromise is established, violence will probably continue to increase.

WHOSE BEHAVIOR SHOULD BE CONTROLLED?

Society now has the power to change the behavior of anyone it chooses. Who should be chosen? Should it be only those whose unacceptable behavior is caused by clearly demonstrable brain pathology or only those whose behavior is so disturbing to others that it cannot be tolerated by or absorbed into society? Why not change even normal behavior to make it more normal? Would not life be more pleasant and comfortable if we had fewer neuroses and never had any trouble with interpersonal relationships? Would we like a little computer to carry around so that when we are stuck in a traffic jam or find ourselves on the verge of an altercation we could push a button, calm down, and accept whatever aggravations life offered? There might indeed be fewer heart attacks, and our collective blood pressure would probably drop considerably, but so would the output of work that requires creative energy, pressure, and anxiety. Push the button only when snarled in traffic and never while composing music? Perhaps, but are we willing to risk the crossed signals that will inevitably occur?

There is, of course, no definitive answer to the question of whose behavior is so unacceptable that it should be changed. Even the psychiatric establishment is unable to agree who is mentally ill, who demonstrates unacceptable behavior for which society is to blame, and who is normal. A perfect example of this indecision is the attitude of the American Psychiatric Association toward homosexuality. For decades homosexuality was considered a serious mental illness, an inability to adapt to heterosexual functioning, although no one could agree about the cause of homosexuality. Homosexuals underwent a variety of forms of therapy from aversive conditioning (electric shocks to the genitals when the person became aroused by nude pictures of the same sex) to years of expensive and useless psychotherapy. Then several years ago after experiencing considerable pressure from gay activists and after arguing for years among themselves the APA voted to remove homosexuality from the roster of mental illness. Mental health by ballot! This example demonstrates the capriciousness of the mental health establishment and the political and social pressure on people who have been labeled sick but who do not feel sick and who generally function quite well in society. This kind of approval could be made with some other forms of behavior that are now considered abnormal or unacceptable, such as the alcoholic who remains sober on the job and creates no overt societal problem (drunk driving, creating a public nuisance, and so on), the person who chooses to dress in a way that is noticably different from others, or the person who has an elaborate hallucinatory life but does not share it with anyone else and can function well within the bounds of reality. Mental health is societally defined, and generally those who create the definitions have power to act on them.

There exists in theologic and philosophic thought a strong tradition about the inviolability of the human mind. Plato and Aristotle stressed wholeness of thought and were wary of tampering with mentation. Both Christian and Jewish theology focus on the rationality of the mind; without a fully functioning mind a person is not a total human being and is not eligible for membership in the moral community. It was also thought that unless one had full use of his mind, one could not be free to worship God and would thus be subject to the blandishments of the devil. Consequently those who were seen as insane were treated as heretics or heathens and sometimes even burned at the stake.

Medicine also has a strong religious tradition that urges some to act as their "brother's keeper" for others. As the medical profession grew more enlightened and began to function more on scientific knowledge than on false beliefs, the attitude toward those seen as less than rational changed. The medical establishment began to attempt to help rather than punish the mentally ill. The rationale behind the helping behavior may have changed, but the effect has remained fairly constant: some people in society "need" to have their behavior changed and others do not. The fact that they are now put into state hospitals rather than snake pits and are chemically tranquilized rather than chained to damp cement floors often makes only a superficial difference.

The decision to change or not change a person's behavior can be political as well as sociocultural. After Adolph Eichmann was captured in South America and before he was brought to trial in Israel, he was examined by a number of psychiatrists, all of whom publicly declared him sane, normal, and fit to stand trial. After his execution Gideon Hausner, then Attorney General of Israel, published reports that psychiatrists had found Eichmann to be murderously perverted.[21] To have judged him insane would not have been politically expedient, and the Israelis would not have permitted him to be treated or released.

Elements of unacceptable or "crazy" behavior are found in many brilliant or creative people. Beethoven flew into intolerable rages at the slightest provocation, Van Gogh mutilated himself, Michelangelo lusted after young boys in his studio, Tchaikovsky was so despondent that he deliberately gave himself cholera. All these people would not have been who they were had their behavior been controlled or changed. It is not possible to alter one behavior of a person without the risk of changing much of his personality and thus also altering his acceptable behavior.

Hoagland[20] reports the case of a 22-year-old daughter of a physician who had irresistible urges to attack people. Once she plunged a scissors into her nurse because she did not perform a request, and on another occasion she stabbed in the heart a woman who accidentally brushed against her in an elevator. She was subjected to ESB of the hypocampus, and her violent outbursts were controlled. What Hoagland neglects to mention (the case has been reported in several places) is that the young woman stopped playing the guitar and no longer engaged in intellectual discussions with others on the hospital ward. She had become a different person.

Can society justify changing someone's behavior? Who should be chosen for this change? Aspects of Richard Nixon's behavior may not have seemed mentally healthy, yet no one suggested that he be forced to undergo psychotherapy as a condition for remaining in office. George Patton demonstrated some of the characteristics of a megalomaniac, yet he was not relieved of command. Enough congressmen are alcoholics (although they usually do not admit it openly) to make one nervous about the way the country is governed. It often seems that decisions to change behavior, like so many other health care decisions, are made on the basis of political power or place in the sociocultural establishment. The poor and disenfranchised run a greater risk of being candidates for behavior change than do the wealthy and politically powerful.

Political and social liberty may be defined as the freedom from physical restraints and from having one's mind tampered with in any way. But liberty also means the freedom to use the fullness of one's mind and to have control over one's life. A man who roams the streets talking only to his thumb is at liberty to wander as he pleases, but he is not free. He is as much a prisoner of his delusions as any incarcerated person is physically held prisoner. Szasz and others who would not hospitalize or treat anyone who did not voluntarily seek treatment are indeed advocating physical liberty and perhaps mental and emotional freedom. The point is that one can never know whether treatment is refused freely and rationally or whether the person is not aware of the options open to him and the consequences of his choice. The catch of this situation is that by granting someone freedom we may be condemning him to a mental prison. Internal restraints can throttle the mind and spirit as surely as external restraints can bind the body.

SUMMARY

Acceptable behavior is what society defines it to be, and the definition is often subject to group moods and standards as well as cultural and societal values. Mental illness and deviant behavior are defined differently depending on the purposes for the definition. An attorney might define insanity or mental illness in a way that would not be agreeable to a psychiatrist, and an average person might not concur with either.

Mental illness is frequently defined as behavior that is disliked, misunderstood, or inconsistent with current social standards. Drawing a line between mental health and mental illness is almost impossible. Mental illness can also be seen as a defect in communication. Many people believe that there is no such thing as mental illness except in certain demonstrable instances of a chemical or electrical malfunction of the brain. Szasz and others believe that attaching a label of mental illness to a person automatically revokes his liberty to some degree and is almost always unjustified. Liberty can also be subverted by confusing moral values with health values, that is, by applying moral judgments to health behavior.

Behavior can be changed by a variety of means: (1) chemical interference with thought or emotional patterns, (2) electric shock to the entire brain or stimulation of various parts of the brain by selectively implanted electrodes, (3) surgical destruction of brain tissue (usually in the limbic system or in the temporal lobe) that is thought to be sufficiently diseased to cause unacceptable (usually violent) behavior, and (4) various forms of psychotherapy including verbal and nonverbal communication performed by professional and semiprofessional therapists.

Psychosurgery, which can be used as a paradigm of the ethical problems of behavior change, has had a somewhat checkered history and has both devoted proponents and opponents. With good reason people generally are in awe of and frightened by psychosurgery, and it has received a great deal of bad publicity in recent years, much of which accused neurosurgeons and psychiatrists of evil intentions. Almost nothing is known about the short- and long-term effects of psychosurgery; federal controls have made experimentation almost impossible. Thus it is likely that psychosurgery will remain in the gray area of behavior control.

There are several major ethical issues involved in behavior control. The first concerns who defines normal behavior and what that definition will be. Who is a mental health expert, and what standards should be placed on behavior? Another issue concerns whose goals should take precedence during behavior therapy—the client's, therapist's, or society's? If goals conflict, whose best interest will ultimately be served?

The issue of power and coercion poses another moral problem: the history of behavior control indicates that those with social and political power have elected to make behavioral choices for those who are in some way disenfranchised. Coercion has always been a strong factor, particularly in terms of involuntary commitment to mental hospitals for a usually indeterminate period.

More and more people are asking why behavior should be changed if the person does not wish it to be. Autonomy and paternalism come into conflict when behavior control is at issue. A person who is drugged or incarcerated has lost autonomy, but the paternalism of the state may be justified if he is deemed dangerous to others. The decision concerning when if ever it is legally and morally permissible to restrain another person is a hotly debated issue, particularly in view of the principles of informed consent. The act of changing behavior is not necessarily immoral, but a strong justification is needed, particularly if the person does not volunteer.

It is difficult to determine whether violent criminal behavior should be treated as evil or sick and whether such a person should be sent to prison or a mental hospital. Many of the decisions made involve political overtones and reflect the class system of society. Theoretically a person's ability to think is protected by the Constitution, but if he uses that capacity to engage in acts of violence, what legal and political protections should he be permitted to claim? The issues involve the degree of threat the person poses and whether he or others are likely to be harmed.

Other issues involved in behavior control concern the social class of people who get into trouble because of unacceptable behavior. Many believe that the social system itself causes and condones violent behavior and that unless society is reformed violence will continue to increase.

The issue of whose behavior should be controlled or changed must be addressed. Again, social class plays a role, as do sociocultural standards and values. Almost anyone's behavior can be changed or "improved," but *should* it be? On the other hand, a person who is the prisoner of his own delusions cannot be considered free; does society have an obligation to grant him a greater liberty of thought by changing his behavior?

REFERENCES

1. Szasz, Thomas: The insanity plea and the insanity verdict. In Wertz, Richard W.: Readings on ethical and social issues in biomedicine, Englewood Cliffs, N.J., 1973, Prentice-Hall, Inc.
2. Szasz, Thomas: The theology of medicine, Baton Rouge, 1977, Louisiana State University Press.
3. Szasz, Thomas: Law, liberty, and psychiatry, New York, 1963, Macmillan, Inc.
4. Mill, John Stuart: Utilitarianism, New York, 1962, The New American Library, Inc.
5. Skinner, B. F.: Beyond freedom and dignity, New York, 1971, Alfred A. Knopf, Inc.
6. Skinner, B. F.: Walden two, New York, 1976, Macmillan, Inc.
7. Dedek, John F.: Contemporary medical ethics, New York, 1975, Sheed & Ward, Inc.
8. Annas, George J.: Psychosurgery: procedural safeguards, Hastings Center Report 7(2):11, April 1977.
9. Mark, Vernon: The case for psychosurgery, Boston University Law Review 54(2):217-230, March 1974.
10. Chorover, Stephen L.: Psychosurgery: a neuropsychological perspective, Boston University Law Review 54(2):231, March 1974.
11. *Kaimowitz v. Department of Mental Health*, Civil No. 73-19434-AW, Circuit Court, Wayne County, Mich., July 10, 1973.
12. Mason, John R.: *Kaimowitz v. Department of Mental Health:* a right to be free from experimental psychosurgery, Boston University Law Review 54(2):301, March 1974.
13. Beauchamp, Tom L., and Childress, James F.: Principles of biomedical ethics, New York, 1979, Oxford University Press.
14. Dworkin, Gerald: Autonomy and behavior control, Hastings Center Report 6(1):24, February 1976.
15. Beauchamp, Tom L.: Paternalism and bio-behavioral control, The Monist 60(1), January 1977.
16. Shapiro, Michael H.: Legislating the control of behavior control, Southern California Law Review 47(2):240, February 1974.
17. Dershowitz, Alan M.: Psychiatry in the legal process: "a knife that cuts both ways," Judicature 51:370-377, May 1968.
18. Veatch, Robert M.: Case studies in medical ethics, Cambridge, Mass., 1977, Harvard University Press.
19. Researching violence: science, politics, and public controversy: proceedings of a conference spon-

sored by the UCLA Center for the Study and Reduction of Violence and the Hastings Center, Hastings Center Report 9(2): special supplement, April 1979.
20. Hoagland, Hudson: Biological considerations of aggression, violence and crowding. In Williams, Preston N., editor: Ethical issues in biology and medicine: proceedings of a symposium on the identity and dignity of man, Cambridge, Mass., 1973, Schenkman Publishing Co.
21. Szasz, Thomas: Ideology and insanity, New York, 1970, Doubleday & Co., Inc.

BIBLIOGRAPHY

Annas, George J.: Psychosurgery: procedural safeguards, Hastings Center Report 7(2)1:11-13, April 1977.

Beauchamp, Tom L.: Paternalism in Bio-behavioral control, The Monist 60(1), January 1977.

Beauchamp, Tom L., and Childress, James F.: Principles of biomedical ethics, New York, 1979, Oxford, University Press.

Bedau, Hugo Adam: Physical interventions to alter behavior in a punitive environment: some moral reflections on new technology, American Behavioral Scientist 18(5):657-678, May/June 1975.

Breggin, Peter R.: Lobotomies are still bad medicine, Medical Opinion 8(3):32-36, March 1972.

Chodoff, Paul: The case for involuntary hospitalization of the mentally ill, American Journal of Psychiatry 133(5):496-501, May 1976.

Chorover, Stephen L.: Psychosurgery: a neuropsychological perspective, Boston University Law Review 54(2):231, March 1974.

Dedek, John F.: Contemporary medical ethics, New York, 1975, Sheed & Ward, Inc.

Dershowitz, Alan M.: Psychiatry in the legal process: "a knife that cuts both ways," Judicature 51:370-377 May 1968.

Dworkin, Gerald: Autonomy and behavior control, Hastings Center Report 6(1):23-28, February 1976.

Hoagland, Hudson: Biological considerations of aggression, violence and crowding. In Williams, Preston N., editor: Ethical issues in biology and medicine: proceedings of a symposium on the identity and dignity of man, Cambridge, Mass., 1973, Schenkman Publishing Co., Inc.

In the service of the state: the psychiatrist as double agent: proceedings of a conference on conflicting loyalties, March 1977, Hastings Center Report 8(2): special supplement, April 1978.

Klerman, Gerald L.: Behavior control and the limits of reform, Hastings Center Report 5(4):40-45, August 1975.

London, Perry: Behavior control, New York, 1969, Harper & Row, Publishers, Inc.

Mark, Vernon H.: The case for psychosurgery, Boston University Law Review 54(2):217-230, March 1974.

Mark, Vernon H., and Neville, Robert: Brain surgery in aggressive epileptics, Journal of the American Medical Association 226:765-772, 1973.

Mason, John R.: *Kaimowitz v. Department of Mental Health:* a right to be free from experimental psychosurgery, Boston University Law Review 54(2):301, March 1974.

Michels, Robert: Ethical issues of psychological and psychotherapeutic means of behavior control, Hastings Center Report 3(2):11-13, April 1973.

Mill, John Stuart: Utilitarianism, New York, 1962, The New American Library, Inc.

Researching violence: science, politics, and public controversy: proceedings of a conference sponsored by the UCLA Center for the Study and Reduction of Violence and the Hastings Center, February 1978, Hastings Center Report 9(2): special supplement, April 1979.

Scoville, William Beecher: Only as a last resort, Hastings Center Report 3(1):2-4, February 1973.

Shapiro, Michael H.: Legislating the control of behavior control, Southern California Law Review 47(2):240, February 1974.

Silverman, Mervyn F., and Silverman, Deborah B.: Medical ethics and psychotropic drugs. In Visscher, Maurice B.: Human perspectives in medical ethics, Buffalo, 1972, Prometheus Books.

Skinner, B. F.: Beyond freedom and dignity, New York, 1971, Alfred A. Knopf, Inc.

Skinner, B. F.: Walden two, New York, 1976, Macmillan, Inc.

Szasz, Thomas: Law liberty and psychiatry, New York, 1963, Macmillan, Inc.

Szasz, Thomas: Ideology and insanity, New York, 1970, Doubleday & Co., Inc.

Szasz, Thomas: The insanity plea and the insanity verdict. In Wertz, Richard W.: Readings on ethical and social issues in biomedicine, Englewood Cliffs, N.J., 1973, Prentice-Hall, Inc.

Szasz, Thomas: The theology of medicine, Baton Rouge, 1977, Louisiana State University Press.

Vaux, Kenneth: Biomedical ethics, New York, 1974, Harper & Row, Publishers, Inc.

Veatch, Robert M.: Case studies in medical ethics, Cambridge, Mass., 1977, Harvard University Press.

Wertz, Richard W. Readings on ethical and social issues in biomedicine, Englewood Cliffs, N.J., 1973, Prentice-Hall, Inc.

9

Informed consent and human experimentation

HISTORY

Professor Carl Clausberg, physician of the woman's clinic at a hospital in Upper Silesia, established an experimental block at Auschwitz to perfect his proposed technique of sterilizing female prisoners. After having told them they were being artificially inseminated, he injected an irritant into their uteruses. He planned to sterilize a thousand women a day with this process.

Viktor Brack of the Fuhrer chancellery proposed the "cleanest" way of sterilizing both men and women. While standing at a counter filling out forms, prisoners would be unknowingly subjected to x-rays. He thought that 3000 to 4000 could be sterilized each day. Himmler proposed that millions of Jewish slave laborers at Auschwitz be prevented from reproducing before they were exterminated.[1]

Freezing experiments were carried out next. Prisoners were forced to stand naked out-of-doors from 9 to 14 hours in below-freezing temperatures. They were then "warmed up" in a variety of ways, including the use of the most obscene sadism, to see at what point they showed vital life signs. The victims either died in the tests or were killed immediately afterward. (One of the most prominent Nazi scientists who gave conceptual guidance to the tests was Dr. Hubertus Strughold. He came to the United States after the war to pioneer in the development of American space medicine.)*

August Hirt added to his collection of shrunken skulls by ordering those specimens he thought would look well in the collection. These people were put to death at Natzweiler and then delivered to Hirt for anatomic research.

SS doctors amputated bones and muscles from living prisoners for transplantation purposes. Cancer was introduced into subjects and the progress of their agonizing deaths recorded.[2]

Medical research on unsuspecting and nonconsenting human subjects did not begin with the Nazis, but in the history of the world no other group of people

---

*Excerpt from page 132 of Never to Forget: The Jews of the Holocaust, by Milton Meltzer, New York, 1975, Courtesy of Harper & Row, Publishers, Inc.

honed torture to such degree of scientific sophistication in the name of medical research. We must never forget what they did, why they did it, and how they gained the cooperation of tens of thousands of seemingly nonpolitical private citizens.

Experimentation has been going on since the ancient Greeks first became curious about the workings of the human body. In ancient Persia, in the Ptolemies' Egypt, in Italy during the Renaissance, and in almost every civilization since, including ours, condemned criminals have been used as subjects in scientific experiments. Hippocrates the Greek began studying neurologic and mental disease; Galen the Roman added experimentation to observation and began to formalize it about 1800 years ago. Vesalius in the 16th century dissected cadavers to disprove Galen's theory of blood circulation, and in 1628 William Harvey published the first measurements of blood volume and velocity.

In 1722 prisoners at Newgate Prison in England chose participation in experimental smallpox innoculations as an alternative to hanging. Davy in 1799 and Horace Wells in 1844 experimented on themselves with anesthesia. When Morton in 1846 conducted the first public demonstration of human anesthesia at the Massachusetts General Hospital, almost no experimentation had preceded it. Roentgen used radiology as a clinical tool after only a few weeks of experimentation. Thousands of women died of puerperal sepsis even though Semmelweiss had demonstrated rudimentary aseptic technique to colleagues.

In 1905 William Fletcher experimented on lunatics in an asylum at Kuala Lampur. He gave half of them plain rice to eat and the other half rice laced with Vitamin B. A significant number of the inmates eating the vitaminized rice were prevented from developing beriberi. It was an important nutritional discovery, but no thought was given to the rights of the subjects.

In 1908 President Roosevelt appointed a board to carry out human experiments with benzoic acid and saccharine. The group that protested most loudly about the morality of the experiment was antivivisectionists.[3]

One of the most famous examples of racism in research with complete disregard for the rights of subjects is the Tuskegee syphilis study.[4] Darwinian scientists in the United States provided a new rationale for racism by believing that blacks were essentially primitive people who could not be assimilated into a complex white industrialized society. They believed blacks could not be helped by education of any kind or by philanthropy and were doomed to degeneration. Many members of the medical profession supported these beliefs, frequently using differences in anatomy in an attempt to prove inferiority. They believed that blacks had insatiable sexual appetites and that black men had strong desires for white women. Dr. W. T. English at the turn of the century wrote that the gray matter of the Negro was about a thousand years behind the development of the white brain and that his sexual organs were overdeveloped.[4]

According to these physicians, lust and immorality, unstable families, and reversion to barbaric tendencies made blacks especially prone to venereal disease. One doctor estimated that over 50 percent of all Negroes over the age of twenty-five were syphilitic. Virtually free of disease as slaves, they were now overwhelmed by it, according to informed medical opinion. Moreover, doctors believed that treatment for venereal disease among blacks was impossible.*

This was the medical and social climate when the Tuskegee syphilis study began.

In 1929 the United States Public Health Service (USPHS) conducted studies in the rural South to determine the extent of syphilis. Macon County, Alabama, where Tuskegee is located, was found to have the highest syphilis rate. In 1932 Dr. Taliaferro Clark, Chief of the USPHS Venereal Disease Division, decided that the high rate of syphilis in Tuskegee merited attention. The Tuskegee study was regarded as a "study in nature" rather than an experiment because it was thought that since so many blacks had syphilis anyway, it would be an excellent opportunity to study the natural course of the disease. No formal protocol was written, but letters between Clark and his colleagues indicated that they primarily wanted to observe the effects of untreated syphilis on the "human economy." They also wished to prove that antisyphilitic treatment was unnecessary because many of the victims experienced a spontaneous cure and 70% of the remainder did not seem inconvenienced by the disease. The other 30% were acknowledged to be seriously affected and highly contagious. It was also acknowledged that syphilis could be treated (at that time with arsenic and bismuth), but the USPHS chose not to treat the men of Tuskegee.

The doctors who devised and directed the Tuskegee study accepted the mainstream assumptions regarding blacks and venereal disease. The premise that blacks, promiscuous and lustful, would not seek or continue treatment, shaped the study. A test of untreated syphilis seemed "natural" because the USPHS presumed the men would never be treated; the Tuskegee study made that a self-fulfilling prophesy.*

The design of the study called for male subjects between the ages of 25 and 60 who were diagnosed to have syphilis. Finding sufficient subjects proved more difficult than anticipated for several reasons: (1) men suspected the physical examination was for the military draft and refused to appear at the health center, (2) fewer men actually had syphilis than was originally thought, and (3) many men refused to participate without being offered treatment, which the USPHS eventually promised but did not provide. The men were not told they were participating in an experiment; they thought they were being treated for "bad blood," a southern colloquialism for syphilis, and were under the impression that their syphilis was being cured. The spinal tap that was part of the diagnosis was not explained beforehand; when it was performed, the subjects were told it was part of the treatment.

Originally designed to last 6 months, the study continued indefinitely so that the subjects could be followed until they died and the clinical effects of syphilis could be studied through autopsy. The subjects were not informed that they were to have a postmortem examination. Dr. Eugene Dibble, Director of the Tuskegee Institute Hospital joined the study so that the subjects could die in his hospital

---

*Brandt, Allan M.: Racism and research: the case of the Tuskegee syphilis study, Hastings Center Report 8(6):22, December 1978. Reprinted with permission of The Hastings Center,© Institute of Society, Ethics and the Life Sciences, 360 Broadway, Hastings-on-Hudson, N.Y. 10706

where they felt secure and trusting. During the entire 40-year period of the study the subjects were kept participating by various incentives such as ineffective "medicinals," transportation to the place of examination, hot meals, and the like. When men started to die of syphilis and others became suspicious and wanted to discontinue participation, the USPHS provided an incentive of $50 per man for burial expenses.

Articles about the study began to appear in the medical press in 1936, and over the years they grew increasingly hostile and critical, especially when it became known that the USPHS went to great lengths to ensure that the subjects did not receive treatment from another source. When several of the subjects were drafted in 1941, the USPHS sent the Army a list of 256 names of men who were not to be treated for syphilis; the Army complied. By the early 1950s many of the men had obtained treatment on their own, and by 1965 the study was still going on.

In July, 1972, when the first article about the study appeared in the national press, data were still being collected and autopsies performed. Finally the Department of Health, Education, and Welfare (DHEW) formed an ad hoc committee to respond to criticism in the press. The committee was concerned with three issues. (1) Was the study justified, and had the men given informed consent? (2) Should the subjects have been provided with penicillin when it became available? (3) Should the study now (in 1972) be terminated? The report was issued in June, 1973, and was filled with misinterpretations and misconceptions. The committee made the following points. (1) Failure to provide penicillin was the major ethical misjudgment. (2) It had been implied that no treatment for syphilis existed in 1932 even though medical authorities firmly believed that arsenic was an effective treatment. (3) The committee believed that the men of Tuskegee had volunteered for the study but acknowledged that informed consent was not obtained. The committee failed to place the report in a historic context, thus minimizing its racist aspects, and made no mention that the entire study was based on nontreatment and deceit of the subjects.

The committee's whitewash of 40 years of racism by the government and the continued defense by many who participated in the study gives one pause to wonder about professional self-regulation and the government's humanity. In the 35 years that the study was reported in the medical press, no hue and cry was raised; only reports in the public press started the wheels in motion that ended the study.

In retrospect the Tuskegee Study revealed more about the pathology of racism than it did about the pathology of syphilis; more about the nature of scientific inquiry than the nature of the disease process. The injustice committed by the experiment went well beyond the facts outlined in the press and the HEW *Final Report*. The degree of deception and damages have been seriously underestimated. As this history of the study suggests, the notion that science is a value-free discipline must be rejected. The need for greater vigilence in assessing the specific ways in which social values and attitudes affect professional behavior is clearly indicated.*

*Brandt, Allan M.: Racism and research: the case of the Tuskegee syphilis study, Hastings Center Report 8(6):22, December 1978. Reprinted with permission of The Hastings Center,© Institute of Society, Ethics and the Life Sciences, 360 Broadway, Hastings-on-Hudson, N.Y. 10706

The Tuskegee Study was carried out not by mad scientists like those one sees in old movies but by Americans at the behest of a branch of the federal government and with tax money. It was halted less than 10 years ago but may have continued if the press had remained silent.

Human experimentation existed in the United States long before the Tuskegee Study was initiated. Large-scale public health experiments in North America first began in 1718. The Reverend Cotton Mather of Boston knew that certain Africans recognized that smallpox scars meant they would never get the disease again and that sometimes Africans deliberately gave the disease to each other. Boston was ravaged by smallpox, and Mather wanted to try experiments (even though the word immunity was unknown to him, he had an inkling of the concept). No physician would consent to what was considered a very dangerous experiment, but Mather found Zabdiel Boylston, who though the son of a physician had no medical training of his own, who agreed to the experiment. Boylston innoculated his son first, who developed smallpox but recovered, and then went on to innoculate (not vaccinate) many others. The results of his work were published in London in 1726 and in Boston 4 years later. General Washington used the Boylston innoculation method in the Revolutionary Army; it thus paved the way for more sophisticated experiments. Though the experiments were hazardous and primitive, nowhere in Boylston's writings does he mention the ethics of how he conducted his research.[5]

Between Boylston's experiments and those of the Nazis are thousands of human beings who participated in medical research completely unaware or without fully understanding the procedure and consequences of the experiment. Some of the researchers had nothing but the most noble intent; some, like the Nazis, had nothing but the most evil. Most, like the vast majority of human beings, had mixed motives.

We concentrate on the Nazis because no human action before or since parallels that degree of evil, because we can use their action as a yardstick to measure the depths of depravity to which medical researchers can sink, and because the Nazi experience was a catalyst for change and a turning point in the way medical research is conducted. It marked the beginning of formal codes of ethics regarding the establishment of research protocols and experimental conduct. Most important, it raised the consciousness of the public about what human beings are capable of doing to each other in the name of medical science; it made the medical establishment more wary and pointed out the possibilities for evil in uncontrolled research.

This is not to say that every research experiment may end like those conducted at Auschwitz or Dachau unless the researchers are constantly watched but that the potential exists. Evil does not always result from evil motives. Reinhold Neibuhr said, "Not much evil is done by evil men. Most of the evil is done by good people who do not know they are not good." The Nazi experiments are frequently used as an analogy for all evil, and one encounters this analogy in bioethics literature. The analogy is often used to show what can happen when research goes too far, to warn of impending moral disaster, to impose guilt, to suggest the lesson of experience, and to question why many German scientists and physicians, people dedicated to the principle of nonmaleficence, participated in the horror. How could it have happened? How could these doctors who the year before had patted children on their heads in their offices have poured caustic substances into women's uteruses and listened to their shrieks of agony—and then do it again? How could they have cut off a man's leg while his mouth gaped and his eyes rolled and he watched his body being torn apart? Why did these physicians move so far from the humanitarian principles of their profession into depravity? Various theories have been postulated; the most common is that the physicians were afraid not to obey their Nazi superiors. That, however, cannot explain the extent of this evil. Will it happen again? How can it be prevented? This is why we study and analyze the Nazis, why we immerse ourselves in the pain of remembrance.

The Nazis committed atrocities out of a sense of principle; all that horror had a purpose. They believed that racially pure Aryans were destined to rule the world and that to accomplish this goal everyone else had to be exterminated. Continuous anti-Semitism in Germany over the centuries and its primary place in the German consciousness marked Jews as the logical place for Hitler to begin. He had no intention of stopping there; they were simply first on his list of non-Aryans destined for extinction. The "final solution" for Jews was only one part of Hitler's master plan for the world, which began with the 1939 invasion of Poland and was planned to continue to ultimate world dominance. Hitler and the Nazis believed in what they were doing—it is important to understand this point. Nazis used the word *euthanasia* in a context other than how we have come to understand it today; euthanasia to them was a code name for the mass murder of specific categories of non-Aryans, starting with deformed children and insane adults and proceeding from there.

Not all people agree that the study of the Nazi experience has a bearing on today's bioethical dilemmas. Lucy Dawidowicz, a historian of the holocaust, says,

I do not think we can usefully apply the Nazi experience to gain insight or clarity to help our problems and dilemmas. If we wish to draw generalizations and make analogies between the Nazi experience and our dilemmas, we must first be clear about basics. One: definition of terms. I have tried to show that what the Nazis meant by certain terms is not at all comparable to what we mean. Two: we must clarify the differences (or similarities) with regard to ends and goals. Three: we must compare (contrast) means as well as ends. Only then can we make comparisons or generalizations with sufficient intellectual rigor.*

The Nazis believed in an evil end, and thus the means they used to achieve the end were necessarily evil because one cannot use good means to achieve evil ends. But the converse is not necessarily true; evil means can be used to achieve a good end. Every scientist currently engaging in cancer research hopes he will find its cause and a cure; he believes his goal is good. It is possible, however, that the zeal to reach a good goal may encourage the use of evil means. A scientist is not nec-

---

*Biomedical ethics and the shadow of Nazism: a conference on the proper use of the Nazi analogy in ethical debate, April 1976, Hastings Center Report 6(4):Special Supplement, August 1976. Reprinted with permission of The Hastings Center, © Institute of Society, Ethics and the Life Sciences, 360 Broadway, Hastings-on-Hudson, N.Y. 10706

essarily evil though his actions might be. Milton Himmelfarb disagrees with Dawidowicz and believes we should study the Nazi experience.

I want to agonize about these things. Part of the agony should be the knowledge that there was indeed Nazism . . . Today we think of Nazis as representing a political thought which is remote from us. Yet Lord Francis Crick, the great Nobel Prize winner in genetics, has proposed that society may have to consider seriously that no neonate should be declared legally human until it is a few days old and has passed a genetic test. Disposing of an infant which fails that test would be different from killing a human being. Again, not that we should be quick to label everything Nazi, but that Nazism should complicate our thinking about such matters.*

Crick and James Watson won the Nobel Prize for their work in discovering the genetic role of DNA. Crick believes that the disposal of a genetically imperfect neonate is not the same as killing a human being. His goal of genetic perfection may be seen by some as good, but his means are evil. Can it begin again? Can it happen here? It can, and thus we must be careful that it does not.

Nuremberg trials

The Nuremberg medical trials took place as a result of evidence brought out at the major war crimes trials. Hermann Göring, an air force pilot who founded and headed the Gestapo, was implicated in Luftwaffe high-altitude experiments in which prisoners died.[6] This revelation led to others, and the examination of vast numbers of German documents and plans brought into focus the monstrousness of the whole episode. By 1946 when the general trials ended, Jewish refugees who were still wandering around Europe began to tell their stories. The documents and stories implicated many German physicians, 23 of whom were tried for war crimes. The trial charges read like a psychotic's nightmare[6]:

1. From March to August, 1942, at Dachau experimental subjects were placed in low-pressure chambers and subjected to a simulated high altitude. Many died or suffered great injury.
2. From August, 1942, until May, 1943, at Dachau prisoners were severely chilled or frozen by forcing them to remain in a tank of ice water for 3 hours or naked outdoors at below freezing temperatures.
3. From February, 1942, until April, 1945, at Dachau inmates were infected with malaria by mosquitos or by injections. The subjects were treated with various drugs to test their efficacy.
4. From July, 1942, until September, 1943, at Ravensbruck wounds were deliberately inflicted on prisoners, infected with *Streptococcus*, gas gangrene, and tetanus, and then aggravated by forcing ground glass or wood shavings into them. Blood vessels leading to the wound were tied off, and the wounds were then treated with sulfanilamide to test its effectiveness.

---

*Biomedical ethics and the shadow of Nazism: a conference on the proper use of the Nazi analogy in ethical debate, April 1976, Hastings Center Report 6(4):Special Supplement, August 1976. Reprinted with permission of The Hastings Center, © Institute of Society, Ethics and the Life Sciences, 360 Broadway, Hastings-on-Hudson, N.Y. 10706

5. From June, 1943, until January, 1945, at Sachanhausen and Natzweiler prisoners were infected with hepatitis to investigate innoculation procedures.
6. From December, 1941, until February, 1945, at Buchenwald and Natzweiler prisoners were injected with spotted fever virus to keep it alive.
7. In December, 1943, and October, 1944, at Buchenwald, poisons were secretly added to prisoners' food. Autopsies were later performed to determine the effect of the poison. Prisoners were often shot with poison bullets for the same purpose.

The Nuremberg prosecution was conducted by American lawyers, many of whom had recently graduated from law school and had little experience with the ethical issues presented. The prosecution was put together hastily, and the trial had a somewhat improvised and impromptu flavor. One of the most interesting and unusual aspects of the trial was that the defendants were given permission to question the American expert witnesses about the ethical standards for conducting research in American prisons. The German physician defendants were trying to prove that what they had done was not criminal but merely *different* from standard medical procedures. During the medical trial the prosecution wanted to know how respected members of the German medical community could have participated in the horror. The answer most frequently given concerned "defense of superior orders and duress": they did what they did because they were under military orders and would have suffered grave consequences if they had refused.

Most of the defendants were found guilty and sentenced to death or long prison terms. The verdicts acknowledged the guilt of those who tortured in the name of medical science. We will never know if the victims who lived found any satisfaction in knowing that their torturers were punished. The most significant result of the trials was the establishment of the Nuremberg Code, which defined moral, ethical, and legal concepts and set guidelines for conducting scientific research on human subjects. The 10 principles are as follows:

1. Voluntary consent of the human subject is absolutely essential. The person should have the legal capacity to give consent, and there should be exercise of free will with no element of force, fraud, or coercion. All the elements of informed consent must be present, and the duty for ascertaining the quality of consent rests with the individual who directs or conducts the experiment; it cannot be delegated.
2. The experiment must be designed to yield fruitful results for the good of society that are not procurable by other means and that are not random or unnecessary in nature.
3. The experiment should be based on the results of animal experimentation and on a knowledge of the natural course of the disease or problem. Anticipated results should justify performing the experiment.
4. The experiment should be conducted so as to avoid all unnecessary physical and mental harm.
5. No experiment should be conducted in which there is reason to believe that death or disabling injury will occur, except perhaps those in which the experimenting physicians also serve as subjects.

6. The degree of risk to be taken should never exceed the humanitarian importance of the problem to be solved.
7. Precautions should be taken to protect subjects from even a remote possibility of injury or death.
8. The experiment should be conducted only by scientifically qualified persons who demonstrate the highest degree of skill and care throughout all stages of the experiment.
9. During the course of the experiment the subject must always be at liberty to discontinue participation if he has reached a point beyond which continuation will be physically or mentally harmful.
10. The scientist in charge must be prepared to terminate the experiment at any stage if he has probable cause to believe that continuation will result in injury, disability, or death of a subject.

The Nuremberg Code is important because it was the first such effort to establish principles and guidelines for human experimentation. It serves as a basis for other codes of behavior in medical and scientific practice, but it has serious flaws. The most obvious and pervasive flaw is that it depends solely on the self-regulation and self-determination of the person carrying out the experiment. This is particularly evident in Article 1 about the duty of ascertaining the quality of informed consent. If this duty cannot be delegated, then the scientist has total control over the conduct of the experiment and the welfare of the subjects. The amount of control this gives the experimenter is ethically questionable.

The second weakness is the subjectivity of the code; its tone implies that as long as the scientist has good intentions, no harm will come to the subject. For example, what results are fruitful for the good of society? Who determines what knowledge will benefit society and by what process that knowledge should be achieved? The degree of risk is compared to the humanitarian importance, but comparisons of this type are difficult to make and are subject to wide interpretation and debate.

The third major flaw concerns the question of who monitors the scientist and passes judgment on his ethical judgment. According to the Nuremberg Code no one does, implying that the scientist has complete autonomy. One might point out that a professional is responsible for his own behavior and should be able to practice with autonomy, but the Nuremberg Code, which was established as a result of history's most flagrant abuse of professional autonomy, does not consider the possibility of uncontrolled professional behavior.

The code is, however, the beginning of a humanitarian consciousness about the rights of human subjects; it is the first step in protecting those rights.

GENERAL ETHICAL CONSIDERATIONS

Human experimentation involves two basic phenomena: observation of what occurs in nature and then alteration of some condition or variable to affect what occurs in nature. An experiment starts with a hypothesis about what will change if certain conditions are altered and then proceeds to test the hypothesis. All experiments involve some degree of risk, depending on the variables to be altered and the hypothesis to be tested. In the strictest sense of this concept every procedure carried out on a human can be considered an experiment. When a nurse goes into a client's room to take a rectal temperature, she is conducting a kind of experiment. She hypothesizes that his skin is warm and flushed because his body temperature is elevated. She seeks his consent for testing the hypothesis by asking him to ex- pose his buttocks. He gives consent by complying and permitting the nurse to insert the thermometer into his rectum. She warns him of possible risk by saying, "Don't roll over until I return." This is a rather elementary example of human experimentation compared to complicated double-blind studies of antimetabolic agents, but the client's body has been invaded and the principles are the same for that experiment as for pharmaceutical testing in which hundreds of people may risk their lives.

The justification for human experimentation rests on the premise that the med- ical and scientific community has an obligation to advance knowledge and to erad- icate or prevent disease and suffering. This can be done only by using the scientific process in the appropriate laboratory, the human body. Many human diseases can be studied to a degree in animals, but all useful knowledge comes from determin- ing how human beings are affected by disease and by intervention in the disease process. Human experimentation is basically a good and worthwhile pursuit and should not be discontinued. It must, however, be done only within certain pre- scribed humanitarian guidelines. I and many others believe that any societal good that may result from human experimentation in which subjects are deliberately made to suffer is not worth the price paid in human pain. No ultimate good, not even a cure for cancer, is worth what happened to the black men of Tuskegee or to Jews of Europe during World War II.

Although informed consent and research on specific groups of people will be discussed later, the general ethical principles can be enumerated here. The first is the principle of consent. When we speak of consent in human experimentation we assume it to mean informed, or understanding, consent. The subject alone has the right to grant or deny consent based on an explanation of the procedure and the known or suspected risks. In addition to this explanation, consent is made valid by the subject's assurance that the experimenter (1) has legitimate and justifiable ends in mind and is not conducting the experiment out of caprice or whim, (2) is well qualified, (3) will closely supervise the experiment even if he himself does not perform all the actual procedures, (4) has performed preliminary tests in vitro or on animals, and (5) is prepared to stop the experiment if unmanageable side effects develop.

The second principle is the determination of whether an experiment is purely experimental or is also therapeutic. In other words, can the subject himself expect to benefit from the research? This is a double-pronged issue. First, in double-blind experiments in which half the subjects receive a chemically active substance and the other half, chosen at random, receive a placebo, the latter group although un- aware of it at the time will receive no therapeutic benefit, whereas the former may benefit. Second, if a person has a condition that has no known treatment, or if the usual treatment has not been successful for this person, the physician may suggest experimental treatment. In a sense every treatment is a sort of experiment, but the matter of degree is important.

A third principle in human experimentation concerns what the medical and scientific community and the general public deem acceptable at any time. These two groups frequently differ on what they believe is acceptable. Moral climates change with varying political and economic moods and social values. It is less likely that the Tuskegee study could have been instituted today because "liberal" people are no longer willing to admit their racism publicly. The public now is hesitant about in vitro fertilization research, but in 20 years this may be as generally accepted as birth control research is today.

A fourth principle involves the security of and protection for subjects. Simply because an experimenter adheres to an ethical code, has the best and most humane intentions, and is possibly subject to peer review, subjects will not necessarily be protected from harm. Although the scientist is responsible for protecting the subjects to the greatest possible extent, subjects do participate on a voluntary basis and are responsible for volunteering in the first place and for withdrawing from the project if they choose.

The fifth principle, involving coercion, hinges on the fourth. It is safe to say that no participation in research involving human experimentation is 100% voluntary; some variety of coercion always exists to some degree. All coercion is not blatant. Sometimes it stems from the research subject himself, from his need to be relieved of disease or pain. It can come from the subject's desire to please his family. It may be vaguely societal in that the subject may feel a need to do something for humanity. Money or other forms of payment may be involved. The subject may see himself caught between two evils, for example, between serving out his entire prison sentence and participating in research in exchange for a shorter sentence. The researchers themselves may coerce subjects in a manner ranging from the very obvious to the very subtle.

Another issue concerns the ease with which volunteers and their consent are obtained. The experimenter needs some knowledge of his subjects and can and should require that they submit to verbal and physical examination. It would be useless for a researcher studying the effect of music on natural sleep patterns to have as a subject a person who routinely takes two Valiums every night and cannot sleep without them. A subject is not likely to volunteer for research that he does not believe in or thinks is useless, even if he understands the purpose and risks of the experiment. A woman who does not believe in artificial birth control would not be likely to wear an experimental intrauterine device.

There is also the problem of the overzealous volunteer who wants to sign the consent form without listening to or understanding the explanation and may make a "career" out of volunteering for human experimentation. This phenomenon is seen most frequently in research on psychotropic drugs and procedures. The problem of this kind of volunteer results in part from the blind faith of much of the American public in the scientific and medical community. The attitude that a physician will not do anything that is not good for one is prevalent in general and is potentially more serious when transferred to a researcher. This kind of childlike adoration and trust is often misplaced and always counterproductive. One of the ways in which nurses can participate meaningfully in human experimentation is to act as advocate for the subject to make certain that this attitude does not result in harm.

The essential philosophic argument about human experimentation concerns its justification. Any experiment will necessarily violate the privacy of one's body, but without experimentation medical and scientific progress would be considerably hampered, to the ultimate detriment of humankind. When is human experimentation justified, under what circumstances, and on whom?

These questions can be examined from a variety of perspectives. The first concerns the rights of the individual versus the common good. In some instances individual rights may be superseded by societal rights, especially in matters of safety and the common public good. Is human experimentation one of those instances? We have seen that voluntary participation is not always completely voluntary: thus one cannot say that the individual is not forced to give up his rights by participation because in some instances he may be. Is society ever justified in requiring that an individual participate in human experimentation? If one takes the position that at certain times an individual must give up his right to privacy by participating in human experimentation because he owes an obligation to society, then it follows that consent is not required. Consent, on the other hand, means that the individual, although not giving up all his rights, does give up the right of total privacy of his body (the researcher must touch, invade, and measure his body to conduct the experiment). Most people will not accept the premise that some individuals must volunteer their services in this way, because it is not consistent with the American concept of individual rights. There is a difference between a moral claim of society and a right of society to a certain good or benefit. A moral claim can be requested, and consent is required to meet the claim, but a right can be demanded without consent. This does not, however, solve the problem of determining when human experimentation is permissible.

Another view of the problem concerns sacrifice:

The primordial sacrificial situation is that of outright human sacrifice in early communities. These were no acts of blood-lust or gleeful savagery; they were the solemn execution of a supreme, sacral necessity. One of the fellowship of men had to die so that all could live, the earth is fertile, the cycle of nature renewed. The victim often was not a captured enemy, but a select member of the group. "The King must die." If there was cruelty here, it was not that of men, but that of the gods, or rather of the stern order of things, which was believed to exact that price for the bounty of life. To assure it for the community, and to assure it ever again, the awesome *quid pro quo* had to be paid ever again.*

We cringe at the thought of equating human experimentation in a hospital with decapitation of a sacrificial victim surrounded by members of the community chanting prayers. But philosophically and perhaps morally there may be little difference. Today's volunteers are not having their throats slit, but they are exposing them-

---

*Jonas, Hans: Philosophical reflections on experimenting with human subjects. In Wertz, Richard W.: Readings on ethical and social issues in biomedicine, Englewood Cliffs, N.J., 1973, Prentice-Hall, Inc., p. 19.

selves to danger and possible death for the good of the community and to assure the continuation of that community. In a very real sense they are offering themselves as human sacrifices.

Political theory, especially as it applies to democracy, provides a kind of circular social contract. The basic premise concerns the privacy of the individual who derives benefits from the public good. For the individual to obtain benefits, certain of his freedoms must be curtailed for his ultimate advantage. For example, my observance of traffic laws will help assure my own safety, and curtailment of an individual's right to move about will help protect my property from damage done by trespassers. There are, however, certain actions that fall outside this general obligation; for example, no one can be forced to die for the public good, certain private actions cannot be controlled or curtailed, and we cannot be forced to work except in stated emergencies such as war. By the same token we are obligated to do certain things to maintain the general good, such as educating our children, observing personal property laws, and conforming to certain safety restrictions (for example, having an automobile inspected or going through a metal detector before boarding an airplane). Human experimentation seems to fall somewhere between societal obligation and societal protection. What a subject can be asked to do and what benefits he can be expected to reap are delicately balanced. Health is generally considered to be a public good or benefit, and almost all of the technology that exists to protect and maintain health has come about at least partly through human experimentation.

The ethical considerations in human experimentation can also be viewed through examining pharmaceutical research. When animal studies have been completed, it must be determined that the drug is worth pursuing for human use. Are the potential benefits of the drug worth the experimental risks? Will an existing drug perform essentially the same function, or is the drug in question an entirely new or significantly better way to solve the problem? Many pharmaceutical companies manufacture similar products, particularly in the area of diuretics, antibiotics, and tranquilizers. In many instances the primary reason for the development of a drug is to capture a share of the huge market. If diuretic B is essentially the same as diuretic A, is it ethically correct for the manufacturer of diuretic B to request human volunteers to submit to experimentation that will not significantly alter society's knowledge of disease or provide a new way to cure it? What methods are ethically acceptable for a pharmaceutical company to use to achieve a profit?

An issue in testing drugs involves the amount of preclinical testing that is required. Before drugs are tested on humans, their toxic levels are established in animals (toxic levels include severe side effects as well as death). How many animals must be used, and how certain must researchers be before they begin human experimentation? How much can be known about the human reactions to a drug if animals are used for testing? This is a particularly crucial issue in psychotropic drugs, when human feelings and behavior are involved. If an overwrought cat becomes placid and docile as a result of an experimental drug, will a human being react the same way?

Once certain facts are established about the toxicity and metabolic effects of a drug, they must be applied to humans. Which ones? To use the sick who might benefit from the drug could skew the results of the experiment by introducing too many variables. To use it on healthy people would deprive the sick of possible benefits and might not give an accurate idea of how a specific disease reacts to the drug. Early human experimentation is the most dangerous because it involves establishing safe dosage levels and measuring metabolic activity and excretion rates. Should it be done on prisoners, volunteers recruited from the general population, people with a specific disease or their families, or medical or nursing students? What indications of the severity of a disease would justify the development of a new drug when there already is an acceptable treatment? No pharmacologic treatment is perfect, but guidelines must be established concerning what side effects will be tolerated before allowing the development of yet another drug. For example, most of the remedies on the market for treating the common cold contain antihistamines that produce drowsiness. This is not a serious side effect unless someone is harmed by it. If a factory worker cannot get his hand out of the way of a machine or if a person's eyelids droop as he is driving on the turnpike and he smashes into another car, the relatively minor side effect then produces a serious result. But would it be justified to engage in human experimentation to find a remedy without such a side effect to treat the common cold? By the same token is it ethical to trivialize the cold, a condition that causes discomfort to many and is enormously devastating to American industry in terms of days missed from work? Against what standard should a new drug be compared—an existing drug, a complete cure of the disease, or its degree of side effects? How much better does a new drug have to be in comparison to an existing one to justify human experimentation? How much good has to result? Will the attitude of the researcher affect how well the drug seems to work or the subject's reaction to it? All these questions require answers if pharmaceutical research is to conform to ethical standards.

RELIGIOUS VIEWS

The ancient Greeks and Romans viewed a person as dualistic: that is, they saw the mind and body as separate. Many philosophers held the body in low regard because they thought the soul resided in the mind, which was imprisoned by the body. Medical attention was given to the physical body only if it was thought that one's mind or soul could also be improved.

The Judeo-Christian view of the mind-body dyad is that it was created in God's image and that the mind expresses itself through the body. Thus both mind and body are equally important and should be prevented from suffering. Life is believed to be valuable and was created for a purpose; therefore some actions are obligatory to increase the value of human life. Although the Old Testament makes no specific reference to human experimentation, one could interpret the many instances of God's requirements for sacrifice as a demand to reduce suffering and improve the value of life.

The Catholic Church has given much thought to the subject of human experimentation. In 1952 Pope Pius XII expressed the view of the Church in "Moral Limits of Medical Research and Treatment" in which he examined the issue by using three principles.[3] The first principle, involving the interests of medical science, stated that knowledge and scientific research are not morally objectionable and in fact are in accord with the moral order. It does not, however, mean that every method used is moral or justified simply because it increases knowledge. Science is not the highest value to which all others are subordinated; therefore defined limits exist beyond which science cannot go before violating higher moral rules. The second principle, involving the interests of the patient as justification, revolves around the patient's or volunteer's right to place himself in jeopardy. Catholic belief holds that a person is not absolute master of his own body and soul and therefore cannot dispose of himself as he pleases. He can, however, allow parts of his body to be destroyed or mutilitated for the ultimate good of the whole. The Church states that a person has no right to subject himself to experiments that entail a serious risk of destruction. The researcher can use only those rights given to him by the subject, but the subject can give away only those rights he possesses in the first place. The third principle, involving the interests of the community as justification, is concerned with the view that the individual is subordinate to the community; individual good must be sacrificed for the common good. The Church believes that God intended community life to be a means of exchange of mutual needs among individuals and that it is not a separate entity in and of itself. The community does not possess a right to an individual's body and thus cannot exercise a right it does not have.

It is obvious that the application of new methods to living man must be preceded by research on cadavers or experimentation on animals. Sometimes, of course, this procedure is impossible, insufficient, or not feasible from a practical point of view. In such a case, medical research must work on its immediate object, the living man, in the interests of science, in the interests of the patient, and in the interests of the community. Nevertheless, the limitation established by moral principles must be borne in mind. One cannot ask that any danger or risk be excused before giving moral authorization to the use of new methods; that would exceed human possibilities and would paralyze serious scientific research, and not infrequently be to the detriment of the patient. In such cases, the weighing of the danger must be left to the judgment of the tried and competent physician.*

This position seems an effort to morally balance the needs of the scientific and general community and rights of the individual. Its most serious drawback is its reliance on the professional judgment of the physician or scientist.

Jewish law states that there is no higher commandment than the saving of a human life as long as that act does not involve murder, public idolatry, incest, or adultery. Any experiment designed to save life is permitted, as are those that are not expected to leave the subject harmed or in any way worse off than before. The care of people has a higher priority than pure science in Jewish ethics, and thus therapeutic research is more highly regarded than nontherapeutic. Controlled experiments in which the outcome is uncertain are a different matter; the permissibility of a given experiment is determined on an individual basis depending

---

*Beecher, Henry K.: Research and the individual: human studies, Boston, 1970, Little, Brown and Co. p. 196.

largely on the harm the subject might be expected to endure or the harm another person might suffer if the experiment were not conducted. An experimental drug might be used if the probability is that the person will be helped rather than harmed. Giving a placebo poses a more difficult problem. Jewish authority states that the Eighth Commandment, "Thou shalt not steal," includes the theft of knowledge from the person receiving the placebo. By the same token, however, if everyone receiving a placebo were informed of that fact, the results of the experiment would be skewed, giving an imperfect answer to the research question, and this also would be a theft of knowledge. Again, each case is decided individually.

INFORMED CONSENT
General components

Consent means agreement or approval and in the context of this chapter will always mean informed consent. In terms of human experimentation, the concept of informed consent means that the scientist or investigator will give the subject all the information he has about the purposes of the experiment, the uses to which it will be put, its value to society, and all present or possible risks. The problem with informed consent is that because it is impossible for the researcher to know everything about the experiment, the subject cannot give consent that is fully informed. The moral dilemma occurs not with the fact that the consent is only partially informed, for there is no solution for that, but with the balance between what the researcher knows and what the subject knows and understands.

Most subjects are not able to grasp every complex detail of an experiment, but on the other hand most are able to understand an explanation that is carefully and patiently translated into lay terms. The amount of information to be given poses a serious problem. If too much detail is presented, the subject may become confused and stop listening. He may then either withdraw from the experiment or sign the consent form because of embarrassment that he does not fully understand the explanation or simply to be done with the confusing discussion. It should be noted that this eventuality cannot occur if the subject is required to repeat the explanation in his own words—a fail-safe mechanism.

When is consent truly informed: that is, how much does the subject need to know before he can give consent? For example, if an experiment requires cardiac catheterization, must the subject know every single vessel of the route the plastic catheter travels or is it sufficient that he be told that a tube will be passed from his arm to his heart? Does he need to know the generic name of the dye that will be used and the number of persons who developed a reaction to the procedure and died during it? Does he also need to know the number of cardiac catheterizations that have ever been performed so that he can calculate the risk to him? At the University of Saskatchewan a student volunteered to participate in testing a new anesthetic, for which he was paid $50.[7] During the experiment he suffered a cardiac arrest, was unconscious for 4 days, and experienced a consequent decrease in memory and concentration. He sued and was awarded $22,500. The judges maintained that although he had been informed that a catheter would be inserted into his arm vein, the physicians had neglected to explain it would be advanced to his heart into a position in the pulmonary artery; thus informed consent had not been obtained.

Though this case occurred in Canada, DHEW used it as a basis for a formulation of guidelines for consent in the United States.[8] The necessary elements are as follows:

1. Fair explanation of the procedure to be followed, including identification of experimental methods
2. Description of attendant discomforts and risks
3. Description of the benefits to the subject that are expected
4. Disclosure of appropriate alternative procedures that might be advantageous to the subject
5. Offer to answer any inquiries concerning the procedure
6. Instruction that the subject is free to withdraw consent and discontinue participation in the project at any time

In addition the consent form should not contain any exculpatory language or statements through which the subject waives or appears to waive any legal right or releases the institution or its agents from liability for negligence.

Omissions are evident in this list. First, the explanation should be given in terms the subject can be expected to understand. Even the most intelligent and informed lay person cannot be expected to know technical jargon used by most health professionals, and it is often difficult for a person to admit he does not know what the physician or scientist is talking about. Second, provision must be made to ensure that the subject understands what he has been told. The fact that one signs his name to a consent form does not mean the consent is informed. If a mechanism were instituted whereby it could be made absolutely certain that the subject understands all the terms and ramifications of the experiment, this problem could be eliminated. There is also no provision to prevent subjects from giving consent while undergoing emotional or physical stress. Moreover, the subject has a right to know why the experiment is being conducted and what the researcher's personal stake is in the experiment because this information could affect his willingness to participate. For example, if the purpose of the experiment is to test the efficacy of a new oral agent for the treatment of diabetes, a prospective subject may be particularly anxious to participate if he has a family history of diabetes. If he is told that the experiment is designed to test people's chemical reactions to stressful situations (intense heat and humidity, for example), he might see no useful purpose and refuse to participate.

The problem of necessary deception frequently arises in experiments, usually in the context of double-blind studies. An experiment funded by Syntex Laboratories and the United States Agency for International Development was conducted at a San Antonio clinic, to determine whether the reported side effects of birth control pills were mainly psychologic or actually physiologic.[9] Most of the subjects were poor Mexican-American women who had come to the clinic for contraception. Half the women were given birth control pills and half placebos, although all were instructed also to use a vaginal spermicidal cream in case the pill was ineffective. Ten of the 76 women (13%) who were given placebos became pregnant. None of the women had been told about the research or that she might receive a placebo. The women were obviously deceived, but because of the nature of the experiment full disclosure would have rendered the results useless. What could have been done to solve this problem? Could some information have been given though not enough to destroy the experiment? For instance, the women could have been told that the pill was being tested for its efficacy, which was in doubt, and that therefore they should be certain to use the spermicide to provide added protection. This also is deception, but it is not quite as blatant. If the women had been told that there was a strong possibility of becoming pregnant even though they were taking the pill, many might have refused to participate. Offering to pay for an abortion or to support the child if pregnancy occurred would not have solved the problem because the women had come to the clinic to prevent pregnancy and had every reason to believe they were doing so. If deception is thought necessary for success of an experiment, should it be cancelled? What if the anticipated knowledge will improve or enhance health? Which is more important, and how much deceit is permissible in informed consent if the consent is not to become totally invalid?

Are there arguments against informed consent? Lasagna[10] thinks there might be. A person in the terminal phase of illness might not benefit from a frank discussion of an experimental drug, although one wonders why the dying should be singled out in this manner. The investigation of psychotropic drugs poses a special problem because being fully informed may affect the way the subject reacts to the drug and his relationship with the attending physician. If absolutely candid explanations were given to subjects about every detail of the experiment, it is likely that fewer subjects would consent, because

there are some experiments which lose their entire point if all the cards are laid on the table. Take, for example, the investigation of the impact of a placebo. Although some patients report benefits from placebos even when they are told they are receiving "sugar pills," the full power of suggestibility and the patient-doctor relationship would almost certainly be affected by a discussion of the experiment with the subjects. This would be the medical equivalent of "bugging" a jury room to study the jurors' deliberations and then showing the jury the hidden microphones.*

Beauchamp and Childress[11] describe a case that exemplifies flagrant disregard for subjects' rights, although this case involved social and psychologic research and was more observational than participatory. The investigator, Laud Humphreys, believed that the public in general and law enforcement authorities in particular held many erroneous stereotypes about male homosexuals and their behavior in public places, particularly bathrooms ("tearooms"). He thought it would be beneficial to discover why some men found quick impersonal sexual encounters in tearooms gratifying. As research for his doctoral dissertation at Washington University (published in 1970 as *The Tearoom Trade: Impersonal Sex in Public Places*) he stationed himself in various tearooms and offered his services as "watchqueen," the person who keeps an eye out for police. He was thus able to watch hundreds of acts of

---

*Lasagna, Louis: Some ethical problems in clinical investigation. In Hunt, Robert, and Arras, John, editors: Ethical issues in modern medicine, Palo Alto, Calif., 1977, Mayfield Publishing Co., p. 309.

fellatio, and eventually he gained the confidence of some of the regulars. To them he disclosed his role as scientist, and he persuaded many of them to talk about their motivations for tearoom sex and about their lives in general.

In other instances he was not so open. He secretly followed some of the men out of the tearoom, copied their car license numbers, and thus learned their names and addresses. A year later he went in disguise to the men's homes claiming to be a health services interviewer and questioned them about their lives, jobs, marriages, and so on. His findings were extremely interesting and important in that they destroyed some widely held stereotypes. He found that more than half the subjects were married, living with their wives, and leading generally exemplary lives. Of all the men, 38% were neither bisexual nor homosexual but had marriages characterized by tension and rare conjugal sex. These men wanted sex without emotional entanglements and without jeopardizing their positions as fathers and respected community members. They also sought something less lonely than masturbation. A second group, 24% of all the men, were bisexual, happily married, well educated, and economically successful. Another 24% were single and covertly homosexual, and only 14% were openly homosexual.

Although the study persuaded many police to stop harrassing homosexuals in tearooms and increased society's knowledge about homosexual behavior, informed consent was not obtained from the subjects. They did not know they were participating in a research study, and their identities became known, though they were not published, through less than ethical means. The research proposal had been reviewed only by members of Humphreys' dissertation committee, and when the rest of the sociology department found out, a furor erupted. After the study was published there was considerable public outrage about Humphreys' unethical conduct, and many people speculated how individuals' privacy could be protected from social scientists and psychologists who study behavior for a variety of legitimate academic and social reasons but who fail to seek consent from their subjects.

Freedom with which consent is given

Internal and external constraints affect the freedom with which people give consent. A study at Harvard Medical School revealed that over 60% of all experimental volunteers were diagnosed as seriously maladjusted in adapting to their social environments.[7] Whether one is maladjusted or has difficulty adaptating is admittedly open to interpretation that is often culturally influenced; in fact the subjects may have been volunteering freely with no internal constraints, but it seems incumbent on the investigator at least to make a cursory examination of the volunteer's motives before accepting him as a subject, especially if the experiment involves procedures or drugs that have a psychotropic effect. Many volunteers, such as those in prison, the military, or other institutions, participate because of external constraints. The special problems with these volunteers will be discussed more fully later. Jonas[12] proposes a "rule of descending order": the less knowledge, motivation, and freedom of decision a person has, the further down the list of available human subjects for experimentation he should be. A scientist or college professor should be chosen as a subject before a prisoner or a mentally retarded person. This is the opposite of the social utility standard that the more expendable a person is to society, the sooner he should be chosen as a research subject. In this view convicted murderers and the hopelessly insane should head the list.

Should the dying be used as research subjects? One might think they could make a valuable contribution to science if only because they have less to lose if the experiment goes awry or if they react negatively to it. A researcher might feel entitled to use a dying person and thus might put considerable pressure on a person to volunteer as a last gift to humanity. This is exploitation in its purest sense, taking advantage of a person's vulnerability. There is in addition the practical consideration that bodies of the dying are frequently so debilitated by disease that their physiology would not respond to an experimental substance the way a more healthy person's might, thus rendering the experiment ineffective.

Other groups of people are also especially vulnerable in terms of medical experimentation. For this reason women in labor may not be asked to participate in experiments unless they have consented prior to the onset of labor. But there is no automatic protection for clients who are poor and uneducated (and often receiving public health care) and who are more likely to be experimental subjects because they are relatively unsophisticated and tend to be intimidated by the system. It is a primary nursing responsibility to determine whether a client is especially vulnerable in this way, to assess the risk to the individual, and then to take steps to protect the client's rights.

Double-blind studies

The principle governing a double-blind study is simple and statistically logical. By random selections half the subjects are given the experimental substance, the other half are given a placebo, and the results are compared. The term "double-blind" means that neither the researcher nor the subjects know who receives the chemically active substance and who the placebo. Double-blind studies result in greater accuracy than those in which the experimenter knows which are the treated subjects because the results are less skewed by psychologic and physical variables and personal biases are eliminated.

The procedure is almost perfect in theory and works well in practice, but it is fraught with ethical problems. The following example illustrates some of those problems. The National Institute of Allergy and Infectious Diseases (NIAID) reported in August, 1977, that adenine arabinoside (ara-A) had been found effective in the treatment of herpes simplex viral encephalitis, an extremely severe and virulent disease that has a mortality of 70%.[13] Of the 30% who survive many are left with severe neurologic aftereffects and frequently require institutionalization. The symptoms begin quickly and violently; it is a particularly vicious disease that can be diagnosed definitively only by brain biopsy. Ara-A had been found effective with other forms of herpes simplex infections. The 1977 project, conducted at 22 institutions and coordinated at the University of Alabama at Birmingham, was designed as a typical double-blind study. Biopsy of the brain was performed on 28 patients with the disease. Ten patients were given placebos, and the other 18 received ara-A; both drug and placebo were administered intravenously for 10 days. Of the 18 people treated with the drug 5 (27.8%) died, 7 (38.9%) recovered to lead reasonably normal lives, and 6 (33.3%) had serious neurologic damage. Of the 10 who received the placebo 7 died, and only 2 recovered sufficiently to lead a normal life.

The ethical dilemma involved in this study concerns whether the researchers were justified in giving placebos to 10 people who suffered from such a serious disease. Since no other known treatment existed for viral encephalitis, giving only a placebo could be seen as harmful or even as a cause of death. Some diseases, because there is no treatment, follow a predictable pattern, usually ending in death. This is true of human rabies, reticulum cell sarcoma, and others, including viral encephalitis. Since the patients receiving placebos could be counted on to die at the rate of 70%, why were they given *only* a placebo? Why was the study designed in part to prove what was already established, that 70% would die? Could not those 10 people have been given a different dosage of ara-A or a combination of the drug and another experimental treatment? The 10 patients who received only placebos could be compared with the men of Tuskegee. One reason for a double-blind study is to test the toxicity of a substance. Since ara-A had already been proved to be relatively safe (previous studies had been done on herpes simplex infections in newborns), the study again seemed designed to prove what was already known.

There appears then to be little if any ethical justification for use of the randomized clinical trials in this study. Since standard care of herpes encephalitis patients results in death 70% of the time, ara-A, already proven relatively safe, should have been administered to all patients involved in the study. Historical controls should have been used to determine whether or not the drug was effective. In fact, some patients who could have been saved were allowed to die in the process of gathering data which could have been generated by a methodology that might have proved more cumbersome and time-consuming, but would have incurred fewer fatalities in its outcome.*

The placebo plays an important role in the double-blind study; it is a substance with interesting effects. Because it is chemically inert, commonly referred to as a sugar pill, its clinical effect results from the faith and belief of the person taking it. In some studies the placebo was half as effective as the active substance to which it was being compared when it was used to control pain.[14] An imaginary drug controlled real pain.

Placebos have been used since the time of Hippocrates and Galen; they figure prominently in the practice of folk medicine. The placebo effect in large measure results from faith, suggestibility, or some other nonphysical phenomenon, but these are not the only factors involved in controlling pain. Beecher[3] reported that two thirds of the soldiers he observed on Anzio beach during World War II refused pain medication for very severe wounds. He later observed patients with similar wounds in civilian hospitals who required large doses of painkillers. He theorized that the soldiers on the beach were occupied with other thoughts, such as thank-

---

*McCartney, James J.: Encephalitis and ara-A: an ethical case study, Hastings Center Report 8(6):6, December 1978. Reprinted with permission of The Hastings Center, © Institute of Society, Ethics and the Life Sciences, 360 Broadway, Hastings-on-Hudson, N.Y. 10706.

fulness or euphoria about being alive and relief at being removed from combat. The soldiers in the hospital, on the other hand, had time to think about their wounds and the consequences of them. Perhaps it is not only the existence of a condition that causes pain but also its meaning.

RESEARCH ON SPECIFIC GROUPS OF PEOPLE

If the Tuskegee Study is the most famous case involving informed consent, the Willowbrook experiment is the most famous regarding human experimentation on a group of people who are especially vulnerable.[8] The principles and ethical issues in this case can be easily transferred to many groups of vulnerable people.

Willowbrook State Hospital in Staten Island, New York, is an institution for the mentally retarded that in 1972 held 5200 residents, 3800 of whom had IQs of less than 20. In 1954 Dr. Saul Krugman was appointed pediatric consultant and noted that infectious diseases, especially measles and hepatitis, were prevalent at Willowbrook. From 1956 until 1970 Dr. Krugman and his colleagues conducted studies on hepatitis. Four times a year they admitted 12 to 15 children to their research unit, for a total of 700 to 800 children from the 10,000 hospital admissions during that period. The researchers injected live hepatitis serum into the subjects to produce the disease. The objective was to understand the disease better and possibly develop new methods of immunization.

The research was funded and approved by the Armed Forces Epidemiological Board, the Committee on Human Experimentation of New York University, and the New York State Department of Mental Hygiene. The researchers defended their decision to deliberately infect mentally retarded children with hepatitis on the following grounds: (1) the children were bound to be exposed to the same strains of the disease in the natural conditions (overcrowded and with poor sanitation) of the hospital, (2) they would be admitted to a special unit that was well equipped and isolated from exposure to the many other infectious diseases at Willowbrook, (3) after deliberate injection of the hepatitis serum they were likely to have a subclinical infection followed by immunity to that particular strain of hepatitis, and (4) only children whose parents gave informed consent would be included.

If those reasons to engage in the Willowbrook experiment sound like hollow rationalizations, they are. The ethical issues are numerous and serious. If the researchers thought that the subjects were bound to be exposed to hepatitis or other infectious diseases merely by living at Willowbrook, why were funds not diverted to clean up Willowbrook and establish an environment that would be less conducive to transmission of disease? How would a mentally competent person react if a researcher said, "You're going to die of something sooner or later anyway, so why don't I just infect these cancer cells into your body and give you only a *little* cancer. I promise to take good care of you during your illness." That kind of logic was used on the parents of the Willowbrook subjects.

If the subjects were admitted to a clean, well-lighted place, could it be said that the other thousands of Willowbrook residents were denied that basic standard of hospital care? Why were they living in such wretched conditions? Three institutions gave their approval for and funded the experiment, but no mechanism existed for an ongoing review. The very nature of these experimental subjects—the facts that they were children, were mentally retarded, and were institutionalized—made them especially vulnerable. The approval and review procedure should have been particularly rigorous in light of these special circumstances. One wonders about the way consent was requested and given. Was there a degree of coercion in the fact that research subjects were to be better treated than the other Willowbrook residents? Did parents who put their children into Willowbrook feel guilt, especially in view of the abominable conditions at Willowbrook in the 1950s and 1960s, and did this guilt influence their decision to give consent? One can hardly think that it would not.

There is no doubt that the research subjects received better care than other Willowbrook residents, and it is quite likely that they received some personal benefit such as better treatment of hepatitis and immunity to that strain of the disease. But whatever benefit accrued them resulted from their isolation from the substandard conditions of the institution. The justification for the experiment would have collapsed had Willowbrook not been such a deplorable place. Recruiting volunteers because the alternative to volunteering is more negative than the risk of being a subject is also unethical because it is based on a choice between two evils. Having to volunteer to receive decent care is being coerced as surely as the men of Tuskegee were coerced.

What might have been the alternatives to the Willowbrook experiment? Although the available research funds might not have benefitted all Willowbrook residents, surely a greater number could have been helped by meeting the primary health needs of the entire institutional population. If a researcher finds that his subjects are volunteering only to improve or escape the conditions in which they are living, does he have a moral obligation to first improve those conditions before continuing his experiment? Should Dr. Krugman and his associates have cleaned up Willowbrook, observed the effect this had on the incidence and prevalence of infectious disease, and then reevaluated need for the experiment?

One might argue from a morally rigorous position that there is always a duty to alleviate social conditions producing suffering when one has the skill and is directly involved in a relationship with those suffering. This view is "rigorous" in that it has a utopian quality. Everyone would certainly be better off if all in such positions throughout the world indeed fulfilled their obligation, but in a less than utopian world there will always be those in need for whom research on, say, hepatitis immunization might, once developed, relieve much suffering. A rigorous moral position might lead to the conclusion that it is impossible ever to develop drugs to treat a socially caused disease, just as research on a "clean" nuclear bomb might be considered inherently unacceptable.*

Another position is that participation in a research experiment by vulnerable volunteers can be seen as a kind of moral trade off. One sees this frequently in prisons where prisoners are given privileges such as cigarettes, better food, and even time off their sentences in exchange for their participation. In a capitalistic society based essentially on the barter system, this might seem a natural or morally

---

*Veatch, Robert M.: Case Studies in medical ethics, Cambridge, 1977, Harvard University Press, p. 277.

acceptable position. It does, however, suggest coerced individual sacrifice for the good of the whole, a position that is morally debatable. The Willowbrook researchers and other like them try to create a rational balance between kinds of evil, between social conditions that are evil and an intentional personal risk of harm that may be equally evil in degree if not in kind.

Children

The National Commission for the Protection of Human Subjects of Biomedical and Behavioral Research (hereinafter referred to as the Commission) was established in 1974 to establish guidelines to protect vulnerable people as they became subjects for human experimentation. Children were included partially as a result of the Willowbrook experiment.[15] With regard to informed consent and children the Commission sought to determine (1) that the information given to parents or guardians before consent was obtained was adequate and (2) that the person who actually gave consent met at least minimal standards of competence. Before the Commission made its recommendations to Congress, it surveyed institutional review board practices for research on children, visited a school for the retarded, and sponsored a national conference to engender debate on the subject. Recommendations were sent to the Secretary of DHEW in September, 1977. The following is a summary[15]:

1. Research on children is important and can be conducted subject to the conditions set forth in these recommendations.
2. Research on children may be conducted provided that it is scientifically sound, that prior research is done on animals and adults, that risk is minimized wherever possilbe, that provision is made to protect the privacy and confidentiality of the children and their parents, and that subjects are selected in an equitable manner.
3. Research that involves more than minimal risk may be conducted provided that the risk is justified by an anticipated benefit for the subject, that the relative risk is at least as favorable as alternative approaches, and that consent is given by the children if possible and their parents.
4. Research that involves more than minimal risk and does not hold a prospect of direct benefit for the subject may be conducted provided that such risk represents a minor increase over minimal risk, that the results should lead to generalizable knowledge about the subject's disease or condition, that the anticipated knowledge is of vital importance to ameliorate the subject's condition, and that consent is given.
5. Research that cannot be approved under the preceding recommendations may be conducted provided that it presents an opportunity to understand, prevent, or alleviate a serious problem affecting the health of children, that a national ethical advisory board has reviewed the proposal and determined that it would not violate respect for persons or the principles of beneficence and justice, and that consent is given.
6. All research must be preceded by informed consent of the children if possible and their parents or guardians. In addition, at least one parent or guardian should be involved in the conduct of the research. A child's refusal to

participate is binding unless it can be shown that he will receive a direct benefit from the research that is available only by participation in the research.

7. Parental consent may be waived if it is not reasonably required to protect the subjects. There must be an alternate mechanism for protecting the children depending on the nature of the research protocol.

8. Children who are wards of the state should not be included in the research unless it is related to their status as orphan, abandoned child, and so on or unless it is conducted in a group setting in which a majority of the children subjects are not wards of the state. An advocate for each child subject must be appointed and given the same power to intercede as is provided to parents.

9. Institutionalized children may participate only if all other conditions regarding research on institutionalized people are met.

One of the crucial issues in the Commission's deliberations involved establishing mechanisms of protection for those unable to protect themselves rather than assuring informed consent to protect the autonomy of the child, since a child is not legally autonomous. Another issue involved the concept of the family as a social unit and the right of parents to make decisions on behalf of their children. Some believed that the entire family should be required to participate in the research as a protective measure for the child; others pointed out that because parents make other potentially risky decisions for their children (for example, allowing them to participate in contact sports), they should be permitted to decide about research. Even though children are not legally autonomous, the Commission recognized that as they grow older they do develop autonomy, and this is the reason why children over age 7 must themselves give consent and why their veto in participation in research must be viewed as binding.

The Commission had difficulty applying the principle of beneficence, including nonmaleficence, to research on children. One problem lay in differentiating between therapeutic (directly benefitting the individual) and nontherapeutic research. The Commission decided not to use these terms and instead to spell out precisely what was meant by benefit to the subject. The result is recommendations that are very specific but also cumbersome and perhaps confusing. Defining minimal risk also posed a problem. One proposed definition was that the research should involve no more than "mere inconvenience," and another was that the child should not be exposed to risks any greater than he would normally encounter in his daily life. The latter definition was adopted, but it involves an unmeasurable risk and is proving to be far too subjective to be of much practical use.

The Commission also had to grapple with the principle of justice when dealing with equitable selection of subjects. The burdens as well as the benefits of research had to be distributed to all segments of society, thus preventing another Willowbrook experiment. Sick children could not be put into a morally separate class even if they might be used to increase medical knowledge and might in some instances be ideal subjects; it would be unjust to single them out.

The Commission never agreed what should be considered "slightly more than minimal risk"; perhaps sick children or those who had social or nutritional deficiencies could be placed in that category. Minimal risk need not be defined solely in terms of the research procedure; the same procedure performed on different individuals may entail a different degree of risk.

On July 21, 1978, DHEW adopted the Commission's guidelines with three exceptions: (1) a child's objection to participation will not be held as binding, (2) no specific age should be set for a child's consent to be mandatory, and (3) the Secretary may appoint an ad hoc panel rather than a national commission to consider difficult proposals. These three exceptions drastically weaken the guidelines and defeat some of their purposes, especially regarding the consent of children.

Ethics of experimenting on children. Ramsey has a particularly negative view of children as subjects in nontherapeutic research.

From consent as a canon of loyalty in medical practice it follows that children, who cannot give a mature and informed consent, or adult incompetents, should not be made the subjects of medical experimentation unless, other remedies having failed to relieve their grave illness, it is reasonable to believe that the administration of a drug as yet untested or insufficiently tested on human beings, or the performance of an untried operation may further the patient's own recovery.*

In Ramsey's position the relationship between a proposed procedure and the child's benefit is crucial, especially as the experimental procedure is compared to other methods that could or should be used. The judgment about likely benefits tends to be subjective at best because it is based on what the researcher believes will occur. When the child cannot benefit from the experiment, he should not be made a subject regardless of how much good will accrue to society at large or to other children. Ramsey thinks that nonadherence to this moral rule constitutes a "sanitized form of barbarism" and is a break of faith between the researchers and the sick or dying child. He also finds fault with the concept of parental consent.

To attempt to consent for a child to be made an experimental subject is to treat that child as not a child. It is to treat him as if he were an adult person who has consented to become a joint adventurer in the common cause of medical research. If the grounds for this are alleged to be the presumptive or implied consent of the child, that must simply be characterized as a violent and false presumption. Nontherapeutic, nondiagnostic experimentation involving human subjects must be based on true consent if it is to proceed as a human enterprise. No child or adult incompetent can choose to become a participating member of medical undertakings, and no one else on earth should decide to subject these people to investigations having no relation to their own treatment. This is a canon of loyalty to them.*

Ramsey's view differs sharply from that of the Commission that permits or even encourages experimentation on children. Which view is morally correct? If one follows Ramsey's reasoning, no nontherapeutic research on children would ever be done. Only therapeutic research would be allowed because the subject child must

---

*Ramsey, Paul: The patient as person, New Haven, Conn., 1970, Yale University Press, pp. 11-12, 14.

benefit directly from the research. There are, however, some instances in which it would be impractical or impossible not to use healthy children as research subjects, particularly in experiments dealing with primary health care and preventive medicine. The Commission's recommendations, although more permissive than Ramsey's view, are not so lax that the issue of benefit to the subject is ignored. Indeed, the Commission took a firm position that the child should benefit if at all possible. By the same token, a child is a human being, and even though he may not be legally autonomous, one seriously wonders if anyone, even the child's parents, has the right to submit him as a research subject. One might agree with Ramsey with one's whole heart to leave the child in peace, but the mind acknowledges the need to forge ahead to increase humankind's knowlege. The problem is how to adequately protect the child while gaining knowledge that might now or ultimately benefit him or other children. What one thinks about the ethics of using children as research subjects may be a matter of conflicting principles, but it is a personal and professional obligation to protect that child at all costs, no matter how beneficial is the ultimate outcome. If a cure for leukemia is just around the corner but one child would be harmed in its discovery, the experiment must cease and leukemic children must wait a bit longer.

Mitchell[16] believes there are several categories in which experimentation on children can be allowed: (1) an experimental treatment with the immediate aim of curing the disease, (2) an experiment on an ill child to learn more about his condition or the disease from which he suffers, (3) an experiment on a child who is well or who suffers from a different disease to learn more about a particular disease, and (4) an experiment on a healthy child to learn more about children in general.

This position is even more permissive than the Commission's, but Mitchell establishes limits by suggesting that researchers should not cause pain, create a risk that is greater than that which occurs in daily living (unless the child is ill and can be expected to benefit), choose some children as more desirable research subjects because of their social conditions (orphans, mental defectives, and the like) or use children in hospitals simply because they are more accessible. Mitchell believes that even if the principle were set forth in writing that experiments should be carried out only on those children who can be expected to benefit directly, too much abuse would occur through rationalizing the purpose of the experiment. Instead he prefers to establish conditions to restrict experimenters from engaging in procedures that would be likely to harm or cause pain to the child. His position does not differ as much from Ramsey's in its intent as in the amount of latitude given the person performing the experiment.

Proxy consent. The major issue involved in proxy consent for children (and other incompetents) concerns whether parents or other proxies have a right to consent to experimentation that will not benefit the child. If the experiment is expected to be beneficial, it can be seen as therapeutic and parents can give consent as for other therapy *with the proviso* that they understand the procedure is experimental.

The Nuremberg Code (1947) does not mention children, and the International Code of Medical Ethics (1949) specifically excludes children and other incompetents from nontherapeutic research. The Declaration of Helsinki (1964) specifically states that the consent of a parent or guardian should be obtained for nontherapeutic research on children. In 1966 the AMA in its "Principles of Medical Ethics" endorsed the Helsinki statement: "Consent, in writing, is given by a legally authorized representative of the subject under circumstances in which an informed and prudent adult would reasonably be expected to volunteer himself or his child as a subject."[3,p.223] This statement gives parents almost total freedom to volunteer their children as research subjects in any kind of nontherapeutic experiment for any reason the parent thinks prudent. This is frightening because parents are thus permitted to use their children as they see fit. In 1963 the Medical Research Council for Great Britain in its "Responsibility in Investigations on Human Subjects" stated that parents cannot give consent for nontherapeutic research. The most recent American statement on proxy consent is that of the Commission discussed earlier.

It is sometimes difficult to distinguish between the legal and moral principles involved in proxy consent, but in the 30 years between the Nuremberg Code and the Commission's report it can be seen that the medical establishment is moving toward a more permissive attitude. Major ethicists disagree about the morality of proxy consent. One parameter by which a decision can be made is based on the nature of the experiment, that is, whether it is mainly observational or whether measurements must be taken and invasive techniques used. For example, the Denver Developmental Screening Test is a valuable tool for pediatric clinicians and parents to determine how a child is developing socially and physically compared to others in his age group. To establish norms for the test, experiments were performed that consisted of observation and noninvasive measurement. It is difficult to morally object to a parent consenting to have his 6-month-old play pat-a-cake and peek-a-boo with a researcher. But if the research involves an invasive procedure that causes even minor pain or discomfort (a venipuncture or gastric analysis, for example), the moral determination is more complex. Even if the experimental procedure does not cause pain but invades the child's privacy or personal space (for example, a rectal temperature), it could be construed as immoral for the parents to consent to this invasion unless there may be a direct benefit for the child. In all these examples, no matter how benign the experimentation is, the child is used as a means to an end and many see this as immoral. Any law that permits proxy consent for nontherapeutic research could then be seen as unethical.

The advantages and disadvantages of proxy consent are argued on two fundamental bases: the individual integrity of the researcher and parents and the risk-benefit ratio. McCormick[17] makes a fascinating case for proxy consent in nontherapeutic experimentation. His premises are that there are certain identifiable values that as moral human beings we ought to support and never directly suppress and that the knowledge of these values springs from human reason and does not require revelation. Proxy consent in the case of therapeutic procedures is morally permissible because health and well-being are desirable values and it is assumed that were the child able, he would embrace these values and give consent himself for a therapeutic procedure, experimental or not. Therefore the parent may given consent because it is assumed that the child would choose these values for himself because as a human being he would choose self-preservation. McCormick then says that because one would choose life and health for himself, he should choose the same for others because life and health are values that as a moral human being he ought to embrace. This is the point at which McCormick makes the crucial jump from the self to others. In his opinion individuals ought to make efforts on behalf of others because we are social beings and the good we contribute to society we also derive from it. It is therefore good to participate in nontherapeutic research, and if one ought to do it oneself, then one's child ought to do it also. McCormick says the child "would choose to do so because he *ought* to do so."[18] Sharing in the general burden of health maintenance is part of the growth and responsibility of a moral human being. McCormick takes a position that is diametrically opposed to Ramsey's.

Concretely when a particular experiment would involve no discernible risks, no notable pain, no notable inconvenience, and yet hold promise of considerable benefit, should not the child be constructed to wish this in the same way we presume he chooses his own life, because he *ought* to? I believe so. He *ought* to want this not because it is in any way for his own medical good, but because it is not in any realistic way to his harm, and represents a potentially great benefit for others. He *ought* to want these benefits for others.*

McCormick makes an assumption about what should be in the mind of a child, and many would find this position to be unwarranted if not dangerous.

Legal considerations. In terms of pharmacologic research children cannot be considered simply "little people." Their metabolic, muscular, and circulatory systems differ so markedly from those of adults that a drug proved safe for an adult cannot be considered safe for a child even if the dosage is altered proportionately. That is, one third of a safe dose for a 75 kg man would not necessarily be safe for a 25 kg child. Consequently pharmacologic research to determine a drug's efficacy and toxicity in children must be carried out. Regardless of the ethics of nontherapeutic research (pharmacologic testing is almost always nontherapeutic), it *is* being done and one should be aware of the legal ramifications. There is no firm legal precedent on the issue of pharmacologic research, but in *Bonner v. Moran* the court ruled that a 15-year-old boy could donate a skin graft without parental consent if he was capable of understanding and appreciating the consequences of his act.[19] In two other cases courts decided that a well child could donate a kidney to an ailing sibling because the well child would benefit psychologically by not losing the sibling.[19]

Common law fixes the age of consent at 21, but statutory law has modified that rule. The American Law Institute has said that if a child is capable of appreciating the nature, extent, and consequence of a procedure, his consent prevents liability even if the consent of his parent or guardian was not obtained or was expressly refused.[19]

Many drug companies state clearly in labeling that a drug is not to be used with

---

*McCormick, Richard A.: Proxy consent in the experimentation situation. Reprinted in Beauchamp, Tom L., and Walters, Leroy: Contemporary issues in bioethics, Belmont, Calif., 1978, Wadsworth Publishing Co., Inc., p. 463.

children because the clinical evidence is insufficient to establish its safety. There are two dangers in this: a physician may prescribe a drug anyway (the FDA had no way to regulate how an individual physician prescribes a drug), and a child may be deprived of a much needed treatment because a drug has not been tested sufficiently to be prescribed even though it may be particularly indicated.

Capron[19] acknowledges that the problem of testing drugs in children is insolvable and proposes the following approximations and questions to limit and define the problem by degrees rather than abandon it altogether:

1. How many drugs exist that are not approved for use in children but that appear to offer significant help in the treatment of a disease or condition? Is the drug to be tested necessary in that it differs markedly from those already approved? Does the drug need to be tested in children immediately, or can these tests wait until more is known about its effect on adults?

2. The risk of each drug to be tested must be evaluated. It is impossible to establish an acceptable level of risk in all situations, but steps can be taken to limit the risk. A drug should not be tested with children until its safety has been established for adults.

3. Participation in the research should be limited by excluding those children in institutions and those whose freedom is severely curtailed in some other way. Only children who are selected by their parent or guardians should be used in research, the assumption being that the parent will have the greatest emotional tie to the child and will protect his interests most vigorously. Random selection should be used when choosing children from a group already limited by the procedures above.

4. The possibility of harm to a child through unforeseen accidents should be limited by monitoring the experiment at all stages by a peer review board. If an accident occurs or harm befalls a child, it is the responsibility of the investigator to provide full compensation.

Prisoners

To some, prisoners seem ideal subjects for experimentation. They are a captive audience, their physical and psychologic reactions to the experiment can be easily monitored, they do not need to be paid much, their situation is coercive in itself and thus tends to produce many volunteers, and they are out of the sight and mind of most authorities and commissions that regulate human experimentation. Bars, barbed wire, and armed sentries tend to give an atmosphere of autonomy to what goes on behind prison walls; few people ask, and fewer talk. Most members of the health establishment never venture into or know much about prisons.

What is most important is not so much the means by which prisoners are recruited and used as human subjects but the ethics of using them at all. Is it morally correct to use a prisoner in human experimentation no matter how freely he volunteers?

Drug companies use prisoners to a large extent when engaging in human clinical trials; if they find this morally reprehensible, they also find it scientifically and economically practical. Many people think that prisoners can be subjected to greater pain, discomfort, risk, and inconvenience than nonprisoner subjects, because in this way they can at least partially expiate their crimes. One wonders if this approach to sin and guilt is not tinged with revenge. If a prisoner suffers pain, serious illness, or even death as a result of serving as an experimental subject, who is to know? Prison records can be easily falsified and the cause of death ascribed to prison violence or natural means.

Prisoners are paid a meager stipend for their services (usually a dollar or two a day) that would have little effect on someone else's decision to volunteer. To a prisoner, however, a dollar a day is a significant amount of money and can be a definite coercive factor. Would it be more ethical to ask for volunteers without paying money? Does the money change the morality, or does it merely provide a rationale for recruitment? A prisoner at Vacaville, California, put up with anorexia (he lost 35 pounds in a year), severe burns, and pain as a volunteer for continued topical application of dimethylsulfoxide because he was paid $30 a month. "Thirty is a full canteen draw [maximum credit allowed] and I wish the thing would go on for years—I'd be lost without it."[20]

Prison sentences are frequently reduced for those who volunteer, sometimes having been promised as an inducement before the experiment begins and sometimes done afterward as a reward. Even if no actual promise is given beforehand, most prisoners know the system well enough to realize that earlier parole may be in the offing, particularly if the experiment is risky or hazardous.

The morality of this situation can be viewed in several ways. If a prison term is seen as a way of forcing a person to pay a debt to society for having committed a crime, then that debt can be reduced by contributing one's services as an experimental subject; thus a reduction in sentence is not only moral but obligatory because society owes something to the person who risked his health for society's good. If a prison term is seen as a particular punishment for a particular crime, then no amount of volunteering should reduce the sentence because the two things are unrelated. In actuality, however, many variables affect both the sentencing and the eligibility for parole, such as the number of times the offense was committed, the person's prior record and age, the circumstances under which the crime was committed, and the person's general behavior. It would be unjust to eliminate volunteering as a research subject as a variable. A prisoner might have purer motives for volunteering than money or a shorter sentence; he might sincerely regret his crime and want to repay society in this way. Should he not be rewarded for this improvment in character if other prisoners have won early parole by demonstrating their rehabilitation in other ways?

Do prisoners who volunteer and thus reduce their sentences have an unfair advantage over those who do not? Can it be said that the latter are discriminated against because they choose not to volunteer? If two people committed a crime together, stood trial together, and were given the same sentence, is it fair to shorten the sentence of one simply because he volunteered?

If the purpose of a prison sentence is thought to be the removal of a criminal from society, thus for a time protecting society from his actions, why should society expose itself to the criminal earlier than it has to simply because the criminal volunteered his body for research? If a person is stripped of his liberty because he has shown that he cannot or will not live peaceably with others, should he be returned to the outside world sooner because he performs an act of which society approves? Can the two concepts be balanced on the same scale? Is a reduction in sentence an appropriate reward for selflessness?

Under the parole system, a reduction of prison sentence is recognized as encouraging and rewarding good conduct and industry, and it is also allowed for exceptional bravery or fidelity in a good cause. The purpose of the use of prisoners in medical research is reformative to the prisoner and constructive in terms of the advancement of medical knowledge. It is assumed that service in a medical experiment is consonant with the parole system's statutory "good time," "merit time," and "industrial credits."*

Rewarding a prisoner with money or time off a sentence for volunteering can be seen as a bribe or an incentive depending on the amount of the reward. Most writers on the subject are vague about how much reward should be given, suggesting that if it is too much it would be unduly coercive and if it is too little the money would not matter. Does it make any moral difference whether the reward is a dollar a day or a full year off the sentence? Is not payment of any reward coercive in itself? Many prisoners will volunteer not because the promise of a reward is an incentive but because they see volunteering as a positive action and often want to do something to help society or atone for their crime. Participation invariably improves a prisoner's self-image and gives him a sense of importance. More practically, it breaks the monotony of prison life, gives the prisoner a sense of purpose, and provides him with something to talk and think about besides the misery of his condition. Some may even see it as an adventure. In addition, participation in a research study could absorb some of the pent-up energy that might otherwise be released in a destructive way.

Many people believe that under no circumstances should prisoners be used as experimental subjects. No matter how ethical the design of the study is, how humane the researcher is, and how much attention is paid to the rights of prisoners, the situation remains in itself coercive and immoral. This position is ethically pure and cannot easily be dismissed. But because prisoners *are* being used as research subjects and will likely continue to be, an effort could be more practically directed at improving the ethical standards with which prison experiments are conducted.

Capron[21] reports a series of horrendous and unnecessary experiments conducted in prisons, such as testicular injections of radioactive thymidine to study spermatogenesis in Oregon; the study of the aversive conditioning effects of succinylcholine chloride (Anectine), which creates muscle paralysis and a sensation of suffocation, on violent prisoners in California; the artificial creation of typhoid fever in Maryland; and the experimental introduction of scurvy in Iowa. Because of these and other useless and scientifically insignificant prison experiments, Capron calls for a moratorium on all research using prisoners as subjects. He thinks that a moratorium is the only way to reevaluate the process by which research protocols are

---

*Beecher, Henry K.: Research and the individual: human studies, Boston, 1970, Little, Brown and Co., pp. 70-71.

approved and to determine whether each experiment is indeed necessary. If a moratorium were called, research would certainly become more expensive, volunteers would be harder to find, and the penal system would be deprived of some of its financial support. Capron points out that Great Britain gets along well without using prisoners. He suggests that the following problems should be solved before the moratorium is lifted:

1. A distinction should be made between general research and research from which prisoners might benefit, for example, behavioral or psychiatric research with a specific goal for the prisoner participant. The major question concerns who benefits from the experiment—the prisoner, the prison itself (researchers pay for using the prison's facilities), or society.

2. Review committees have not satisfactorily safeguarded the rights of prisoners or supervised their safety during the experiment. Another system of review if needed that is not composed of people whose function it is to guard the prisoners or administer the prison system; perhaps a committee of prisoners or interested community members would be better.

3. The kinds of institutions that are used and the prison population from which volunteers are recruited need to be examined.

4. The matter of informed consent is inadequate because controls are insufficient to ensure that the prisoners fully understand what will be done to them and what risks they will be taking.

5. Most prisoner consent forms contain an exculpatory clause that releases the researcher from liability in the event of a mishap or harm to the subject; prisoners need to be protected against undue harm and to have legal recourse in the event that harm occurs.

Some reflections on coercion. Coercion varies in kind and degree. At one extreme is mild coercion that provides some amount of choice. For example, an executive for a large company is offered a promotion, but if he accepts, he will have to relocate. If he refuses to move, he does not receive the promotion, but neither is he directly punished by losing his present job. Some might think this is undue influence rather than coercion. Another example: if I wish to teach at certain state universities, I must be willing to sign a loyalty oath. If I refuse, I am not hired, but I am not directly punished in any way. These are forms of coercion that may be seen as benign, but they are powerful in their effect.

Slightly further along the continuum is less benign coercion with the threat of minimal punishment, for example, requiring college professors to obtain a doctorate before granting tenure. The punishment is not granting tenure and the subsequent lack of job stability. Parents use this kind of coercion all the time: "Eat your vegetables or you won't get any dessert" or "No television if you don't finish your homework." Withholding the desired end can be seen as punishment for not acting in a certain way, and the threat of this punishment is coercive.

The degree of coercion depends on the undesirability of the threatened outcome if a requested action is not performed. For example, if a woman is kidnapped and her captors demand that she perform fellatio, the degree of coercion differs depending on the outcome if she refuses. If the captors threaten to lock her in a room, the coercive factor is less than if they threaten to beat her. If the executive's refusal to move causes no change in his present job status, the coercive factor is relatively weak. But if he knows that his company subtly punishes people who refuse opportunity by gradually decreasing their responsibility and status, the coercion is considerably stronger.

The ease with which it can be resisted is also a factor in the degree and kind of coercion. If the executive is a highly competent person and receives many excellent job offers, he can easily resist his company's efforts to transfer him. If the child dislikes ice cream, he can easily resist his mother's exhortation to eat the vegetables.

There are forms of coercion in which a person performs an act against his will because he lacks the strength or will to resist or does not resist because the coercive threat is too strong. This situation is seen frequently among prisoners of war. Soldiers inform on their comrades because torture has broken all their resistance. This is the basic principle behind psychic and physical torture, and a similar form of coercion is used to recruit prisoner volunteers for experimental studies. Direct physical coercion is no longer used; neither is overt psychologic torture. The fact that the prisoner is in prison is exploited, however, and to some degree he is unable to resist the request for volunteers. If he refuses, he will serve his full sentence, he might not be able to buy everything he wants, or he might have to endure the hostility and derision of fellow inmates. Whatever the threat, whether it is real or imagined, he fears it and finds it difficult to resist.

Another measure of coercion concerns how freely an action is taken. If I give $100 to a friend to pay a doctor bill, I do it because I like her and want to help. If I give $100 to a mugger on the street, I do it to avoid getting killed. One act is free and the other is coerced, even though in both instances I am doing what I *want* to do. I could refuse the mugger, but I want to avoid harm and therefore will take an action that I hope will lead to that end. A person volunteers for an experiment for a variety of reasons, most of them altruistic in some form. He wants to volunteer. A prisoner also wants to volunteer, but his altruistic motives may be secondary to his pragmatic reasons. He could refuse, but he may want those benefits enough that he takes an action that will result in his obtaining them. Both actions are taken voluntarily, but the amount of freedom behind the action differs and this changes the coercive factor.

Another way of measuring the coercive factor is by distinguishing between a threat and an offer. The difference lies in the consequences. If a threat is made, the probable consequence of not acceding to the demand is that the person will be worse off than in the natural course of events. If an offer is made, the probable consequence of performing the action requested is that the person will be better off than in the natural course of events. Sometimes the difference is not easily determined. In a prison situation one would have to determine what the natural course of events would be—usually a maintenance of the status quo. If a prisoner is promised early parole for participation, an offer is made. If he is told that he has no chance of parole if he does not volunteer, a threat is made. But if he volunteers and his situation remains the same, has he been threatened or given an offer? The determination is almost impossible to make because so many other variables exist. One can therefore assume that the presence of a threat implies coercion, but one cannot assume in the case of prisoners that the presence of an offer means there is no coercion. An offer may be as coercive as a threat although in a different way and to a different extent, depending on the circumstances of the prisoner's life and probable future.

Because a prison is a closed, secret place, everything that occurs there is to some degree coercive. The control of prisoners and the security of the prison are of prime importance; protecting the rights of prisoners is secondary if it exists at all. To believe that coercion does not exist in the recruitment of prisoners as subjects for human experimentation is dangerously naive. When the gates clang shut behind the prisoner he knows he has lost liberty. Loss of liberty automatically implies the presence of coercion.

PUBLIC POLICY
Codes of ethics

Public policy about human experimentation is generally determined by both statutory and case law, both of which are strongly influenced by codes of ethics that have been established for the purpose of protecting subjects. No matter how detailed, legalistic, or stringent, any code of ethics has one central purpose: to protect the health and safety of subjects. The FDA, although it requires human experimentation for all drugs proposed for use in human beings, is subject to DHEW guidelines, which are in turn derived from codes of ethics.

Scores of codes have been formulated for many reasons and as a result of hideous abrogations of human rights. Some have sprung from public outcry, and others were devised by individuals. Beecher[3] lists 100 pages of codes of ethics, and even his are only a small portion of the total. The following discussion is intended to provide a representative sample of codes of ethics to show the development of responsibility in human experimentation. This history can be seen perhaps as a comment on human development.

Perusal of a considerable number of such codes can be useful in indicating troublesome areas that others have encountered. On the other hand, rigid codes can never anticipate all of the possible contingencies in any given situation, and if trouble arises, an endless vista of possible legal actions opens up.*

The Hippocratic Oath (470-360 B.C.) is the first recorded effort to control the ethical behavior of physicians. In language and intent it can still be applied today, but certain passages, such as those involving not giving a deadly medicine (as in active euthanasia) and not performing abortion, are so hotly protested by medical students that they are no longer required to take the oath before receiving the degree of Doctor of Medicine. The oath is still administered by medical schools, but a graduate may remain silent if he chooses.

The oldest American oath is that of William Beaumont, drawn up in 1833 when

---

*Beecher, Henry K.: Research and the individual: human studies, Boston, 1970, Little, Brown, and Co., p. 215.

he used Alexis St. Martin, a Canadian trapper, as a subject in a series of experiments on the physiology of digestion. St. Martin was accidently shot in the stomach, and Beaumont saved his life. St. Martin was so grateful, though he had to receive food via a tube inserted into his stomach from the outside, that he permitted Beaumont to make periodic recordings and analyses about his digestive processes. The code was basically a personal contract between Beaumont and St. Martin, but it embodied all the basic principles of human experimentation, including voluntary consent. It is simple and beautifully written.

The American Medical Association (AMA) adopted its first code of ethics in 1847 and has updated it six times since, the latest in 1980. It is interesting to note that after the original code was written, the first revision did not take place for 99 years. In regard to human experimentation, the first revision in 1946 required only three things of the physician: (1) the voluntary consent of the subject (2) animal experimentation prior to that on humans to determine the "danger," and (3) performance of the experiment under "proper" medical management and protection. The entire statement about human experimentation took only six lines and was more vague than Beaumont's agreement 130 years before. In 1949 the AMA published a booklet, "Principles of Medical Ethics," in which *nothing* was said about human experimentation. In 1966 the AMA endorsed the ethical principles set forth in the 1964 revised Declaration of Helsinki of the World Medical Association (WMA) concerning human experimentation.

In a 1952 addendum to the AMA code the House of Delegates made the following statement about using prisoners as subjects:

> Resolved, that the House of Delegates of the American Medical Association express its disapproval of the participation in scientific experiments of persons convicted of murder, rape, arson, kidnapping, treason, or other heinous crimes, and also urges that individuals who have lost their citizenship by due process of law be considered ineligible for meritorious or commendatory citation.*

The Declaration of Helsinki (originally written in 1962) was established, in addition to stating general ethical principles of conduct in human experimentation, to distinguish between therapeutic and nontherapeutic research. The code is divided into three sections: basic principles, clinical research combined with professional care, and nontherapeutic clinical research. Although the code does mention informed consent, it is treated superficially and no mention is made of how much information is to be given and how the consent should be obtained. The important contribution of the Declaration of Helsinki, one of the first major codes after the Nuremberg Code, was its distinction between therapeutic and nontherapeutic research.

In 1954 the General Assembly of the WMA established "Principles for Those in Research and Experimentation," which is divided into five sections: (1) Scientific and Moral Aspects of Experimentation, (2) Prudence and Discretion in the Publi-

---

*Beecher, Henry K.: Research and the individual: human studies, Boston, 1970, Little, Brown and Co., p. 225.

cation of the First Results of Experimentation, (3) Experimentation on Healthy Subjects, (4) Experimentation on Sick Subjects, and (5) Necessity of Informing the Person Who Submits to Experimentation of the Nature of Experimentation, the Reasons for the Experiment, and the Risks Involved. Judging by these subtitles and the august nature of the WMA, one would expect a definitive and detailed document, but it is so short and vague that one gets the impression that it was written more to assuage the consciences of those performing the research than to protect subjects.

In 1957 the American Hospital Association (AHA) published a statement of principles involved in the investigational use of drugs in hospitals. It is more procedural than protective, and not once does it mention protection of the research subject. The U.S. Department of the Army in 1962 drafted regulations concerning the use of volunteers as subjects of research. It is detailed and protects subjects' safety and rights more than any other code at that time. The 1962 Kefauver-Harris amendment to the federal Food, Drug, and Cosmetic Act, though a law rather than a code of ethics, should be mentioned here because prior to that time *no federal or state law required that a physician inform a person that he was using an experimental drug or treatment*.

The American Psychological Association in 1963 wrote a code of ethics that was concerned in great detail with the responsibility of the investigator, public statements, maintaining confidentiality of subjects, client welfare, investigational test security and interpretation, research precautions, and other aspects of experimentation.

The most detailed code and the one that appears to be the most humane and thoughtful is "Responsibility in Investigations on Human Subjects" of the Medical Research Council in Great Britain (1963). The protection of the subject is its underlying concept, and its tone implies much deliberation and recognition of the ethical dilemmas involved.

The 1966 code established by the National Institutes of Health (NIH) is similar in tone and content to the Declaration of Helsinki, especially as it differentiates between therapeutic and nontherapeutic research. The same year the U.S. Public Health Service wrote a code with special emphasis on the welfare of children, as did the FDA about experimentation with new drugs.

The 1960s in the United States was a time of great racial strife, counterculture movements, and a tremendous interest in individual civil rights. It is more than likely that this atmosphere affected those agencies that required human beings for research. The Tuskegee Study and the Willowbrook experiment were still going on. Organ transplantation was beginning, the Harvard Ad Hoc Committee was meeting to define irreversible coma, and new drugs were being marketed. It was the beginning of the great boom in health technology as well as a time for change in the mores of society in general. The women's movement was beginning, blacks had been moving toward civil rights, and homosexuals were beginning to protest their persecution. It was a time when people were clamoring for rights that had been denied for years. Human research subjects were no exception; they simply were not as public or vociferous. But agencies engaged in human experimentation heard them and began to provide for their rights.

Public policy ethics

Codes of ethics are suggestions for moral and correct behavior. Most have an ethical intent and were established to protect human subjects, though some are more straightforward than others in this statement of intent. They have at least two drawbacks: stated intentions provide no legal protection for subjects, and for the most part the physician or investigator is entirely self-regulated with nothing to prevent him from engaging in unethical behavior. Legal protection for subjects involves written informed consent with a declaration that the investigator is liable for untoward damages resulting from negligence. Existing malpractice laws are insufficient to cover the conditions involved in human experimentation.

Individuals and society as a whole are used to accepting serious risks. Much in life involves calculated risks: we ride in elevators hoping the cables are not faulty, and we drive with our eyes open and hope to spot trouble before it happens. But if the elevator cable does snap, we know whom to blame and whom to sue, and if another car crashes into us, we know that insurance will cover the damages. This should also be true in human experimentation. Every subject should have a clear idea of who is responsible for the experiment and accountable for its results, what the expected outcome is (if it would not destroy the experiment to disclose this), and what steps one can take if negligence occurs.

One of the best ways to protect the subject's safety and ensure that he knows his rights is to appoint a subject advocate who does not work for the investigator (but who works in cooperation with him) and is not paid by the agency that funds the research. A nurse, by virtue of her professional education and her role as client advocate, is well equipped to perform this function. Not only can she do this service, but she is obligated to. The International Council of Nurses in its 1973 code, "Ethical Concepts Applied to Nursing," maintained that "The nurse takes appropriate action to safeguard the individual when his care is endangered by a co-worker or any other person." The Code for Nurses of the American Nurses Association states in Article 4, "The nurse acts to safeguard clients when their care and safety are affected by incompetent, unethical, or illegal conduct of any person." Article 6 states, "The nurse participates in research activities when assured that the rights of individual subjects are protected." This statement has the correct intent, but it is too passively stated. It implies that the nurse must wait for someone else to ensure the safety of subjects before participating. This is not sufficient. The nurse must *actively* ensure subjects' rights and safety. If she is to consider herself a professional and is to be regarded as such by other health professionals, then she must break out of this passive role. She is obligated to do this as a professional and as a human being. If she were to adhere rigidly to Article 6, how would she be assured that the rights of subjects are protected? If she simply accepts the declaration of the chief investigator, she has actually done nothing, but if she satisfies herself by direct investigation that subjects are protected, then she moves out of the passive role of occupational helper and into the active one of professional participant and colleague.

The nurse who actively assumes the role of advocate may find herself in an uncomfortable position. If she is aware of areas in which subjects' rights are in jeopardy, she may come into direct conflict not only with the researchers but also with the agency funding the research. In addition nurses themselves are becoming researchers and are as likely to lose sight of subjects' rights as physician and scientist researchers. Because of their generally higher consciousness about clients' rights they have a special obligation to serve as their own advocates and as positive research role models for other nurses.

Why do physicians and scientists, who are trusted by the public as much or more than any other group, sometimes grow careless about the ethics of research? How can they in good conscience ignore the basic rights of subjects? This is not meant to imply that researchers are heartless, insensitive fiends. Most scientists are ordinary human beings who are no more or less ethical and sensitive than the rest of the population. Therein lies the trouble. It is not sufficient for them to be merely ordinary in this regard. They must deliberately and conscientiously go beyond the usual for they are not doing ordinary things even though they are ordinary people. It is difficult to put this raised ethical consciousness into practice. One way to understand the concept is to imagine a small circle surrounded by a much larger one. The small circle is an ethical rule or commandment, for example, informed consent. The larger circle represents all behavior necessary to achieve informed consent, for example, explaining the procedure, finding out what questions the subject has, allowing him time to think it over, using lay terms instead of technical jargon, and so on. The actions in the outer circle, if consciously and deliberately carried out, will lead to fulfillment of the inner circle rule. The outer circle must be closed, that is, all the actions accomplished, before the inner circle rule will be met. This process is by no means haphazard or unconscious but requires a deliberate and sensitive effort by the investigator.

Scientific peer review is gaining in popularity and practice and is even mandated by federal agencies that fund research, notably NIH and DHEW. The effectiveness of the review committees is questionable, however. Of 300 clinical investigators 34% stated that the review committee had never required revisions of a research proposal or rejected a proposal for ethical reasons. Only 31% reported revisions, and 32% rejections.[22] It is difficult to believe that the remainder of the proposals were ethically perfect; one wonders how carefully the committee reviewed them.

It is no secret that the scientific establishment places a premium on publishing research. The more research a scientist does, the greater collegial rewards he receives, such as university tenure, important grants, lucrative consultant positions, and the admiration and respect of the scientific community. It is no wonder that priorities frequently become confused in the rush to perform and publish research, that the rights of the subject are seen as less important that the career of the scientist. The pursuit of knowledge, both for its own sake and for the aggrandizement of the researchers, is all too often emphasized more than the pursuit of ethics. When the 300 respondents were asked what three characteristics they would look for in a researcher before entering a collegial relationship with him, only 6% listed anything that could be classified an ethical concern for the subjects.[22]

A possible solution. Since 1974 it has been federally mandated that every institution that conducts research funded by DHEW must have an institutional review board (IRB) whose function is to determine whether subjects will be placed at risk, and if so, to ensure that three criteria are met: (1) risks to subjects are outweighed by the sum of the benefit to the subject and the importance of the knowledge to be gained, (2) the rights and welfare of the subjects will be protected, and (3) legally effective consent will be obtained.[23] The overseer of all these IRBs is the National Commission for the Protection of Human Subjects of Biomedical and Behavioral Research, which was discussed earlier in relation to children as subjects. In 1978 the Commission issued a report on the effectiveness of the various IRBs and made recommendations. Some of the recommended changes from existing DHEW regulations are as follows:

1. Twenty-eight federal entities outside DHEW authority conduct human experimentation, including the military, the Bureau of Standards, and the Department of Agriculture. Some accept DHEW guidelines as is, some use them in modified form, and some use their own. Though the DHEW regulations themselves are confusing and ambiguous, the recommendation is that all human experimentation conducted by any federal agency be subject to DHEW jurisdiction in regard to ethical standards. This would not cover all research done in the United States because a significant portion is funded by private organizations that do not receive federal funds, but more would come under a single rubric than now occurs.

2. Under current regulations only subjects at risk are controlled by an IRB. The definition of risk is ambiguous, and thus some subjects will not be protected. It was recommended that all human subjects regardless of the degree of risk be protected by an IRB.

3. Public attendance at IRB meetings and public access to the records have never been established because it has not been determined whether an IRB is a government agency and thus subject to sunshine laws or a committee of a private institution (the one doing the research). The Commission recommended that this jurisdictional problem be solved.

4. It was recommended that the selection of subjects be more equitable, although no specific suggestions were made about how this might be accomplished. The IRB would have to justify any disproportionate use of institutionalized subjects or ethnic minorities.

5. In regard to informed consent the Commission recommended that subjects be given sufficient information about the experiment so that they can make an autonomous decision about participation.

Robertson[24] suggests ways to clarify jurisdiction and improve the performance of IRBs:

1. Each IRB should have an explicit statement of its function and powers and the source from which the power is derived.

2. The rights of investigators should be clarified in their relationship to the IRB. This could prevent the current charges in some quarters that IRBs are

    limiting academic freedom and the ways in which research is carried out. Some restrictions must be placed on scientists, but the IRB cannot unfairly prevent them from doing their work.

3. It needs to be clarified which research categories are subject to review. Too many gaps in IRB coverage now exist; some experiments receive too much scrutiny and some not enough.

4. Public involvement in the IRB system should be increased, as should the proportion of nonscientists on the boards.

5. No subject surrogate or advocate now appears before the IRB when a research proposal is presented, and therefore the board tends to be biased in favor of the researcher. This should be remedied.

6. Consent forms should be made clearer and contain more specific information.

7. The recruitment of subjects and the explanation of the procedure are as important as the consent form itself. IRBs need to devote more time to these aspects of research protocol and should monitor the recruitment process.

8. Risk and inconvenience to subjects should be further minimized through closer scrutiny of subjects and better overall supervision of the project.

9. IRBs should embark on a plan of public education about scientific research.

Since research subjects are the most valuable resource the scientific investigator has, he is morally and professionally obligated to protect subjects at all costs.

SUMMARY

    Human experimentation has gone on since people first became inquisitive about how their bodies worked. Not until the full horror of the Nazi holocaust became known, however, were codified efforts made to protect research subjects. Even as the Nuremberg trials were being conducted in postwar Germany, the Tuskegee Study, an experiment demonstrating flagrant racism, was being conducted in the United States at the request of the U.S. Public Health Service. Atrocity in human experimentation knows no national boundaries.

    There are certain ethical considerations involved in all research using human subjects. The first and most important is that participation by the subject must be voluntary and that his consent must be fully informed and freely given. This is not easy to accomplish. People volunteer for research for a variety of reasons and can be subject to internal and external coercion of which the researcher is unaware. The problem of consent revolves around how much information should be given and how the subject's understanding can be ensured.

    Another consideration concerns whether the experiment is therapeutic or nontherapeutic; that is, can the subject be reasonably expected to benefit directly from the research or will he simply be contributing to a general fund of knowledge?

    The element of coercion may be present in the recruiting of human subjects. It can range from the very subtle (convincing a prospective volunteer that he will be helping medical science) to the very obvious (promise of some reward such as a shortened prison sentence).

    Another issue concerns the justification for the experiment. Is the knowledge necessary, can the research be done without using human subjects, and how much benefit can it be expected to produce? Will the public good be enhanced by the experiment. Does an individual have an obligation to donate his services as a volunteer to further the public good? How much if any sacrifice can society demand of an individual? Should sick or healthy people be used as research subjects? What about those who are terminally ill?

The Catholic Church permits human experimentation but does not believe that scientific knowledge is the highest human value. Although it permits human beings to volunteer, there is some debate in the Church about the extent to which a person is permitted to sacrifice a part of his body. Jewish law holds that there is no higher commandment than saving a human life, but the permissibility of human experimentation is decided on an individual basis.

Double-blind studies are the most effective way to test an experimental drug, but serious ethical issues are involved. Is it moral to give a placebo to subjects who may be under the impression that they could receive therapeutic benefit? Could the drug be tested by any other method, for example, by historical data or by comparing the experimental drug with one already in use to determine the differences?

Using vulnerable groups of people as human subjects for research poses ethical problems because of the ease with which they can be coerced. Children, the mentally retarded, and prisoners are such groups. The major issues here concern informed consent and coercion. Some ethicists maintain that a child should not be used as a subject unless he will directly benefit from the experiment because he cannot freely give informed consent and no one has the right to consent for him. Others believe that children should participate because there are some things that people ought to do if they are to embrace desirable human values. Prisoners are particularly vulnerable to all kinds of coercion, and some ethicists believe that a moratorium should be placed on using prisoners as human subjects.

Codes of ethics for the conduct of physicians and scientists in relation to human subjects have existed since Hippocrates, but they are no more than professional suggestions to colleagues about how to behave. Most depend almost entirely on self-regulation and give the investigator almost complete autonomy. Although the intent of most codes is admirable, they provide little legal protection for subjects.

Institutional review boards required of all institutions receiving DHEW funds are an improvement, but there is not enough public participation and subjects are not represented when the research proposal is presented for funding. One of the most effective ways of protecting subjects' rights is to appoint an advocate, and a professional nurse is well equipped to fill that role. Many think it is her moral obligation to protect subjects in this way.

REFERENCES

1. Rubenstein, Richard: The cunning of history, New York, 1975, Harper & Row, Publishers, Inc.
2. Holocaust, Jerusalem, 1974, Keter Publishing House.
3. Beecher, Henry K.: Research and the individual: human studies, Boston, 1970, Little, Brown and Co.
4. Brandt, Allan M.: Racism and research: the case of the Tuskegee syphilis study, Hastings Center Report 8(6):21-29, December 1978.
5. Moore, Francis D.: A cultural and historical

view. In Experiments and research with humans: values in conflict, National Academy of Sciences conference, Washington, D.C., February 1975.

6. Biomedical ethics and the shadow of nazism: a conference on the proper use of the Nazi analogy in ethical debate, April 1976, Hastings Center Report 6(4):special supplement, August 1976.

7. Pappworth, M. H.: Ethical issues in experimental medicine. In Cutler, Donald R., editor: Updating life and death, Boston, 1969, Beacon Press.

8. Veatch, Robert M.: Case studies in medical ethics, Cambridge, Mass., 1977, Harvard University Press.

9. Nelson, James B.: Human medicine: ethical perspectives in new medical issues, Minneapolis, 1973, Augsburg Publishing House.

10. Lasagna, Louis: Some ethical problems in clinical investigation. In Hunt, Robert, and Arras, John, editors: Ethical issues in modern medicine, Palo Alto, Calif., 1977, Mayfield Publishing Co.

11. Beauchamp, Tom L., and Childress, James F.: Principles of biomedical ethics, New York, 1979, Oxford University Press.

12. Jonas, Hans: Philosophical reflections on experimenting with human subjects. In Wertz, Richard W.: Readings on ethical and social issues in biomedicine, Englewood Cliffs, N.J., 1973, Prentice-Hall, Inc.

13. McCartney, James J.: Encephalitis and ara-A: an ethical case study, Hastings Center Report 8(6):5-7, December 1978.

14. Evans, Frederick J.: The power of a sugar pill. In Hunt, Robert, and Arras, John, editors: Ethical issues in modern medicine, Palo Alto, Calif., 1977, Mayfield Publishing Co.

15. McCartney, James J.: Research on children: national commission says "yes, if . . . " Hastings Center Report 8(5):26-31, October 1978.

16. Mitchell, Ross G.: The child and experimental medicine, British Medical Journal 4(1):721-727, March 21, 1964.

17. McCormick, Richard A.: Proxy consent in the experimentation situation, Perspectives in Biology and Medicine 18(1):2-20, Autumn 1974.

18. McCormick, Richard A.: Proxy consent in the experimentation situation. In Beauchamp, Tom L., and Walters, Leroy: Contemporary issues in bioethics, Belmont, Calif., 1978, Wadsworth Publishing Co., Inc.

19. Capron, Alexander M.: Legal considerations affecting clinical pharmacological studies in children, Clinical Research 12(2):141-150, February 1973.

20. Mitford, Jessica: Experiments behind bars: doctors, drug companies, and prisoners. In Gorovitz,

Samuel, et al., editors: Moral problems in medicine, Englewood Cliffs, N.J., 1976, Prentice-Hall, Inc.

21. Capron, Alexander M.: Medical research in prisons: should a moratorium be called? Hastings Center Report 3(3):4-6, June 1973.

22. Barber, Bernard: The ethics of experimentation with human subjects, Scientific American 234(2):25-31, February 1976.

23. Veatch, Robert M.: The National Commission on IRBs: an evolutionary approach, Hastings Center Report 9(1):22, February 1979.

24. Robertson, John A.: Ten ways to improve IRBs, Hastings Center Report 9(1):29-33, February 1979.

BIBLIOGRAPHY

Abrams, Natalie: Medical experimentation: the consent of prisoners and children. In Spicker, Stuart, and Engelhardt, Tristam: Philosophical medical ethics: its nature and significance, vol. 3, Boston, 1977, D. Reidel Publishing Co.

Ayd, Frank J., Jr.: Drug studies in prisoner volunteers, Southern Medical Journal 65(4):440-444, April 1972.

Barber, Bernard: The ethics of experimentation with human subjects, Scientific American 234(2):25, February 1976.

Beauchamp, Tom L., and Childress, James F.: Principles of biomedical ethics, New York, 1979, Oxford University Press.

Beauchamp, Tom L., and Walters, LeRoy: Contemporary issues in bioethics, Belmont, Calif., 1978, Wadsworth Publishing Co.

Beecher, Henry K.: Research and the individual: human studies, Boston, 1970, Little, Brown and Co.

Biomedical ethics and the shadow of Nazism: a conference on the proper use of the Nazi analogy in ethical debate, April 1976, Hastings Center Report 6(4):special supplement, August 1976.

Bok, Sissela: The ethics of giving placebos, Scientific American, November, 1974.

Brandt, Allan M.: Racism and research: the case of the Tuskegee syphilis study, Hastings Center Report 8(6):21-29, December 1978.

Capron, Alexander M.: Legal considerations affecting clinical pharmacological studies in children, Clinical Research 12(2):141-150, February 1973.

Capron, Alexander M: Medical research in prisons: should a moratorium be called? Hastings Center Report 3(3):4-6, June 1973.

Cutler, Donald R., editor: Updating life and death, Boston, 1969, Beacon Press.

Dedek, John F.: Contemporary medical ethics, New York, 1975, Sheed & Ward, Inc.

Evans, Frederick J.: The power of a sugar pill. In Hunt, Robert, and Arras, John, editors: Ethical issues in modern medicine, Palo Alto Calif., 1977, Mayfield Publishing Co.

Experiments and research with humans: values in conflict: proceedings of a conference, National Academy of Sciences, February 18-19, 1975, Washington, D.C.

Gorovitz, Samuel, et al., editors: Moral problems in medicine, Englewood Cliffs, N.J., 1976, Prentice-Hall, Inc.

Holocaust, Jerusalem, 1974, Keter Publishing House.

Hunt, Richard: Entering the future looking backwards: "Holocaust" and the Nazi experience, Hastings Center Report 8(3):5-6, June 1978.

Hunt, Robert, and Arras, John, editors: Ethical issues in modern medicine, Palo Alto, Calif. 1977, Mayfield Publishing Co.

Jonas, Hans: Philosophical reflections on experimenting with human subjects. In Wertz, Richard W.: Readings on ethical and social issues in biomedicine, Engelwood Cliffs, N.J., 1973, Prentice-Hall, Inc.

Lasagna, Louis: Human experimentation. In Visscher, Maurice B.: Humanistic perspectives in medical ethics, Buffalo, 1972, Prometheus Books.

Lasagna, Louis: Some ethical problems in clinical investigation. In Hunt, Robert, and Arras, John, editors: Ethical issues in modern medicine, Palo Alto, Calif., 1977, Mayfield Publishing Co.

Lipsett, Mortimer B., et al.: Research review at NIH, Hastings Center Report 9(1):18-22, February 1979.

Marston, Robert Q.: Medical science: the clinical trial and society, Hastings Center Report 3(2)1-4, April 1973.

McCartney, James J.: Encephalitis and ara-A: an ethical case study, Hastings Center Report 8(6):5-7, December 1978.

McCartney, James J.: Research on children: national commission says "yes, if . . ." Hastings Center Report 8(5):26-31, October 1978.

McCormick, Richard A.: Proxy consent in the experimentation situation, Perspectives in Biology and Medicine 18(1):2-20, Autumn 1974.

Meltzer, Milton: Never to forget, New York, 1976, Harper & Row, Publishers, Inc.

Mitchell, Ross G.: The child and experimental medicine, British Medical Journal 4(1):721-727, March 21, 1964.

Mitford, Jessica: Experiments behind bars: doctors, drug companies, and prisoners. In Gorovitz, Samuel, et al., editors: Moral problems in medicine, Englewood Cliffs, N. J., 1976, Prentice-Hall, Inc.

Moore, Francis D.: A cultural and historical view. In Experiments and research with humans: values in conflict, National Academy of Sciences conference, Washington, D.C., February 1975.

Neslon, James B.: Human medicine: ethical perspectives on new medical issues, Minneapolis, 1973, Augsburg Publishing House.

Pappworth, M. H.: Ethical issues in experimental medicine. In Cutler, Donald R., editor: Updating life and death, Boston, 1969, Beacon Press.

Ramsey, Paul: The patient as person, New Haven, 1970, Yale University Press.

Ramsey, Paul: Children in institutions. In Gorovitz, Samuel, et al., editors: Moral problems in medicine, Englewood Cliffs, N.J., 1976, Prentice Hall, Inc.

Ramsey, Paul: The enforcement of morals: nontherapeutic research on children, Hastings Center Report 6(4):21-30, August 1976.

Robertson, John A.: Ten ways to improve IRBs, Hastings Center Report 9(1):29-33, February 1979.

Rubenstein, Richard: The cunning of history, New York, 1975, Harper & Row, Publishers, Inc.

Rutstein, David D.: The ethical design of human experiments, in Beauchamp, Tom L., and Walters, LeRoy: Contemporary issues in bioethics, Belmont, Calif., 1978, Wadsworth Publishing Co.

Sabin, Albert, et al.: The military/the prisoner. In Experiments and research with humans: values in conflict, National Academy of Sciences conference, Washington, D.C., February 1975.

Spicker, Stuart, and Engelhardt, H. Tristam: Philosophical medical ethics: its nature and significance, vol 3., Boston, 1977, D. Reidel Publishing Co.

Thomas, Lewis: The benefits of research. In Experiments and research with humans: values in conflict, National Academy of Sciences conference, Washington, D.C., February 1975.

Vaux, Kenneth: Biomedical ethics, New York, 1962, Harper & Row, Publishers, Inc.

Veatch, Robert M.: Case studies in medical ethics, Cambridge, Mass., 1977, Harvard University Press.

Veatch, Robert M.: The National Commission on IRBs: an evolutionary approach, Hastings Center Report 9(1):22-29, February 1979.

Wojcik, Jan. Muted consent: a casebook in modern medical ethics, West. LaFayetts, Ind., 1978, Purdue University Press.

10

Informed consent in nonexperimental procedures

AUTONOMY AND PATERNALISM
Autonomy

Most people will not serve as subjects in human experimentation, and most practitioners of nursing will not participate in any way in this kind of research. But many people will at some time in their lives, and often several times, subject themselves to medical procedures that are not experimental but for which consent must be given in writing. All nurses will be in a position to request consent from clients and provide information on which consent is obtained. Informed consent, the foundation of the relationship between clients and health professionals, is based on one of the most fundamental human principles, autonomy.

Autonomy is a form of personal liberty of action when the individual determines his or her own course of action in accordance with a plan chosen by himself or herself. The autonomous person is one who not only deliberates about and chooses such plans but who is capable of acting on the basis of such deliberations, just as a truly independent government has autonomous control of its territories and policies. A person's autonony is his or her independence, self reliance and self-contained ability to decide.*

A person whose autonomy is diminished for some reason has a decreased capacity for acting and is dependent on others to some extent. No human being is completely autonomous in that he is free to act with no constraints whatsoever; that kind of autonomy would result in anarchy and the collapse of society. When we refer to an autonomous person, we generally have in mind someone who has set an independent life course and has the ability to take those actions that will keep him on course or to take a new course if the need arises. Autonomy involves being an independent person even though one needs the help, support, and love of others to achieve emotional fulfillment.

All people lose some degree of autonomy several times in their lives; it is usually a temporary situation but is sometimes permanent. Loss of autonomy generally implies being subject to a physical or psychologic constraint that affects both the

---

*Beauchamp, Tom L., and Childress, James F.: Principles of biomedical ethics, New York, 1979, Oxford University Press, p. 56.

will to be independent and the capacity to act on that will. Major long-lasting constraints include mental retardation or severe mental illness, imprisonment, and profound physical incapacity such as quadriplegia or severe full-thickness burns. Most losses of autonomy, however, are not this dramatic or permanent, but they should not be minimized or trivialized because of the observer's perception of their degree. Some losses of autonomy that seem minor at the time can affect the rest of a person's life. Often in physical illness when a decision for a health care procedure must be made, the person's autonomy is so diminished through the illness itself, pain, fear, and anxiety that his ability to make an autonomous decision is decreased. The following case illustrates this problem.

Jim is 44 years old and a successful attorney who has achieved respect among his colleagues for the creative ways he has been able to save money for large corporations. He and his wife were divorced 2 years ago, but their relationship is reasonably cordial. He sees his two children frequently, and they love him. Up until 2 months ago he felt healthy and vigorous, working hard, playing tennis, and enjoying a satisfying love relationship with an attorney in a competing firm. Then be began to feel "rotten all the time" and suffered severe constipation. A barium enema revealed a large mass in his transverse colon that had all the earmarks of cancer. The physician recommended exploratory surgery and said it was likely he would wake up with a colostomy. Jim asked about the chances for survival with and without a colostomy. The surgeon said that without the colostomy he would be "a dead man in a year" but with it there was no way to predict until exploratory surgery had been done.

Jim's legal training warned him not to make an immediate decision, and he went home to think. He saw three choices: (1) have no surgery and simply let nature take its course, (2) consent to the exploratory surgery but not the colostomy and then make this decision based on the results of the surgery, or (3) give the surgeon permission to do whatever he thinks most appropriate.

In this situation a person has lost a good deal of his autonomy already and will lose more if he enters the hospital. The autonomy is decreased by having to make a blind decision because neither he nor the surgeon knows the full extent of the decision he is facing. His fear of cancer and revulsion at the thought of a colostomy put him in indecision, but his need to know the facts strengthens him. He is subject to external forces that shake but do not collapse his autonomy. The decision for surgery is entirely his although he has discussed it with his former wife and present lover. Jim decides to have the exploratory surgery and refuses to give consent for any other procedure even though he is aware that the surgery itself could increase the risk of metastasis.

The large bowel tumor is malignant, and Jim is now faced with deciding between dying soon with great pain and debilitation and having a colostomy that may add a few years to his life. His autonomy is now further diminished by his present pain, his knowledge of the future, and his temporary physical dependence that will increase no matter what decision he makes. He is still autonomous in that he can and will make his own decision, but external factors have shaken the foundation of his independence.

Jim is now in a situation that Kant described as heteronomy, being ruled by other persons or conditions, as opposed to autonomy, being ruled by the self. Autonomy involves self-imposed moral rules that obligate one to act in a certain way. One acts heteronomously when actions are coerced by external or irrational forces including habit, desire, impulse, and other forces not based on reason. Thus if Jim's decision is guided at least in part by fear or anxiety, he is heteronomous. In other words, Kant applies the maxim of reason to the principle of autonomy.

John Stuart Mill conceptualized autonomy as freedom of action rather than freedom of will and believed that individual social and political freedom is always permissible if harm to others is prevented during exercise of that freedom.

The liberty of the individual must be thus far limited; he must not make himself a nuisance to other people. But if he refrains from molesting others in what concerns them, and merely acts according to his own inclination and judgment in things which concern himself, the same reasons which show that opinion should be allowed, without molestation, to carry his opinions into practice at his own cost.*

Mill believed that the universal promotion of autonomy would maximize benefits for everyone and would serve the greatest utility. The individual freedom of action with the proviso of not harming others will result in a society in which individual productivity and creativity develop more fully. Society benefits in direct proportion to the development of individual talent. Autonomy is supremely important to Mill; a person with "character" takes from the culture only what he finds individually valuable and is not unduly controlled by his social environment.

The ideas of Kant and Mill are not as far apart as one might suppose. Kant held that a person's reasons for action are autonomous, that is, that one acts by reason of one's own moral principles. Mill is concerned with freedom from the tyranny of society; an individual should be completely autonomous except where harm to others might be involved.

It is impossible to disagree with the principle of autonomy unless one is a dictator. It is one of the basic principles of the United States Constitution (Thomas Jefferson and John Stuart Mill were contemporaries) and people have fought and will continue to fight for the right of individual liberty. But paying lip service to the principle is not the same as actually respecting and providing for another person's autonomy.

To represent autonomous agents is to recognize with due appreciation their own considered value judgments and outlooks even when it is believed that their judgments are mistaken. To respect them in this way is to acknowledge their right to their own views and the permissibility of their actions based on such beliefs. And to grant them this right is to say that they are entitled to such autonomous determination without limitations on their liberty being imposed by others.†

Disregard for autonomy is glaringly evident in the health care system. Hospitalized clients lose a good deal of their personal autonomy; they even lose personal

---

*Mill, John Stuart: On liberty. In Utilitarianism, New York, 1974, The New American Library, Inc., p. 184.

†Beauchamp, Tom L., and Childress, James F.: Principles of biomedical ethics, New York, 1979, Oxford University Press, p. 58.

identity when hospital personnel refer to them by their disease (such as "the appendectomy at the end of the hall"). They must eat food they may not like, must go to sleep and wake up at prescribed times, are subjected to strange people touching their bodies in intimate places and in possibly threatening ways, and are not even allowed to leave a small prescribed physical area. They cannot run to the corner for a newspaper or go out for a pizza if they feel hungry in the evening. This loss of autonomy, compounded by the fear and anxiety of being ill, creates a dependency that further diminishes autonomy.

Having respect for the autonomy of clients in the health care system implies providing them with means by which to make decisions about their health; in other words, they must be able to give informed consent. Autonomy also implies respect for the person, that is, the belief that every person is responsible for his own destiny and should have the means to determine that destiny. Health care providers frequently find themselves in a position to affect another person's destiny. The degree of power or authority exerted often depends on how much respect the health professional has for the client's autonomy.

The administration of oral medicines in hospitals is a paradigm of the health care system's respect for individual autonomy. The average person has given himself medication prescribed by a physician or purchased over the counter. The average person can tell time and manage to swallow a pill, but in hospitals medications, even aspirin and other common remedies, are administered one dose at a time by nurses who push a trolly down the hall and hand pills to individual clients. In no hospital except for a few intermediate care units is a client given a bottle of pills with written information about what they contain, what effect they can be expected to have, what side effects are common, and how often to take them. That procedure would respect the autonomy of clients in regard to oral medications. Instead clients are given pills about which they know nothing unless they specifically ask, and even then the information may not be forthcoming or may be incorrect. Pills are doled out as if the client cannot be trusted with a whole bottle, and nursing time, which could be more appropriately devoted to more sophisticated care, is wasted.

It is acknowledged that many people make errors in taking their own medication, some of them quite serious. But the principle of autonomy compels the responsible health professional to teach the client about the medication, its use, how it will affect his health problem, and why it is important to take it at specified times. With this correct and full information the client can make his own decision about whether to take the medicine. Full autonomy implies that the decision to take the medicine belongs to the client rather than the opposite situation of obeying a nurse who comes into his room with a pill, saying, "Here, take this."

Those who argue from a paternalistic point of view say that the hospital has a responsibility to see that the client receives his medicine and that the only way that responsibility can be discharged is to give each dose to each client personally. Those who argue from the principle of autonomy say that the hospital should instead allow the decision to be made by the client and that the hospital can fulfill its responsibility by asking the client if he has taken his medication. This response is characteristic of a pure principle of autonomy, which institutions have not found practical. If autonomy implies a moral demand for noninterference with others (Mill) or a moral demand for respect of the personhood of others (Kant), and if the client is to be autonomous in the matter of oral medications, he must be free to take them or not as he chooses.

Autonomy by nature involves a conflict with authority, and it could be argued that a totally autonomous person never submits to authority. Complete autonomy, however, is impossible in any society, as is total authority. In nondictatorial political theory and practice, persons in authority are expected to give reasons for their exercise of authority; if the reasons are deemed just and rational by the majority, people are then expected to accede to that authority. "In democratic theories of state, for example, authorities are not envisioned as issuing commands without justification. And the legitimacy of any command is regarded as contingent upon the command's not exceeding the limits of autonomously delegated authority."[1,p.61]

Autonomy and authority can be compatible in a society, and moral principles can be upheld. All autonomous actions are not necessarily moral simply because they reflect individual freedom (the decision to murder may be autonomous, but it cannot be considered moral); by the same token, decisions to accede to authority do not imply rejection of autonomy (driving no faster than the speed limit may be an autonomous decision to protect one's safety). The balance of autonomy and authority is particularly delicate in the health care system, especially when informed consent is concerned. If a decision to submit to a certain procedure is to be autonomous, the decision must be made on a rational basis with no interference from those in authority. However authorities in part control the means by which a rational decision can be made. For example, if it is suggested that a person submit to a cardiac catheterization, whether his decision to accede to the suggestion is autonomous depends on the quality of information he has been given to make an informed decision. A physician (authority) has that information; he can partially control the client's autonomy either by refusing to divulge information or by giving so little that the client still cannot make an informed decision. The client-physician relationship can take several forms during the decision-making process: (1) The client can be given complete information about cardiac catheterization so that he can make as autonomous a decision as possible given the circumstances, (2) he can seek his own information by doing extensive research on cardiac catheterization (though if he does not understand what he reads he can be in a worse position than if he had no information at all), or (3) he can leave the decision to someone else, such as the physician or a family member, thus relinquishing his autonomy.

Paternalism

Paternalism is often seen as the opposite of autonomy although many health professionals view paternalism as a protection of autonomy by preventing people from making harmful or ill-advised choices. Paternalism involves the regulation of the activities of a state or individual by another state or individual in much the same way as a father regulates the activities of his child.

When the analogy with the father is used to illuminate the role of professionals or the state in health care, it presupposes two features of the parental role: that the father is benevolent and beneficent, i.e., that he has the interests of his children at heart, and that he makes all or at least some of the decisions relating to his children's welfare rather than letting them make these decisions. Paternalism poses moral questions precisely because it involves the claim that beneficence should take precedence over autonomy, at least in some cases.*

Beneficence, the obligation or duty to promote good, to further a person's legitimate interests, and to actively prevent or remove harm, can include strong elements of paternalism, especially in contrast to autonomy.

If I have a polyp or some other precancerous growth, it is the physician's beneficent duty to tell me about it and suggest strongly that it be removed. It might even be his duty to frighten me a little so that I recognize the importance of the surgery, especially if he sees that I am reluctant. If in my autonomy, however, I refuse to have surgery, I am in a sense thwarting the physician's duty of beneficence. If he says, "You should have the polyp removed for your own safety and protection," and does everything in his power to convince me to consent, he could be accused of paternalism because he seems to have made the decision. However, he knows more about polyps than I do, so I consent to the surgery. Have I given up my autonomy and submitted to the physician's paternalism? The answer depends on how one views paternalism. The situation could be seen as forcing a person to give up his autonomy and as an imposition of one's authority over another. Paternalism can also be seen as the persuasion of a person to make a decision that will ultimately benefit him most, as in the example above.

Paternalism in health care usually involves a health professional's decision in which the client does not participate. In the past when informed consent was not enforced as assiduously, paternalistic decisions were made more commonly, especially when they involved clients who were poor, uneducated, and unsophisticated about health matters. Much surgery was performed on people who had no idea why they were being operated on and who were so intimidated by the power of the system they did not question the decision. Paternalistic decisions are still being made, but more people are asking questions and requesting a second opinion before consenting to procedures.

Beauchamp and Childress[1] present a classic case of paternalism regarding the information offered a client. A woman had a fatal reaction to urography. Two urologists had confirmed the need for the test, and the radiologist said that in the 25 years urography had been performed at that hospital no one had had a fatal reaction. He had not told her before-hand that she had a remote chance of death because he thought this information would not accomplish anything and because he thought that even if he had told her of this small chance of death, she would have had the urography and died anyway. The attitude of the radiologist is clearly based on beneficence, but is it justified? He likely thought there was no point in frightening the woman unnecessarily, especially since there is some evidence that increased anxiety will cause a greater likelihood of a fatal reaction, but she might not have consented to urography even though it was obviously required.

---

*Beauchamp, Tom L., and Childress, James F.: Principles of biomedical ethics, New York, 1979, Oxford University Press, p. 154.

The conflict in this situation involves whether she had the right to know exactly what her chances were. Many health professionals correctly argue that most clients do not *want* to know the statistical danger of every procedure or the exact way the scalpel will cut into flesh. But they have a *right* to know, and it is generally the health professional who makes the decision of how much information to give and how to give it, because most people do not know enough about health care to know which questions to ask. Consider the following dialogue:

Physician: "Good evening, I'm Dr. Cutaway, and I'm going to be taking out your gallbladder tomorrow morning. You have a right to know what's going to happen to your body, so I'm going to inform you of everything before you sign the consent."

Client: "Oh, fine. Please sit down."

Physician: "First the nurse will give you a shot of meperidine hydrochloride to help you relax because we feel your anxiety level will be so high in the morning that it will be difficult for the operating room personnel to take care of you. If you're relaxed, you're more cooperative. The meperidine will be mixed with atropine to help dry up your mucous membrane secretions. You see, we have to insert a tube down your throat, called an airway, and if your mouth is filled with saliva you could choke when we put the airway in. But if your mouth is dry, there is less likelihood that you'll choke. It's for your own safety. Oh yes, about the airway. Well, we need to put it down your throat because that's where we attach the tubes connected to the respirator that will be helping you breathe. All your muscles from head to toe will be completely paralyzed by the curare we inject into you. What? Oh yes, that *is* the poison the Indians used to tip their arrows with to make them more lethal—how interesting that you should know that! The paralysis includes your chest muscles, and since your chest can't move in and out by itself, we have to breathe for you because you *do* need to keep breathing. . . ."

By this time the client has his clothes on and is out the door, though the physician had barely begun to describe the anesthesia, let alone the surgery. It is no wonder that paternalism exists in some spheres of health care; it probably should exist to some degree. The moral issue concerns the parameters of paternalism. Where should it begin and end and when is it justified? Mill defines paternalism as an exercise of power over any member of the community against his will and believes it is justified only when harm to others will be prevented. Preventing physical or mental harm to the individual concerned is not a sufficient reason. Mill might have insisted that the client in the dialogue above had a right to know all the details of his surgery and that the physician cannot be compelled to abrogate the client's rights since no harm would come to another person. The physician might be persuaded to desist if it were known absolutely that the client would be harmed by the information, but because this is not known the client's rights must prevail. This is generally known as Mill's principle of harm and is concerned more with the abrogation of liberty than with paternalism itself.

There are, however, instances in which one may morally engage in paternalism. If a person has made a choice or has embarked on a course of action that is extremely dangerous, it may in some cases be justified to prevent him from carrying it out. The evil to be prevented by paternalistic intervention must, however, be greater than the evil of the interference with liberty, and those instances are rare.

The following is an example of a state's refusal to act in a paternalistic manner even though the individual had embarked on a dangerous course of action.

A 23-year-old woman in Maryland had a 10-year history of severe mental illness that included several suicide attempts.[2] She had been receiving psychiatric care intermittently throughout her adult life and in 1978 she slashed her wrists while talking on the telephone to a social worker at a crisis center. She was admitted to the psychiatric unit of a general hospital and was released after 3 weeks of lithium therapy. While at home she stopped taking the drug and again became suicidal. After another stay in a private hospital, her parents' money ran out and she was admitted to a state hospital so that her parents could have time to decide what course of action would be most appropriate. She remained in the state hospital for 4 days under observation and was then released because a legal officer (Maryland law does not require a physician to be present at a release hearing) thought she belonged in the community and because she could not be committed against her will. Three days later she lay down on the tracks of the Washington, D.C., Metro and waited for a train. She achieved her goal of suicide, and the state had been legally powerless to intervene. Civil commitment laws had been changed after years of charges of paternalism. One could say that this woman had the autonomous right to kill herself, but she had been trying for 10 years and had not succeeded; therefore one might also say that she had not made a definite decision to do so. Should she have been commited to protect her from herself, or was the state correct in not interfering with her autonomous right to continue her suicidal course?

Another justification for paternalism involves an individual's severe limitation or defect that results in an increased probability of harm, as is the case with mental incompetents and children. A person who cannot understand the possibly harmful consequences of an action should be prevented from taking that action. We would no more permit a severely mentally retarded person to keep his own bottle of tranquilizers than we would permit a toddler to wander in the street alone. Preventing harm to such individuals is a greater good than restricting their liberty is an evil. It can be argued that paternalism can be justified on a sliding scale of the potential for harm, that is, the greater risk of harm to the individual, the stronger the case for paternalism. This argument, however, is weak because agreement about the degree of harm cannot be reached and, even more important, because autonomy cannot be morally connected to the degree of harm. An example of this dilemma is the argument of compulsory contraception or even sterilization for the retarded. Does the possible harm of parenthood outweigh the revocation of their autonomy to reproduce at will?

One could also justify paternalism if other methods of persuasion have been tried and found ineffective and if it is seen that great harm will be prevented. The form of paternalism must, however, be the least coercive and insulting to the process of decision making. As in all other justifications, the harm to be prevented must be much greater than the harm of overriding autonomy.

Feinberg[3] distinguishes between strong and weak paternalism. Weak paternalism involves preventing harmful conduct that is substantially nonvoluntary or temporarily intervening to determine if the conduct is indeed voluntary. Strong paternalism involves limiting a person's autonomy or liberty even if his choices are informed and voluntary. Almost everyone acknowledges weak paternalism to be morally correct in some cases, such as preventing an obviously drunk person from driving a car. His decision to drive cannot be said to be completely autonomous and voluntary, because he is temporarily incapable of making a fully informed decision. Strong paternalism is justified by fewer people and involves a more ambiguous moral issue, such as is the case when one wants to give a person a blood transfusion even though it is against his religious convictions and death will result if the transfusion is not given.

The Georgetown College case[4] is an excellent example of strong paternalism. Mrs. Jones lost two thirds of her body blood because of a ruptured ulcer and was brought to an emergency room by her husband. She had no personal physician. Both she and her husband were Jehovah's Witnesses, and they had a 7-month-old child. Without a transfusion death was imminent, but neither the client nor her husband would consent. Judge J. Skelly Wright of the District Court of Appeals was asked by the hospital for a writ to order transfusion. Judge Wright went to the hospital and spoke with Mr. Jones, who refused counsel on the advice of his church. Mr. Jones did, however, say that if the court *ordered* transfusion he would not protest because it would then not be his responsibility, but he would not consent to it voluntarily. Judge Wright visited with Mrs. Jones, who was so weakened by loss of blood that she was not in a condition to make a decision. She did audibly speak the phrase "against my will" and indicated that the decision for a blood transfusion would not be her responsibility if the court ordered it. Judge Wright signed the order.

The difference between strong and weak paternalism can be seen as a function of how voluntary and informed the individual's decision is. Often, however, one cannot be certain about the degree of voluntarism, and thus justification for paternalism is also uncertain. The ultimate issue in the balance of autonomy and paternalism concerns whether paternalism is ever justified or offset by an act of beneficence that results in abrogation of autonomy.

NATURE OF INFORMED CONSENT

In the United States the doctrine of informed consent has arisen in part out of a series of malpractice suits involving the touching of another person's body without consent, which legally qualifies as battery. If a person is capable of consent, it is now considered morally and legally impermissible to perform any procedure that involves touching or invading his body without specific written permission to do so. The person must not only give written consent but also must understand what he is consenting to and not be unduly coerced. The first part of the requirement is relatively easy to satisfy with a signature on a consent form. The second is more difficult and gives rise to most of the ethical dilemmas.

The primary purpose of informed consent is the protection of individual autonomy. This is accomplished by leaving all health care decisions to the client even though the health professional may have far greater knowledge and expertise about what is required to improve or maintain the client's health. No matter what the professional thinks should be done to benefit the client, it is the client who should decide what will be done. Informed consent also protects and promotes autonomy by placing the client in a position in which he *must* make a decision; therefore his thinking and knowledge are heightened along with his individual initiative. The greater the power of the individual in matters of his health, the weaker the power of the institution over the individual.

In addition to promoting individual autonomy, informed consent also serves to protect people from unscrupulous health professionals who may be tempted to make decisions that are not in the client's best interest. If the client decides to submit to a procedure and if his consent is informed (assuming that by obtaining other opinions the client has satisfied himself that the procedure *is* necessary), then the decision is totally his. He is therefore theoretically protected from the risk of unnecessary or dangerous procedures. If he has the opportunity to reflect on the consequences of the decision and to consult others, the client should be protected from duress, coercion, and fraud.

Another function of informed consent is that decisions to perform surgery and other procedures are scrutinized more carefully by professional colleagues for two major reasons: clients tend to seek second opinions before making a decision for surgery (many private insurance companies, as well as the federal government, bear the cost of a second opinion), and as malpractice suits increase, health professionals will tend to seek each other's opinions before recommending surgery or a complex diagnostic procedure.

What if a person desires a particular procedure but does not wish to give consent in writing because he does not want to participate in making a formal decision? (This situation is not as rare as one might think; decision making is a complex process, fraught with emotional peril, and many people shy away from it.) Institutions do not perform procedures without a legal signature, but what justification do they have for requiring the consent of the client? The hospital is justified in assuring itself that it has endeavored to protect the client from harm; this is especially appropriate in a legal context. If a client has given consent, he cannot sue the health professional or institution for battery, and if he feels he has grounds for a malpractice suit, he must show that he incurred damage because of provable negligence on the part of the health professional or institution. A person must give his own consent unless he is not competent to do so, because he alone is in a position to determine what degree of risk he is willing to take, which may be considerably more or less than another person would take on his behalf.

A few legal concepts closely associated with informed consent should be discussed here. Negligence or malpractice can be defined as "the failure of a professional person to act in accordance with the prevalent professional standards or failure to foresee possibilities and consequences that a professional person, having the necessary skill and training, to act professionally, should foresee."[5,p.42] Since informed consent involves foreseeable possibilities, a health professional could be held negligent or be sued for malpractice if informed consent is not obtained. In addition to legal action (a civil or criminal suit), a nurse may be subject to censure or disciplinary action by a state board of nursing on the grounds of dereliction of duty for neglecting to obtain informed consent.

If a client institutes a malpractice suit for failure to obtain informed consent, he will claim physical or mental injury or both. To collect damages the plaintiff (client) must show that his claimed injury would not have resulted if there had been an attempt to seek his informed consent. Although it is frequently difficult to prove a causal relationship between an action or inaction and an injury, the present tendency of society and the increased awareness surrounding clients' rights in regard to informed consent place the health professional on the defensive more often than not unless there is proof that informed consent was obtained.

Legal doctrines

Benjamin Justice Cardozo's statement about autonomy remains the legal foundation for most decisions regarding informed consent: "Every human being of adult years and sound mind has a right to determine what shall be done with his own body; and a surgeon who performs an operation without his patient's consent commits an assault, for which he is liable in damages."[6] In *Natanson v. Kline* an even stronger view of autonomy is expressed: "Anglo-American law starts with the premise of thoroughgoing self determination. It follows that each man is considered to be master of his own body, and he may, if he be of sound mind, expressly prohibit the performance of lifesaving surgery, or other medical treatment."[7]

At present there are no legal guidelines to determine how much risk warrants obtaining informed consent; therefore it is not uniformly required for all procedures. All surgery done in hospitals must have written consent, but many invasive procedures done in private physicians' or dentists' offices do not necessarily require consent. A dentist may perform invasive procedures such as a root canal and minor surgery such as removing gum and may give local anesthesia and inhalation analgesia (nitrous oxide) without first asking the client to sign a consent form. A dentist may say that written agreement is not necessary because by the client's voluntary presence he consents to the procedures , but he may not be able to explain, however, how these procedures legally differ from minor surgery done in a hospital that requires consent. The dentist is not behaving illegally, because there is no way to define or determine the risk. Risk is usually assigned by the individual provider of care. Therein lie many conflicts.

It has become a common practice in some institutions that when risk is sufficient to warrant written consent, so much information and risk-benefit analysis are provided that some clients are not only disturbed but frequently are more confused than before the information was given. Alfidi[8] proposed an alternative solution in his practice of radiology. He gave clients a choice between being informed and not being informed of the risk inherent in certain radiographic procedures, such as intravenous urography, arteriography, transhepatic cholangiography, and so on. He found that most people did not want to know the risk, although he mentions nothing about the clients' desire to have the procedure explained. There is a significant difference between knowing what is to be done and knowing how many people have died as a result of the procedure. The Supreme Court of California in *Cobbs v. Grant* (1972) established precedent for nondisclosure of risk if the person requests that he not be so informed.

It might seem logical to dismiss the discussion of risk by stating that all procedures carry an element of risk and that clients, if they are to have as much autonomy as possible, should be informed of all risks and should consent to each individual procedure. In theory this sounds commendable, but in practice it would be unworkable. Every time a person enters the hospital he would be bombarded by consent forms for all the procedures that might entail risk, including venipuncture (the risk of infection at the puncture site) and every dose of medication (the risk of side effects). To prevent a mountain of paper work the client is asked to sign a blanket consent form that covers all procedures performed while he is in the hospital except those that entail special risks, such as surgery and particularly complex invasive diagnostic procedures such as cardiac catheterization or bronchoscopy. However, the client may refuse any medication or procedure that is covered by the blanket permission.

The degree of risk of a given procedure cannot be determined only by the number of people who have died or been seriously injured by it. Probably more people are allergic to penicillin or other drugs than have died of cardiac catheterization. Yet medications do not require informed consent as does the latter procedure. Courts have settled matters of informed consent in the past, and it is likely that in the future they will be asked to determine what procedures require consent.

Elements of consent

Competence. Since consent cannot be informed if the client is not competent, competence is the foundation on which all other elements rest. Competence can be established on a number of levels; though a person is competent to function in one area of life, he may not be in another. For example, a person of limited intelligence may be considered legally incompetent though he is perfectly able to conduct his personal affairs, maintain a home, and hold a job. If he were to enter a hospital, he might be considered incompetent to sign a consent form, which is a legal document, though he may understand ramifications of the procedure if it is explained in language at his level of comprehension. Sometimes the level of competence varies over time; a person may be competent to decide a matter today that he may not be able to decide in the future if his life situation changes.

Because competence is multidimensional and varies from time to time and from situation to situation, Beauchamp and Childress[1] have proposed the idea of "intermittent" or "limited" competence. This concept would avoid someone being labeled either totally competent or incompetent, would preserve a maximum amount of autonomy, and would justify declaring a person incompetent only in those areas in which his competence is truly questionable. Therefore the person of limited intelligence in the example above would be competent to decide whether to proceed with elective surgery because he could understand the risk-benefit ratio, whereas he might not be competent to understand the details of financial arrangements his attorney has made for him.

Having declared a person incompetent does not mean that he actually is; unless specific criteria are applied each time consent is required, an unfair evaluation of competence is likely to be made. In a large state mental hospital an attendant kicked a client so hard that he died 2 days later of a ruptured liver. The attendant was indicted for first degree murder, but he was not fired or even suspended from his job. The administrator's rationale for permitting him to continue to work was that he was certain to be acquitted of the murder charge. When someone mentioned all the witnesses who could testify to what happened, the administrator replied, "No one would take the word of a crazy person." He implied that because society had declared a person incompetent in one or more areas, he was automatically incompetent in other areas as well. In all likelihood these inmates would not have been considered competent to sign a surgical consent form even though no criteria for competence in this area would have been applied.

Beauchamp and Childress[1] present a rather unusual case that illustrates the concept of limited or intermittent competence. A 27-year-old man was involuntarily committed to a state mental hospital after having amputated his right hand. He had been committed on earlier occasions after having pierced his right eardrum and having removed his right eye. He had spent a total of about 8 years in a variety of hospitals for treatment of physical and mental disorders. The man wanted to leave the hospital, but his family was opposed to his release because they could not control his self-destruction and they feared for their own lives. The client believed that his actions were completely rational because he was obeying the will of God, who demanded this sacrifice. The client believed he was the only one God had selected for his sacrifice and said there was no treatment for him at the hospital because "I would cut off my right foot if God told me to." The question of his competence raises interesting questions. Who can determine that this person does or does not speak with God? Is he competent to live his life of self-mutilation as he chooses (so far he has not harmed anyone but himself, and he gives no indication that this is likely to happen), or has he clearly demonstrated that he is not competent? His actions seem quite reasonable to him; he is merely following his religious convictions. Does the fact that he is a religion of one make him incompetent? How can this man's competence be determined?

Standards can be applied, usually involving the ability to retain information, comprehend its meaning, and process it to arrive at a decision in which both an end and a means to that end are chosen.

A person is competent if and only if that person can make decisions based on rational reasons. In biomedical contexts this standard entails that a person must be able to understand a therapy or research procedure, must be able to weigh its risks and benefits, and must be able to make a decision in the light of such knowledge and through such abilities even if the person chooses not to utilize the information.*

It is important that nurses understand the competence issue particularly as they frequently witness the actual signing. Although it is the physician's legal responsi-

---

*Beauchamp, Tom L., and Childress, James F.: Principles of biomedical ethics, 1979, Oxford University Press, p. 69.

bility to obtain informed consent, the nurse is morally and professionally responsible for ensuring that the client is competent to sign the form. We have been taught and now teach that the most effective way to be certain of this is to ask the client to say in his own words what he understands his consent to signify. But this is not enough. It merely assures the nurse that the client has assimilated some information *for the moment;* the nurse still does not know if the client has used the information to make his decision about the procedure.

For example, a woman consents to radical mastectomy because she has been told her cancerous breast must be removed. She relates this to the nurse, but this simply means that the client has a piece of information. The nurse does not know if the decision to have the mastectomy is based on the client's knowledge of breast cancer and the alternative forms of therapy and on her utilization of this information to choose among the options. The key question for the nurse to ask is *why* the client has chosen radical mastectomy (use of the word *chosen* is important). Only by listening carefully to the answer will the nurse know if the client has made a rational decision.

It is more difficult to establish the parameters of incompetence than the criteria for competence. People who fall into the gray area between obvious competence and obvious incompetence (such as one who is comatose or so disoriented about time, person, and place that he cannot begin to function rationally) present moral dilemmas. Individuals in this indefinite situation usually slip in and out of a "state of competence" or perhaps are only temporarily incompetent because of a physical disability such as a sudden loss of blood or progressive kidney deterioration. Should they be considered incompetent and subject to second-party (proxy) consent, thus attempting to ensure their safety while denying their liberty? Or should they be considered competent to make their own decisions, thus preserving liberty but risking an irrational and thus unsafe decision?

Health professionals often make value judgments when deciding whether an individual is competent. A person who is dirty, unkempt, and smelly is more likely to be considered incompetent than someone is who is well groomed. A person who is volatile, hot-tempered, and loudly emotional is more likely to be declared incompetent than one who is quiet, controlled, and soft-spoken. Those who express radical or deviant opinions are more likely to be considered incompetent. But ignorance or behavior that is thought to be unreasonable or even irrational does not imply incompetence. The absence of rationality should be proved by specific criteria before a person is declared incompetent.

Disclosure of information. The ability to make a decision depends on having information. The dilemma in informed consent concerns how much information is necessary for a client to make a rational decision. Does the doctor have to disclose every cut, snip, and stitch as well as every drug and gas that will be used—all to enable the client to decide whether to have his gallbladder removed? Most people would agree that this much information is not only unnecessary but may be harmful to the client's well-being. The increased anxiety level may even jeopardize his safety. What information can be eliminated? What if the doctor decided not to mention the intubation procedure because it is not part of the surgery and will have no lasting effect? The client will have a sore throat after the operation. If he does not know that it resulted from intubation and will heal in a day or two, he might be thrown into anxiety and turmoil. What if the anesthesiologist is careless and damages the client's larynx such that his voice is permanently changed? Could the client sue because he was not specifically informed that his throat would be invaded? (A famous opera singer undergoing an operation was given general anesthesia completely by mask because of such an eventuality; she was willing to risk not being intubated.)

Most institutions have established guidelines about what kind of information is to be provided. The information should generally include a description of the proposed procedure, the available alternatives, a description of risks and benefits, and an offer to answer questions. The client is generally not given the names of all people who will participate in the procedure, and only sometimes is he encouraged to obtain a second opinion.

The issue of what and how much information should be disclosed is not easily resolved. Beauchamp and Childress[1] have proposed three general standards for determining what information should be disclosed (1) what is operative in the biomedical professions, (2) what a reasonable person would want to know, and (3) what individual subjects of research would want to know. The following discussion concerns the first two standards. The first is rather paternalistic and reflects what physicians think the client should know. What is thought to be in the best interest of the client might actually be in the best interest of the physician. According to this standard the amount of information disclosed depends on the judgment of the physician and not on the client's right to the information. This standard is declining in significance because the amount of information a person needs to make a rational decision is relative to the individual rather than a medical judgment. This standard is losing ground also because more people think that the information given to clients should be as free as possible from medical value judgments, especially as it relates to the risk-benefit ratio and the necessity for the procedure.

Case law has gradually developed a set of considerations concerning the reasonable-person standard. Since it is almost impossible to define this rather amorphous concept, courts have formulated four major principles about what information a person needs to make a decision leading to informed consent:

1. Whether information is necessary must be judged on the basis of what a jury would deem necessary, not a panel of medical experts (*Wilkinson v. Vesey,* No. 1479-1482, Supreme Court of Rhode Island, 1972).
2. The known risks of significant bodily harm and death must be revealed (*Cobbs v. Grant,* S.F. 22887, Supreme Court of California, 1972).
3. A reasonable person is considered a composite of reasonable persons in society rather than the individual in any specific instance (*Canterbury v. Spence,* No. 22099, U.S. Court of Appeals, District of Columbia, 1972).
4. The standards of disclosure of information are no different from those of other professions in which there is a similar fiduciary relationship (*Berkey v. Anderson,* No. 481, Supreme Court of California, 1969).

These standards of disclosure are based on the principle of autonomy and can be coalesced into one basic standard: "the patient or subject should be provided with information that a reasonable person in the patient's or subject's circumstances would find relevant and could be reasonably expected to assimilate. In this way the moral requirement to respect autonomy is translated into a consent standard."[1,p.72] Is information disclosed to clients actually used by them to make a decision? Studies[9,10] have shown that many people generally make decisions about proposed procedures before they receive significant medical information and that, although this information is not irrelevant or unwelcome, the facts do not significantly alter their decisions. Facts may or may not play a role in decision making, usually depending on the emotional significance of the decision, but this should have no bearing on whether they are given to the client, who has a right to the information. What he does with the information is irrelevant. Using the reasonable-person standard might not be sufficient in individual instances, but it is a base with which to begin. A reasonable person might want or need a certain amount of information to make a decision; another person, who is perhaps more inquisitive, skeptical, or hesitant, might require a greater amount. For autonomy to be preserved this greater amount must be provided without hesitation.

It has been said with some truth that fully informed consent cannot exist because no one possesses sufficiently complete information to give to the client. Even had the doctor explained the entire gallbladder operation in all the detail he could manage, he would have left out some information simply because he cannot know everything that could happen during the course of the procedure. The goal of complete disclosure is not realistic; neither is the goal of revealing every fact known to the health professional. An appropriate goal is the disclosure of all information that is relevant to a particular situation with an offer of still more information if the client requests it. If the health professional keeps in mind the *purpose* with which he is disclosing the information, he is less likely to be too sketchy or too detailed in his description. The purpose is almost always to provide the client with facts sufficient for a rational decision.

A landmark case regarding the scope of information to be disclosed in informed consent is *Canterbury v. Spence*,[11] in which Circuit Judge Spottswood W. Robinson III acknowledged in his opinion that full disclosure is unrealistic and said that the client's right of self-determination "shapes the boundaries of the duty to reveal." In other words, the amount of information should be determined by the client's need to have it to make an intelligent decision. Judge Robinson also acknowledged that the physician has no way of knowing exactly how much information the client needs to make this intelligent choice and said that it would not be reasonable to expect him to second-guess the client. But the physician has an idea of what a reasonable person in the client's position would need to know. From these two concepts Judge Robinson made his decision: The scope of the standard is not to be subjective in regard to either the physician or client. Rather it is to be objective "with due regard for the patient's informational needs and with suitable leeway for the physician's situation." Any risk must be disclosed if the physician knows or should know that it would be of significance to a reasonable person in the client's position and that he would need to know it to make a decision.

A line cannot be easily drawn between information that is significant and that which is not; decisions will always have to be made by reason. *Canterbury v. Spence* suggested that the rule of disclosure can be waived (1) when a genuine emergency arises while a person is unconscious or otherwise unable to consent and when spending time giving information to a second party would clearly place the client in jeopardy and (2) when the disclosure of risk would clearly threaten to have a detrimental effect on the client, as when so much distress would be caused that treatment would be impossible. These exceptions must be carefully circumscribed so that the disclosure rule itself is not impeded. "The privilege does not accept the paternalistic notion that the physician may remain silent simply because divulgence may prompt the patient to forego therapy the physician feels the patient really needs."[11] *Canterbury v. Spence* further struck down the notion that the parameters of information to be disclosed should reflect those standards practiced by most members of the health professions at any given time; it increased the strength of the reasonable-person standard and attempted to create objective criteria for disclosure. This change could be interpreted to suggest that a reasonable person wants to know more than an average physician wants to reveal.

Comprehension. All necessary information can be given to a client, but unless he is able to comprehend it, he cannot use it to make a decision. Many health professionals think that no consent is really informed because the client is unlikely to comprehend fully what is about to be undertaken. They argue that the information is so sophisticated and complex that even the most intelligent person is not able to grasp it. This is an unduly pessimistic and paternalistic view and reflects the attitude of some health professionals toward clients more accurately than it reflects the capacity of clients to understand. There is no reason why a person of average intelligence should not be able to comprehend even the most complex procedure if the health professional takes the time and trouble to explain it in language the client can understand without giving so many technical details that the client becomes confused. Health information *sufficient to the purpose of the client* is no more difficult to comprehend than any other information. When a person asks an attorney for legal advice, he is told what he may and may not do within the limits of the law, why the law exists, and what punishment he can expect if he breaks it. The attorney describes various ramifications depending on the complexity of the law and the client's situation, but additional information would simply embellish the basic explanation. The health care client is in a similar position and needs to know similar facts, and the health professional is responsible for helping him to understand those facts. It is a rare client who because of lack of intelligence or severe disorientation cannot be led to comprehension, and it is likely that such a client would be declared incompetent. Comprehension of any problem is based in part on the ability of the person disclosing information to relate it in such a way that facilitates communication. This is not difficult to achieve, but it requires time, patience, and effort to learn the client's level of understanding; this is a communicative art in which sensitivity and intelligence are involved.

What about the client who refuses information and thus cannot possibly comprehend what is about to happen to him or give informed consent? Should the surgery or diagnostic test be cancelled? What about the client who blocks out everything the health professional says and thus comprehends none of it because he simply does not want to hear it? He surely has as little information as the client who says, "Do what you have to do. I don't want to know anything."

Beauchamp and Childress[1] present two ways of dealing with this problem. Either the client should be coerced into receiving the information, thereby circumventing his autonomy, or the client's refusal of information should be taken to mean that he understands what the refusal means and waives his right to the information. The consent he signs will then be *valid* but not *informed*. Both positions present problems. Forcing information is a serious violation of autonomy, and it is difficult to imagine circumstances other than emergencies in which this moral dilemma could be solved while autonomy is ignored. The second alternative runs the risk of enlarging people's already inordinate trust in physicians. A waiver of consent, if it became widely used, would render ineffective all the strides recently made in providing clients with the information they need. The problem of refusal of information presents a moral dilemma. Each case will have to be solved individually, but autonomy must never be sacrificed unless the client willingly gives it up, and even then he must be informed of the rights he is waiving.

It may seem to the health professional that the client is behaving irrationally and should be prevented from doing so to protect his interests. That view, although well meaning, could be seen as paternalistic; that is, if the client wishes to give up his autonomy, the system has no right to coerce him into not doing so. Autonomy belongs to the client; many think that as long as he knows what he is doing, he has made an autonomous decision. It must be determined, however, that the client *does* know what he is doing. "When a patient's or subject's autonomy is clearly limited by his own ignorance, as in the case of false belief, it may be legitimate to promote autonomy by attempting to impose the information."[1,p.80]

Voluntariness. Voluntariness implies choice with freedom of action and without undue influence, duress, or coercion. Avenues of choice must be made available if a person is expected to choose. It does no good to say that one may have any flavor ice cream he wishes if only vanilla is presented; his choice of flavor has been removed and for all intents and purposes does not exist.

The primary meaning of voluntariness in relation to informed consent is the exercise of choice without undue influence or coercion. There is a difference between undue influence and coercion. With the former a substantial reward or a highly persuasive technique is used to make a person reach a certain decision. With coercion an actual threat of physical or psychologic harm is made to manipulate a decision (see Chapter 9 for a more detailed discussion of coercion).

No one decides to undergo surgery or some other health procedure without being subject to some outside influence, much of which is positive. If a person is experiencing chest pain, his anxiety exerts a certain amount of influence to seek a diagnosis and his family may apply even more pressure. A decision to consent to surgery may be influenced by the desire to be rid of a painful or dangerous condition, or it may be the only alternative to certain death, as in amputation of a gangrenous leg. Undue influence, however, is almost always negative and takes a variety of forms. Asking a person to make a complex decision when he is under the influence of central nervous system depressants, as happens if a nurse rushes in to have the client sign a consent form after he has had preoperative medication, is a common example of undue influence. It invalidates the consent and in this case is illegal. Requiring a decision when the person is under emotional stress is also undue influence and is commonly used, for example, by funeral directors when they ask a family to choose a casket. Grief renders them at least partially incapable of making a rational decision, and they tend to agree to whatever the funeral director suggests. A physician can influence a client to consent to surgery by describing the benefits to be gained, but he exerts undue influence if he paints an excessively negative picture of what will happen if he does not consent. He can exert undue influence by appealing to the client's vulnerability ("If you don't have your gallbladder out now while you're reasonably healthy and can plan for it, you'll find yourself in an emergency, and then your wife will have to quit her job to take care of you and you'll be in a mess"). Or he can coerce the client by threatening to discontinue his services or threatening to tell everything he knows on the insurance form, thus creating financial difficulties for the client. The difference among influence, undue influence, and coercion are important to the concept of voluntariness.

REFUSAL OF TREATMENT

Health professionals are not used to having their services refused and are usually shocked when it happens. They sometimes see it as an unflattering reflection of the competence of the client or as a personal affront. The refusal of a competent person to consent to treatment is a function of his autonomy, and health professionals have the basic responsibility to (1) find out why the client refuses treatment and determine if the reason is based on accurate information and rationality and (2) respect the client's right to refuse treatment while at the same time giving him unlimited opportunity to change his mind.

The Patient's Bill of Rights of the American Hospital Association grants a client the right to refuse treatment to the extent permitted by law, and recent court cases have greatly enlarged the latitude of clients in making decisions regarding health care, especially with life and death decisions. Byrn[12] describes several court cases involving refusal of treatment. *Erikson v. Dilgard* (1962) concerned a conscious adult patient brought to an emergency room suffering from intestinal bleeding. Both surgery and blood transfusions were required to prevent death. The client consented to surgery but refused transfusion on religious grounds. The court upheld the client's right to refuse a transfusion, but religious factors were not mentioned in the decision, which was based on the individual's right to make a final medical decision even if that decision would result in death. *In re Yetter* (1973) describes a 60-year-old inmate of a state mental hospital who had a breast discharge. She refused biopsy and surgery because she thought that if she did have breast cancer, surgery would further spread the disease and cause harm. After her initial refusal Ms. Yetter seemed deluded about the problem, but the court upheld her refusal, citing her right to privacy. The court found that even if the prolongation of life appears in the eyes of a third party to be in someone's best interest, the state cannot interfere with an individual's right to privacy if no minor children are involved and if there is no clear and present danger to public health and safety. *Palm Springs General Hospital, Inc. v. Martinez* (1971) concerned a 72-year-old woman with terminal hemolytic anemia who refused further cutdown transfusions because she wanted to die in peace and who begged her family not to "torture me any more." Her refusal was not based on religious reasons; she simply want to be left alone. The court ruled that she could not be forced to undergo the cutdown surgery and she died within a day. The court stated that she had the right to acquiesce to imminent death.

Courts are definitely leaning toward noninterference in clients' decisions even when death seems inevitable. Prevention of suicide (if this issue can be viewed in relation to suicide) is not within the power of the state, nor can a person be compelled to submit to medical treatment, whether his life is in jeopardy or not. According to Byrn, unless there is compelling state interest to the contrary, "a patient's decision to reject treatment ought to prevail in every case," even when (1) the prognosis is poor but the client's life is not in imminent danger, (2) the client wants to live and his choice to refuse treatment does not seem reasonable, and (3) treatment is particularly hazardous or painful and the person would remain seriously incapacitated even after treatment.[12]

An exception to Byrn's rule of universal client autonomy might be the person who can be easily and inexpensively treated with no undue risk and who can be expected to benefit from treatment; it is this person who, if he refuses treatment, does so *only* because he wishes to die. Even then it is not legally or morally clear that autonomy should be abrogated. One might want to consider the ramifications of the person's refusal for the same reason one would want to temporarily restrain a person from committing suicide: to determine why the person has chosen this course of action. If he has thought through the decision and made it rationally, it would be a serious violation of his autonomy to interfere with an action that results from that decision.

If a physician or any other health professional ignores a client's refusal of treatment, he is liable for battery. Many acts of refusal may seem small and do not involve lifesaving procedures. Nurses are confronted with them every day and frequently do not know how to handle them. Angry confrontations can be avoided if the problem is seen as a moral dilemma rather than an example of fractious behavior by the client. When the chief resident enters the client's room with a group of eight or nine staff and medical students and the client refuses to be examined, the resident usually responds by applying undue influence ("How else are these students going to learn if you don't cooperate?") instead of recognizing the client's right not be be touched by people to whom he has not given permission.

Veatch[13] presents two cases in which refusal of treatment is complicated because the clients were considered mentally unbalanced. The first involves Mary Malone, who voluntarily admitted herself to a psychiatric ward of a private hospital. The diagnosis was severe depression, and a series of electroshock treatments was prescribed. She was told that the treatments would be unpleasant, but she agreed in writing. She found the treatment worse than she had anticipated because when the shock was applied, she experienced a convulsion similar to a grand mal seizure. When it came time for her next treatment, she refused further electric shock. She tried to leave the room and was quickly surrounded by the staff. The psychiatrist tried to explain why the treatments, although they were unpleasant now, would prove ultimately beneficial. She was adamant in her refusal. The staff had a heated argument, and many paternalistic statements were made about Ms. Malone not being able to discontinue shock therapy "with her lack of control." Ms. Malone was dragged back to the shock therapy room by nurses and attendants under the direction of the psychiatrist.

The second case concerns Robert Watson, a 22-year-old student who suddenly dropped out of school and spent his time locked in his room or taking long walks. On one of these walks he was stopped by two policemen who asked him why he was swinging a large stick. Robert gave an answer that the police thought was insufficient, and a scuffle ensued during which Robert was shot in the shoulder and thigh. He appeared rambling and inconsistent to his attorney and seemed not to understand the seriousness of the charges against him. His behavior in court was so strange that the judge committed him to a state hospital for observation, and there he was diagnosed as paranoid schizophrenic. The physicians prescribed chlorpromazine hydrochloride (Thorazine) which Robert refused to take, and his mental condition deteriorated drastically. It was thought there would be no improvement without medication. Robert was quite clear and rational when discussing his reasons for refusing the drug and continued to refuse even when it was pointed out that it might speed his release. The physician wanted to have the medication forced, a feat that would have required five attendants, but the state had no law about forcing medication on committed mental patients.

The dilemma of consent with mentally ill people is complex. One wants to give them as much autonomy as possible for ethical reasons and because the more sanely a person is treated, the more sanely he is likely to behave. On the other hand, treatment should be both beneficial and desirable to the person. Mentally ill people are, however, frequently unclear about what they want and inconsistent about their needs and feelings. Arguments can be made for and against forcing people to accept treatment for mental illness. Jack Himmelstein, an attorney for the NAACP legal defense fund, argues that because we permit "normal" individuals to make all kinds of unhealthy and self-destructive decisions the diagnosis of mental illness is not a justifiable basis for forcing pschiatric treatment.[13] Himmelstein concedes that in some cases the person is obviously unable to make a choice and therefore cannot be compared with "normal" people in that regard. Most mentally ill people, however, like Robert Watson are not so divorced from reality that they cannot understand the implications of drugs. The detention of Watson or anyone else involuntarily committed for an indeterminate period is unjustified if he had no chance to prove his innocence, and thus forced medication is also unjustified. A rule that would allow physicians to force medications without a legal check on their power could subject mentally ill people to serious abuses. Allowing courts to simply rubber-stamp medical opinion is also useless in protecting the client. Perhaps after a person has been hospitalized for a long period of time in which it has been shown clearly that he is unable to make a choice and that his condition has deteriorated severely, medications could be forced. but this condition would need to be determined after long and careful observation and would occur infrequently.

Robert Michels, a psychiatrist at Cornell University Medical College, disagrees.[13] He points out that one of the most striking features of mentally ill people is the difference between what they say and what they mean. If a person who is deranged and whose thought processes may be incoherent refuses a medication, does he really understand the import of the refusal? Can his refusal be taken at face value? Michels thinks it highly unlikely that a deranged mind retains an "island of clarity" for making rational decisions; usually the appearance of clarity is superficial, and close questioning reveals that the person does not have a clear idea of what he is refusing.

The conflict can be understood in terms of rights: the right to health and the expectation that society will assist one to regain health in conflict with the right to liberty, to do what one pleases as long as no one else is harmed.

The mentally healthy majority, with lawyers and politicians as their spokesmen, place liberty first, and are suspicious of the psychiatrist's arcane knowledge which could if abused, give him the ultimate power to determine who shall be free and who shall not. The minority who suffer from psychiatric illness, with their caretakers as their ombudsmen, will suffer if a liberty they cannot enjoy is made superior to a health that must sometimes be forced upon them. For their lives, the preservation of individual liberty rather than the right to treatment is another of the tyrannies of the majority to which they might be subjected.*

Michels believes that the only solution to the dilemma involves the professional competence of the psychiatrist—with judicial review. If a client's mental illness is serious, his right to receive treatment should take precedence over his right to refuse it.

Being a resident in a psychiatric hospital does not automatically make one either competent or incompetent to refuse treatment, nor does a diagnosis of mental illness, a label often attached to people for nonpsychiatric or nonmedical reasons. There is no reason to believe that the same criteria of competence should not be used for a mentally ill person as for "normal" people in the matter of refusing treatment or consenting to it. The criteria are based on a person's ability to make a rational decision by rational means utilizing information provided. As the court decided *In re Yetter*, commitment need not imply incompetence.

RELATIONSHIP BETWEEN HEALTH PROFESSIONAL AND CLIENT

The relationship between a health professional and a client is essentially a contractual one in which both parties enter and maintain the relationship on certain principles. One of the basic principles is veracity, or truth telling. Veracity can be seen as an independent principle in itself or as a derivation from the principle of respect for others. Either way, it is indispensable to any worthwhile human rela-

---

*Michels, Robert, quoted in Veatch, Robert M.: Case studies in medical ethics, Cambridge, Mass., 1977, Harvard University Press, p. 314.

tionship, particularly the professional-client one. Respect for persons also involves the principles of autonomy, beneficence, and nonmaleficence, all of which must be based on truth telling. Veracity also implies a duty of promise keeping or fidelity, which is an integral part of a contractual relationship. The contract implies a general truthfulness and confers on the client specific rights to the truth regarding diagnosis, treatment, and prognosis.

"Relationships of trust between human beings are necessary for fruitful interaction and cooperation."[1,p.203] Trust is essential between health professionals and clients because if one or the other lies, cooperation between them decreases, possibly leading to more lies and the eventual destruction of the relationship. It is interesting to note that none of the codes of ethics discussed in Chapter 9 mentions except in very oblique terms that truth telling is morally demanded of a health professional. The right to an explanation of procedures is granted to clients, and it is implied that the explanation is truthful, but the principle of veracity is not specifically stated.

Novack et al.[14] found that physicians' attitudes about telling clients of a diagnosis of cancer has changed radically in the past 25 years. In 1953 only 31% of 442 physicians surveyed said they always or usually tell the diagnostic truth to a person with cancer. In 1960, 16% of 5000 physicians said they always told the client the truth. In 1977, 278 physicians responded to Novack's questionnaire, and 98% reported that their usual policy was to tell the truth. There were differences between the 1960 and 1977 samples (the latter was a younger population and had a greater percentage of women), but these differences alone are not sufficient to account for the marked change in attitudes toward truth telling. Several factors have been suggested to account for this change. The marked improvement in cancer therapy and better survival rates encourage physicians to communicate more honestly with clients, whereas in the past because of a lack of hope it was thought too depressing to discuss the patient's situation with him. Public awareness about cancer has increased, and public figures are openly discussing their cancer; this may have led to a decrease in stigmatization or to an increase in the awareness of cancer symptoms. The upsurge of interest in death and dying may have led more physicians to be frank with clients. People are increasingly participating in cancer research projects and thus need to know their diagnosis as a requirement for informed consent; even nonexperimental treatment for cancer is complex, and informed consent requires full diagnostic disclosure.

Is deliberate deception always morally wrong in a professional-client relationship? Some believe that providing or withholding the truth depends on a person's right to that truth and that a deliberate lie may sometimes be morally justified. For example, if a friend is a guest in your home and his sworn enemy comes to your door with a gun in his hand and demands to know whether your friend is there, a deliberate lie would be morally correct for two reasons both based on the principle of nonmaleficence: (1) the enemy has no right to the truth because you have every reason to believe that he will use it to harm your friend, and (2) if you were to tell the truth, your friend might be hurt or killed, and you have an obligation to prevent harm from coming to him.[15]

The moral dilemma of truth telling is illustrated by a case presented by Beauchamp and Childress. A 5-year-old girl was dying of progressive renal failure and had been on dialysis for 3 years. A kidney transplant was considered even though it was by no means clear that the transplant would prove beneficial. However, there was enough favorable evidence to proceed with the plans for a transplant. Tissue typing of the immediate family revealed that only the father was histocompatible with the child. The nephrologist met alone with the father and explained that his daughter's prognosis was quite uncertain. The father gave the matter some thought and then admitted to the physician that he did not want to donate a kidney, because of both his daughter's uncertain future and his own lack of courage. He was afraid to face his family with the truth, however, and asked the physician to tell his wife that he could not donate because he was not histocompatible.

Should the physician lie for this man, or can the principle of veracity be overridden by other considerations? If the physician agrees to lie, the father would not have to admit his reluctance to give his daughter a kidney and the family may be able to avoid a traumatic experience. If the physician refuses to lie, the wife and family are likely to discover the truth, which may or may not hurt the family as the man believes. The family may have the opportunity to come closer together if they manage to deal effectively with this crisis. The results of either the lie or the truth could be equally beneficial or harmful to the functioning of this family. When this case was discussed in an ethics seminar, the strong consensus of opinion was that the principle of veracity should take precedence and the physician should not accede to the man's request that he lie.

Can withholding information in the professional-client relationship be considered deception, and if so is it ever justified?

The duty not to lie or to otherwise deceive others is stronger than the duty to disclose information to others. This duty to disclose depends more on special relationships than the duty not to lie or deceive others. In a therapeutic relationship, for example, the patient entrusts his care to the therapist and has a right to information that the therapist would not be obligated to provide to total strangers. It is difficult to conceive of a positive duty to promote the truth by providing information apart from special relationships.*

Special relationships are those in which particular duties and obligations are owed or in which certain duties and obligations go beyond the scope of ordinary social intercourse. Parent-child, friend-friend, and professional-client relationships are special in this sense. A professional may withhold information from a client without actually lying to him, as when giving a placebo in a randomized clinical trial, if the deception does not lead to harm or contribute to breaking the trust between them. When a client asks, "Will it hurt?" the therapist is obligated not to lie, but the expected intensity of pain need not be disclosed. Lying would destroy or damage the relationship of trust whereas not fully disclosing this information would not. This benevolent deception is sometimes morally correct but should be used rarely and judiciously.

---

*Beauchamp, Tom L., and Childress, James F.: Principles of biomedical ethics, New York, 1979, Oxford University Press, p. 205.

Another important principle in the professional-client relationship is confidentiality, which is founded on the principles of trust and respect for persons. At first glance it appears that the rule of confidentiality is not to be broken under any circumstances, but at times social obligations and responsibilities come into conflict with individual confidentiality. Two individuals can have an equal right to the same information, but the information "belongs" to one of them. Can confidentiality be broken to satisfy the rights of the other? The most important case to address this issue is *Tarasoff v. Regents of the University of California*.[16] On October 27, 1969, Prosenjit Poddar killed Tatiana Tarasoff. Tatiana's parents alleged that 2 months prior to the murder Poddar had confided his intentions to Dr. Lawrence Moore, a psychologist employed at a hospital of the University of California at Berkeley. On Moore's request the campus police questioned Poddar but released him because he appeared rational. Nothing further was done, and no one warned Tatiana's parents that Poddar had said he was going to kill Tatiana when she returned from a vacation in Brazil. Poddar was temporarily committed for observation at a mental hospital but was released because he was judged rational. Poddar killed Tatiana shortly after her return from Brazil. The plaintiffs asserted that the defendants (Dr. Moore and his superiors who concurred in the medical judgment) had been negligent in releasing Poddar from police custody and in not warning their daughter that she was in grave danger. The majority opinion in the case maintained that the therapist could not escape liability for negligence merely because Tatiana herself was not also under their care. When a client presents a serious danger of violence to another person, the therapist must use reasonable care in protecting the intended victim from the expressed danger, which may include warning the victim. The therapist has a legal duty not only to his client but also to the intended victim. The majority opinion recognized the right of privacy in a professional-client relationship but stated that this does not outweigh the public's safety. "The protective privilege ends where the public peril begins."[15]

The minority opinion stated that a rule undermining absolute confidentiality would decrease the effectiveness of treatment of the mentally ill. Warning an intended victim would offer little if any benefit to society but would frustrate psychiatric treatment and increase violence by making people hesitant to reveal violent fantasies or plans to the therapist. Having no professional outlet for the violent feelings, they would be more likely to act out those feelings to the ultimate detriment of the public safety. The fear that confidentiality could be breached would tend to decrease a client's trust in the psychiatrist, also lessening the treatment's efficacy. If a duty to warn of impending violence were imposed, more people will be subject to civil commitment—total deprivation of liberty. Most of those who would be committed should not be, as verbalized intentions of violence are usually not carried out, but because the psychiatrist has no way of predicting who will act violently, he would be compelled to commit all those who verbalize violent intentions.

The California Supreme Court set a precedent concerning confidentiality in the case of murderous intent, but most problems with confidentiality are not this dramatic or life-threatening. Less dramatic situations are far more common, such as the dilemma of known genetic defects. For example, Dr. Jenkins has a female client who is a known carrier of hemophilia; two of her brothers have the disease. She plans to marry Tom, who happens to be Dr. Jenkins' brother and close friend. The woman lives in a city far from her family and is not emotionally close to them. Her fiancé is eager to have children. The woman has not yet told her fiancé of her genetic background and does not intend to because she fears the engagement would then be broken. Dr. Jenkins knows of the hemophilia, but the client has repeatedly asked him not to breach the confidentiality because she "could not face life without Tom." Dr. Jenkins knows Tom well enough to realize that he would indeed break the engagement if he knew.

The dilemma hinges not only on the conflict between the social obligation to warn a potential father he may have congenitally abnormal children and the obligation of professional confidentiality, but also on the conflict between the professional-client special relationship and that between brothers and friends. Even if Tom were not Dr. Jenkins' brother, there would still be a conflict in social responsibility. The woman is engaging in a deliberate deception and is therefore behaving in a morally reprehensible way. If Dr. Jenkins does not reveal the information, is he equally morally guilty or does his primary responsibility lie with his client even if he strongly urges her to have a frank discussion with her fiancé? Which special relationship takes precedence, the professional-client or the brother-brother? The latter is closer, more long-lasting, and more emotionally significant, but the former binds him by oath and by his own sense of professional responsibility. The woman client has every reason to expect that when she confides in her physician, he will respect her personhood by respecting her privacy and will share her health problems with no one, not even the person closest to her, unless she gives express permission. Beauchamp and Childress summarize confidentiality as a prima facie duty:

> Anyone who thinks that disclosure of confidential information is morally justified or even mandatory in some circumstances bears a burden of proof. While this approach requires a balancing of conflicting duties, it also establishes a structure of moral reasoning and justification. It is not enough to determine which act will respect the most duties or maximize the good, for the strong presumption against revealing confidences establishes the direction and burden of deliberation and justification.*

In some circumstances when there is a duty higher than that of confidentiality to the client, the health professional may morally divulge information. This can occur when he is required by law to disclose information in the interest of public health of safety, such as reporting communicable diseases, or to protect a client himself, as in child abuse. *Tarasoff* has indicated that a physician must break confidentiality to prevent harm to another person, but the scope of this decision has not yet been determined. Any decision to break confidentiality must be clearly justified; in most instances, except when a distinct harm would be prevented, this act is extremely difficult to justify.

---

*Beauchamp, Tom L., and Childress, James F.: Principles of biomedical ethics, New York, 1979, Oxford University Press, p. 212.

"ROUTINE" PROCEDURES

When clients in hospitals and other health care settings ask questions about procedures, the health professional often answers, "Oh, this is just routine." But *nothing* is "just routine" to the person on whom the procedure is done. A simple blood test may be frightening because it involves a needle puncture and because an unknown disease might be revealed thereby. A person may have had his blood drawn dozens of times, but this time could signal the beginning of the end. Most health procedures are not performed on people when they are feeling perfectly well (even if a general examination is "routine," it is accompanied by nervousness), because they seek help and diagnostic intervention generally only after something has happened to their physical or mental equilibrium. Consequently no diagnostic or therapeutic procedure can be considered routine to the client.

Health care institutions generally define as routine those procedures they perform on a regular basis and those for which a written protocol exists; in other words, they are routine to institutional personnel. The fact that appendectomies are performed frequently does not mean they are all identical or that the risk is less. It is not. An appendectomy and pneumoencephalography may be equally routine procedures, but they carry different degrees of risk, which results from the interplay of forces among the procedure itself, the condition of the client, and circumstances that have nothing to do with either. This interchange is never the same, no matter how many times the procedure is performed, even with the same person.

When a procedure is routine, the quality of informed consent is usually less, especially with diagnostic procedures. A laboratory technician would be suprised if a client wanted to know exactly what was to be done with the blood that had just been removed from his vein and would probably say, "We're going to test it." If the client wanted to know what the tests are, how they are done, and what information can be gathered from them, the technician might flee in a panic or think the client quite eccentric. The client, however, has a right to precise information, and if he does not receive it, his consent will be invalid. The composition of blood may be endlessly fascinating and not at all routine to that particular client.

Because every procedure is unique to every individual, there is no such thing as a routine procedure. If this is recognized by health professionals, it is likely that care will be provided with increased ethical sensitivity.

SUMMARY

Informed consent, the foundation of the professional-client relationship, is based primarily on autonomy, the liberty of personal action that gives one's life direction and permits one to make free choices. Informed consent involves self-reliance and independence.

Paternalism is the regulation of the activities of a state or individual by another state or individual for the purpose of maintaining control. A health care professional may think his paternalistic action is benevolent, but it also causes a decrease in the liberty and autonomy of the client. Autonomy and paternalism frequently conflict in the matter of informed consent; it is from this conflict that most ethical dilemmas arise. These dilemmas usually concern the parameters of paternalism and autonomy and what happens when they overlap.

Paternalism may be justified, usually when the client's safety is in jeopardy and paternalistic action will prevent harm, but these instances are few and far between. Careful deliberation is necessary before paternalism in informed consent can be justified. Restricting liberty is almost never morally permissible.

Informed consent involves a client giving specific written permission to a health professional to touch him in the course of providing care. Consent cannot be considered valid unless it is based on accurate information about the procedure and is given freely without undue influence or coercion. All components of informed consent are geared toward achieving the protection of individual autonomy.

Various court cases have served to increase clients' autonomy, especially regarding the amount and kind of information disclosed and the refusal of treatment even if the only alternative to treatment is death. The basic elements of informed consent are the professional's disclosure of sufficient information so that a rational decision based on facts can be made, the client's competence to make a rational decision, comprehension of the information and the implications of the procedure, and voluntariness—the autonomous decision made as freely as possible.

The relationship between a health professional and a client is a special relationship; that is, duties and obligations are owed beyond what is ordinarily owed in a relationship between strangers or casual acquaintances. The two major elements in the professional-client relationship are veracity, or truth telling, and confidentiality. The application of neither of these principles is clear-cut, and ethical dilemmas arise when a decision must be made about how much truth to tell and when confidentiality can be superseded by a conflicting duty or obligation.

REFERENCES

1. Beauchamp, Tom L, and Childress, James F.: Principles of biomedical ethics, New York, 1979, Oxford University Press.
2. Diehl, Jackson: Do phychiatric laws protect? Washington Post, p. A1, June 4, 1979.
3. Feinberg, Joel: Legal paternalism, The Canadian Journal of Philosophy, 1971, pp. 64-84.
4. *Application of the President and Directors of Georgetown College*, 331 F. 2d 1000 (D.C. Cir.), certiorari denied, 377 U.S. 978 (1964).
5. Murchison, Irene, et al.: Legal accountability in the nursing process, St. Louis, 1978, The C. V. Mosby Co.
6. *Schloendorff v. New York Hospital*, 211 N.Y. 125, 127, 129; 105 N.E. 92, 93 (1914).
7. *Natanson v. Kline*, 186 Kan. 393, 350 P. 2d 1093 (1960), rehearing denied, 187 Kan. 186, 354 P. 2d 670 (1960).
8. Alfidi, Ralph J.: Controversy, alternatives, and decisions in complying with the legal doctrine of informed consent, Radiology 114(1):231-234, January 1975.
9. Faden, Ruth R.: Disclosures and informed consent: does it matter how we tell it? Health Education Monographs 5:198-215, 1977.
10. Fellner, C. H., and Marshall, J. R.: Kidney donors—the myth of informed consent, American Journal of Psychiatry 126:1245, 1970.
11. *Canterbury v. Spence*, No 22099, U.S. Court of Appeals, District of Columbia Circuit, May 19, 1972. 464 Federal Reporter, 2nd series, 772.
12. Byrn, Robert M.: Compulsory lifesaving treatment for the competent adult, Fordhan Law Review 44(1):1, October 1975.
13. Veatch, Robert M.: Case studies in medical ethics, Cambridge, Mass., 1977, Harvard University Press.
14. Novack, Dennis H., et al.: Changes in physicians' attitudes toward telling the cancer patient, Journal of the American Medical Association 241(9):897-900, March 2, 1979.
15. Childress, James F.: Personal communication, July 1979.
16. *Tarasoff v. Regents of the University of Califor-*

nia, California Supreme Court (17 California Reports, 3rd Series, 425), Decided July 1, 1976.

BIBLIOGRAPHY

Alfidi, Ralph J.: Controversy, alternatives, and decisions in complying with the legal doctrine of informed consent, Radiology 114(1):231-234, January 1975.

Beauchamp, Tom L., and Childress, James F.: Principles of biomedical ethics, New York, 1979, Oxford University Press.

Besch, Linda Briggs: Informed consent; a patient's right, Nursing Outlook 27(1):32-35, January 1979.

Byrn, Robert M.: Compulsory lifesaving treatment for the competent adult, Fordham Law Review 44(1):1, October 1975.

Canterbury v. Spence, No 22099, U.S. Court of Appeals, District of Columbia Circuit, May 19, 1972, 464 Federal Reporter, 2nd series, 772.

Diehl, Jackson: Do psychiatric laws protect? Washington Post, p.a1, June 4, 1979.

Dworkin, Gerald: Paternalism, Monist 56(1):64-84, June 1972.

Faden, Ruth R.: Disclosure and informed consent: does it matter how we tell it? Health Education Monographs 5:198-215, 1977.

Feinberg, Joel: Legal Paternalism, The Canadian Journal of Philosophy 1:105-124, 1976.

Fellner, C. H., and Marshall, J. R.: Kidney donors—the myth of informed consent, American Journal of Psychiatry 126:1245, 1970.

Freedman, Benjamin: A moral theory of informed consent, Hastings Center Report 5(4):32-39, August 1975.

Freud, Anna: The doctor-patient relationship. In Katz, Jay: Experimentations with human beings, New York, 1972, Russell Sage Foundation.

Gorovitz, Samuel, et al., Editors: Moral problems in medicine, Englewood Cliffs, N.J., 1976, Prentice-Hall, Inc.

Hegland, Kenney F.: Unauthorized rendition of life-saving medical treatment, California Law Review 53(3):86, August 1965.

Ingelfinger, Franz J.: Informed (but uneducated) consent, New England Journal of Medicine 287:465-466, August 31, 1972.

Kant, Immanuel: Lectures on ethics (Louis Infield, translator), New York, 1963, Harper & Row, Publishers, Inc.

Kelly, Kathleen, and McCelland, Eleanor: Signed consent: protection or constraint? Nursing Outlook 27(1):80-82, January 1979.

May, Katharyn Antle: The nurse as researcher: impediment to informed consent? Nursing Outlook 27(1):36-39, January 1979.

Mill, John Stuart: On liberty. In Utilitarianism, New York, 1974, The New American Library, Inc.

Murchison, Irene, et al.: Legal accountability in the nursing process, St. Louis, 1978, The C. V. Mosby Co.

Novack, Dennis H., et al.: Changes in physicians' attitudes toward telling the cancer patient, Journal of the American Medical Association 241(9):897-900, March 2, 1979.

Tarasoff v. Regents of the University of California, California Supreme Court (17 California Reports, 3rd series, 425), Decided July 1, 1976.

Veatch, Robert M.: Case studies in medical ethics, Cambridge, Mass., 1977, Harvard University Press.

Walters, Leroy: Ethical aspects of medical confidentiality, Journal of Clinical Computing 4:9-20, 1974.

11

Organ transplantation

HISTORY

Homografting, the transplantation of an organ or tissue between members of the same species, has had a long history. Medea in Greek mythology was depicted arranging a blood transfusion between Jason and his father, and autografts (using one's own tissue for grafting) were successfully done in India as early as 600 B.C. The first successful homograft occurred in 17th century Italy, and in 1688 an 80-page transplant textbook on blood transfusions was published. Blood is the most commonly and successfully transplanted tissue, although transfusion is generally not viewed in the same dramatic light as organ transplants. Heterografts, the transplantation of an organ or tissue from an individual of one species to that of another, were performed in Europe prior to World War I by taking kidneys from rabbits, goats, pigs, and primates and attempting to graft them in humans. Homografts of skin between identical twins became successful in the 1920s.[1]

Modern organ transplantation, with its attendant physiologic complexities and moral dilemmas, began in the 1950s. In 1951 Dr. David Hume of Boston performed the first of several kidney transplants, using cadaver organs. The longest survival time was 6 months. In 1954 Dr. Joseph Murray and Dr. John Merrill transplanted a kidney from an identical twin to his brother. That first recipient lived 8 years with his brother's kidney, during which time he married and had a child. He died of a heart attack that was thought to be related to the original kidney disease. Other recipients did not fare as well, however, because of the body's tendency to reject a foreign organ. In 1961 the first effective immunosuppressive drug, azathioprine, was ready for human use, and thereafter kidney transplants were done frequently and with increasing success.

Immunosuppressive drugs paved the way for Dr. Christiaan Barnard in South Africa to transplant the heart of Denise Darvall into Louis Washkansky in an operation on December 3, 1967, that made headlines around the world. Washkansky lived only 2 weeks but this surgery spurred other transplant teams to improve the technique and it was thought that a major solution to heart disease was at hand. However, heart transplants were not as successful as had been originally hoped, mainly because of the rejection problem. By the mid-1970s the number of heart transplants had dwindled to a few, but research into immunosuppressive drugs is as enthusiastic as ever.

It is interesting to note that 3 years before Dr. Barnard's successful heart homo-graft, Dr. James Hardy of Mississippi had unsuccessfully attempted a heart het-erograft from a chimpanzee to a 68-year-old man suffering from terminal hyperten-sive cardiovascular disease.[2] The man was admitted to the hospital in an almost moribund state (his gangrenous leg had to be amputated before the transplant could proceed). No mention was made in the report of adequate informed consent, and the man died an hour after mechanical supports were removed. The next year a sheep heart was used in a transplant attempt that failed, and the medical com-munity acknowledged that heart heterografts were not a practical area for further research.

On April 4, 1969, Dr. Denton Cooley performed the first total replacement of a human heart with a mechanical device. The surgery was designed as a temporary stop-gap until a donor could be found. The recipient's wife made an emotional appeal for a donor heart on national television. A donor was found within 2 days, causing a fear that more public pleas would be made for donors, a situation with serious ethical problems. The recipient died the day after the transplant.

A totally implantable artificial heart (TIAH) seems the most promising area of research concerning heart replacements. Constructed entirely of synthetic materi-als, its pump driven by a small motor powered by a rechargeable battery or a nuclear engine, the entire mechanical system would be permanently installed in-side the body. The cost for each implantation is estimated at about $50,000 to $75,000.[3] The device is now being developed at the National Heart and Lung In-stitute and at various research centers through funding supplied by the National Institutes of Health. No one knows when the device will be ready for human ex-perimentation, although debates about the morality of human testing have already begun.

Other human homografts have been successfully accomplished. Corneas have provided sight for thousands, and bone has been so successfully transplanted that bone banks are fairly common in large medical centers. Bone marrow transplants are used in the treatment of certain kinds of leukemia although rejection is a greater problem with bone marrow than it is with whole blood. It is also thought that the liver and lungs might possibly be transplanted, although the complexities are so monumental that success with either remains in the distant future. The major problem with liver transplants is damage to the transplanted organ. It is highly susceptible to blood clots and hemorrhage and begins to deteriorate about 20 minutes after it has been removed from the cadaver unless it is thoroughly and immediately cooled and perfused. The liver is so perishable that the time it would take to reattach it in the recipient would damage it sufficiently to ensure rejection.

The first lung transplant was performed in 1963 by Dr. Hardy at the University of Mississippi Medical Center on a prisoner serving a life sentence for murder who had chronic kidney disease and lung cancer.[4] He died 18 days after the surgery. Several more attempts have since been made by surgeons in the United States and Europe, and no recipient has survived more than 3 weeks. The two major problems in lung transplantation involve correctly reconnecting the nerve supply and pre-venting massive infection. Part of the recipient's own lungs must be left in place to provide adequate nerve control for breathing, and this usually leads to infection of the donor lungs followed by death. Lungs, however, are relatively easy to preserve and transport. Transplantation has a reasonable likelihood of success if the infection problem can be solved. Dog lungs have been successfully stored and transplanted with the respiritory system working at almost total efficiency a few weeks later.[4]

Organ transplantation is in its infancy and has a bright future, but opinion is divided about the extent to which health resources should be invested in solving the problems of homografts. Since the supply of donor organs is limited and the technologic and medical problems are so great, research into treatment of heart and kidney disease might be more efficiently directed toward mechanical means such as TIAH and portable kidney dialysis machines. The latter would be simple, compact, and automatic enough to be used with no help from others and perhaps even during normal activities or sleep. No matter what directions future research takes, the costs will be enormous.

RELIGIOUS VIEWS

The central issue in the religious view of organ transplantation concerns whether a person has a right to deliberately mutilate his own or another person's body or, in the case of the organ recipient, to cause such mutilation to take place. The liberal view is that parts of the body exist for the good of the whole and that a diseased or nonfunctioning part may be destroyed or removed if the ultimate good is the preservation of health of the whole body. The conservative view is that mutilation of any part of the body is impermissible because the body is a complete entity and should be kept intact. God created the human body and intended each body part to be used in a specific way for a specific purpose. There are wide variations among Western religions between these two views.

In a 1930 encyclical, *Casti Canubii,* which had to do with Christian marriage, Pope Pius XI stated that private individuals had no power over "members of their bodies" and were not free to destroy or mutilate them in any way "except when no other provision can be made for the good of the whole body."[5] Pope Pius XII in 1952 reinforced that view by saying that each body part is integral to the whole and is absorbed by the totality of the organism. In neither statement is organ transplantation specifically prohibited. Because a transplant is never undertaken unless it is the last hope for restoring the person to health, the 1930 encyclical might be interpreted to expressly permit transplants even though the first transplant was not to be accomplished for more than 20 years. The statement by Pope Pius XII was made about 2 years prior to the first kidney transplant. He was probably aware of the research being conducted and knew it would be only a matter of time until it was performed on a human, but he chose not to address the issue directly. Many Catholic theologians thought that because the Pope had not expressly forbidden organ transplant, he tacitly condoned it.

The 1952 statement about the totality of the human organism may have been the Pope's general view of the ethics of human experimentation and a general affirmation of his humanism. Because there has not been specific papal opposition, the Catholic Church has taken the stand that organ transplantation is permissible as long as the recipient stands a reasonable chance of benefit and the donor does not risk his life or is not completely deprived of some vital function (donation of both kidneys is impermissible).

The principle of totality in the Catholic Church neither permits nor prohibits organ transplantation, but the principle of fraternal charity, which states that unity among people makes one's neighbor "another self," allows a person to do for another that which he would do for himself. If he would and should save his own life, he can and should save another's by charitably giving part of himself. The principle of fraternal charity is higher than the principle of totality because the former prevents the latter from becoming a form of selfish self-preservation. "In the Catholic tradition, charity is an infused theological virtue which finds itself in continuity with 'nature,' confirms our experienced bonds of life with life, and elevates and perfects us in our existing direction toward God and toward life with and for our fellow man."[6]

Ramsey[6] reports that liberal Catholic theologians, notably Martin Nolan, believe the traditional view of totality was overly concerned with "physicalism." Totality should not be defined or limited by the physical space of the body because the wholeness of a person is concerned with his mind-body integrity and his "ultimate finality." A person cannot achieve totality only within the confines of his body; there is continuity between physical space and membership in a communion with God. Nolan believes that the debate over permissibility of organ transplantation tends to lend a barter atmosphere to charity. He does, however, impose limits on the extent of physical charity by stating that one's body or organs may not be disposed of arbitrarily, that to do so would be an act of suicide. At the same time he believes that the gift of charity or participation in human experimentation should not be thought of in terms of the merely physical. Even liberal Catholics have not come to a firm conclusion regarding whether charity triumphs over physicalism in the matter of organ transplantation.

> The price paid for this victory, however, is that the human person not only breaks the bonds of physical existence in quelling the emptiness that is the hallmark of his finitude by faith and love toward God. He also overflows the narrow limits of personhood by seeking to fill his own vast emptiness through love for another person as his "other self."*

The concept of the self equated with the other is strong in Catholic theology and is one of the bases of the principle of charity. It does, however, raise an issue: if the self and the other are equated to some degree, where is the line drawn, and how much of oneself can be sacrificed for another without risking the sin of self-mutilation or suicide?

The theme of bodily mutilation is woven into Western religions and gives rise to a taboo against organ transplantation. People have had a strong aversion to mutilating their bodies, even after death, and traditionalists still forbid autopsies because they think the body must remain intact for burial and possibly for the passage into the next life. Judaism, which has no clearly defined concept of an afterlife, forbids autopsies, as does conservative Catholicism.

Both Leonardo da Vinci and Michelangelo were denied access to hospital morgues

---

*Ramsey, Paul: The patient as person, New Haven, Conn., 1970, Yale University Press, p. 186.

because it was known that they were dissecting bodies to study anatomy. In 1788 five people were killed in a street riot in New York after a mob burned the Hospital Society's building because it housed an anatomy collection.[7] When medical education became organized into schools in the 19th century, cadavers were needed for dissection to teach anatomy. Medical schools could not obtain them legally, however, and the number of body snatchers increased. They stole bodies from homes before burial, but they also became proficient as grave robbers. These grotesqueries continued until the law permitted medical schools to collect unclaimed bodies from prisons and poorhouses that would have gone to potter's fields.

Autopsy, which necessarily involves mutilation of the cadaver, is still feared by many. Only about 16% of people who die in hospitals are autopsied despite fairly heavy pressure on the family.[7] In 1967 a group of Orthodox Jews attacked the Knesset in Jerusalem and held public demonstrations there and in Tel Aviv protesting autopsy. The Jewish prohibition against autopsy stems from the Talmudic requirement that a corpse be buried on the day of death because it is seen as unclean. Priests (Kohanim) are forbidden to be in the presence of a corpse, and the Old Testament describes many cleansing rituals for persons who come into contact with a corpse.

This taboo against the mutilation of dead or living bodies creates problems for those who require donor organs. More young people are planning to will their bodies to medical schools to be used as sources of organs or for educational purposes, but the general fear of mutilation remains stronger than the desire to donate organs and a severe shortage exists.

The Protestant position on organ transplantation stems from the principle of charity or *agape* (Christian love). The charitable gift of an organ is seen as an entirely free action that arises out of a state of grace. The gift, however, is not a right that can be claimed or a duty or obligation to be imposed. A person may feel obligated to donate an organ to someone, but he does not need to accede to an obligation placed on him by another. Martin Luther believed that an act is not charity if it is done on a "servile or mercenary principle" by one seeking personal gratification or fulfillment. He thought that those who do good for mercenary reasons are "numbered among the wicked" and are warned not to do good to obtain some benefit, whether material or spiritual.[6]

> True faith is effective in love which seeks the neighbor's good alone and not the self's compensation, fulfillment, or wholeness; self-giving acts should not be done under the false impression that through them you are to come into cosmic communion; this would in fact be a godless presumption and perversity and a godless addition to the self-giving of organs, that personhood and a higher spiritual wholeness is to be sought through such donations.*

Ramsey believes that the Protestant justification for organ transplantation need not depend on a "sticky (psychological or spiritual) benefits theory" but can be translated into the secular concept of informed consent on the part of the donor.

Traditional Jewish ethics expresses a great concern for bodily integrity before and after death and forbids mutilation except to save the person's life, for example,

---

*Ramsey, Paul: The patient as person, New Haven, Conn., 1970, Yale University Press, p. 180.

amputation of a gangrenous limb, or to investigate the causes of a mysterious plague. This ban on mutilation poses a serious problem for organ transplantation. The person with kidney or heart disease might be permitted to receive an organ to save his life, but if no body is to be mutilated, a donor organ would not be available. However, other laws in Judaism can be viewed as overriding the traditional taboo on mutilation. Some interpretations state that if the donor runs no more risk of death than during ordinary surgery, he may be permitted to give up an organ.[7] There is also the tradition of *pikuach nefesh,* which permits breaking moral law if life is in danger. This covers situations such as ill persons eating or taking medications during the 24-hour fast of Yom Kippur, driving on the Sabbath to transport a gravely ill person to a hospital, or bearing arms on the Sabbath if one's territory is being attacked. *Pikuach nefesh* can also be seen as permitting an organ transplantation to save a life, although it is doubtful if this principle covers all situations, such as when a person's life is not in immediate danger because he can be adequately sustained on kidney dialysis or the transplantation of corneas to a person who is blind but not dying. Reform and Conservative Judaism have broken away from the Orthodox view on these matters and permit organ transplantations without restriction.

ETHICAL ISSUES

One might not believe there are strong ethical issues concerning organ transplantation. After all, what could be wrong with the desire to save a human life by the selfless act of giving of oneself? We may see even less of a moral issue in terms of cadaver organs, especially if we do not subscribe to the taboo against bodily mutilation. Nothing in bioethics is as simple as it may seem, however.

One view of the morality of organ transplants is seen in terms of violence done to the body, a kind of war on a limited field. Nelson[1] describes it as a "just war"; that is, we should be concerned not only with the morality of ends (saving a life) but with the means used to justify those ends. Can violence be done to a body to save the life of another? Even if a donor consents willingly and if surgery is the last resort before death, can transplantation be morally condoned? Nelson draws a parallel with military violence and states that if military force is ever justified, it is only for defensive purposes. Therefore a physician may commit physical violence (surgery *is* violent, no matter how well intended) on a person only to save that person's life. This view raises a conflict: if the recipient's life is to be defended and aggression in the form of surgery is therefore morally permissible, what of the donor's life? Is it not in jeopardy? The donor is placed at greater risk than if he had not volunteered his organ. How can violence done to the donor be morally justified? The donor faces certain hazards. The risk of surgery is small, but it does exist, and although a donor can live quite comfortably with one kidney, he has given up a certain margin of safety in the event his remaining kidney should be damaged accidentally or fail to function. Psychologic hazards, which will be discussed later, can be even greater than the physical ones.

Probably the single most pressing ethical issue involves the potential donor's sense of obligation to the recipient. Distinguishing between a donation made to avoid guilt and one made with the moral conviction that donation is a human obligation is difficult, especially because the donor and recipient are almost always blood-related close family members. If we can assume that organ donation is acceptable to all but the most orthodox traditionalists, can we equally assume that a person is morally obligated to give a part of himself to save another? Where is the line drawn between "You *may* donate" and "You *must* donate"? Should there be a line drawn at all, or are the issues entirely different? If there is a natural moral bond between human beings, it would seem that bond implies moral equality. But the request for an organ requires one person to subordinate himself to the other, and the natural order of things is violated because preservation of the other now takes precedence over preservation of the self. "Therefore because of the equality among men in their natural ordination to one another, it does not immediately follow that a donor can rightfully consent to give an organ to his 'other self.' "[6,p.169] In other words, organ donation is not a moral obligation.

Many disagree with this view by pointing to the Christian tradition of self-sacrifice and love. Love probably does require a certain amount of sacrifice, but how much? If love does not exist between a potential donor and recipient, is the sacrifice still required because a family tie exists? The only family member one deliberately chooses is one's spouse, who is not genetically related and therefore is not a candidate for organ donation. One is related to other family members through no choice of his own, and although certain emotional ties exist because of sociocultural tradition, one does not necessarily love one's family as a free choice. Therefore, since the blood relationship was established by chance, does a moral obligation for self-sacrifice exist? If the moral obligation is viewed as a desire to seek a higher moral plane by giving of a part of oneself, and if one believes that this sacrifice is necessary to achieve a particular state of grace, then organ donation may be viewed as obligatory, although probably a relatively small number of people think this is the case. The position could also be seen as a subordination of the physicality of one's being to the perfection of one's total self, the Catholic view of totality.

In 1956 the Massachusetts Supreme Judicial Court had to decide whether a 19-year-old boy could donate a kidney to his identical twin brother.[8] Leon Masden was dying of kidney disease, and his brother Leonard not only consented to donate his kidney but urgently requested it. Both parents also consented. The case came to court because the Masden twins were minors and because there was doubt that the surgery would benefit Leonard; therefore his parents could not legally consent to the assault on Leonard. Judge Edward A. Counihan, Jr., found that Leonard not only understood the implications of what he was about to do but also *needed* to do it. The judge found that Leonard would suffer grave emotional consequences if the transplant were denied and Leon died, as he surely would. Because Leonard would have been adversely affected for the rest of his life, the transplant was seen to benefit both twins; emotional need was equated with physical necessity. In this case it seems that Leonard felt a definite moral obligation to his brother, although the psychology of identical twinship may have played a large part in Leonard's decision. The court approved the transplant.

Some object to the principle of totality as a prohibition for organ transplantation because totality is perfectly egocentric; that is, a person cannot morally sacrifice his totality for another. If totality were viewed only in physical terms there might be no argument here, but much theologic and philosophic thought sees a duality of mind and body and sees the spirit encased with the flesh. Therefore, if totality *is* duality, the principle cannot be used to prohibit organ transplantation. If reverence for life, one's own or another's, is the highest moral principle, then it must supersede the principle of totality. Is one obligated, however, to view the two principles in relation to each other or in competition with each other? If one sees reverence for life as a higher principle than totality, is an obligation for organ donation created? If one believes in the obligation of organ donation for this reason, does it then follow that abortion and the termination of artificial life support must be opposed for the same reason?

Is there another moral principle that opposes allowing one who feels obligated to donate an organ? Although the question cannot be answered to everyone's satisfaction, Ramsey[6] presents a hypothetical example that illustrates the dilemma. The 15-year-old son of Roger Johnson was admitted to a hospital to determine why his physical condition was declining. It was discovered that he was suffering from a progressively deteriorating congenital condition of his heart valves. The son would not live past the age of 20, and there was no known treatment. At first Mr. Johnson tried to resign himself to his son's death, but he began to brood about all the pleasures of adult life that his son would miss. The more he thought about it, the more unwilling he became to accept the inevitability of his son's death. He devised a plan that he confided to a friend who was a physician: given the recent success of heart transplants and the increased probability of success with genetic relatives, he would donate his own heart to his son. He had lived a full life and could provide financial security for his son. His wife had died several years before, and he thought that his own parents had no rightful claim to his continued life. The friend reluctantly found a surgeon who consented to the plan. His son was told that he would receive a heart transplant in an attempt to prolong his life, but if the attempt failed, he would die. He was not told whose heart he would receive. He agreed to the transplant. Preparation for the surgery proceeded, and the father was anesthetized. At this point a nurse informed the hospital chief of staff what was happening (he had no prior knowledge). The chief has the power to halt the procedure or permit it to continue. What should he do?

In this instance a man is willing to sacrifice his life, not just a part of himself, for his son, but the ethical issues are similar. Could the argument of *Masden v. Harrison* be applied in this case, that Mr. Johnson will suffer emotionally if he is not permitted to save the life of his son? Ramsey thinks that such self-sacrifices need to meet several tests. Informed consent must be rationally and freely given and not the result of a "warped or guilt-ridden mind." A self-sacrifice must meet the "prevention of detriment" test; that is, it must be judged that suffering another's death would be more unbearable than one's own death if one thinks the former may be prevented by the latter. It might also meet the "spiritual benefits" test if the donor achieves a higher state of grace by sacrificing himself than by preserving his own life over another's. According to Ramsey, the crucial question is this: "Are a person's consent or his spiritual or psychological wholeness the only right-making considerations to be taken into account in deciding such a question? Are violation of a person's consent or violation of his felt need for spiritual or psychological wholeness the only wrong-making features?"[6,p.190] Is free and informed consent or the fact that all the tests have been passed sufficient to make this kind of self-sacrifice morally correct or even obligatory? Can the avoidance of intolerable sadness or the promise of supreme spiritual benefit justify this degree of self-sacrifice? Is Mr. Johnson in any way morally obligated to give up his life for that of his son? Conservatives would argue that the donation of a heart cannot in any way be compared with any other moral sacrifice, even jumping from an overcrowded lifeboat to save others. The latter illustrates the principle of double effect; that is, the death of the person jumping overboard is foreseen but not purposefully intended. A living heart donor not only foresees but intends his own death. Liberals might see the act as praiseworthy or certainly not blameworthy, as long as it was undertaken rationally and freely.

Ramsey does not address the issues of suicide and murder in this hypothetical situation, but they cannot be ignored. Mr. Johnson's act is certainly suicidal in that he has consciously and deliberately decided to end his own life. But the purpose of his decision lends it a different cast, and although it is still an act of suicide, its moral ramifications differ. Whether one views this suicide as morally permissible depends to a large degree on one's view of the purpose of life and the rights an individual has in regard to the physical disposition of his own body (see the section on suicide in Chapter 12).

Suicide may or may not be morally permissible, but murder is not. The surgeon who removes Mr. Johnson's heart will be murdering him regardless of the rationale or the state of grace to which Mr. Johnson will be elevated. There is no getting around the fact that the physician will be committing an illegal and immoral act. Can it be justified? Conservatives would be unlikely even to look for justification; liberals would need to do some fancy ethical footwork to find moral justification. Few people would debate the issue of whether a person is morally obligated to sacrifice his life for another in this way, no matter how close the relationship or how loved the person. Most would automatically dismiss the notion that such an obligation is required.

Deciding when a transplant is justified is another ethical dilemma. In 1968 the Board of Medicine of the American National Academy of Sciences issued a public statement concerning heart transplant guidelines.[9] The procedure must not be regarded as a routine form of therapy and is therefore justified only under highly restricted conditions. In addition to its being the last hope for the recipient, there must be resources available for "gaining maximum scientific value for the future of medical service." Therefore only certain physicians in certain institutions should be permitted to perform transplants. Strongly implied though not actually stated is the belief that the recipient shall be deemed a suitable candidate so that he can be expected to survive a reasonable length of time to avoid wasting a donor heart and to provide research data.

There is strong feeling in some quarters that a transplant should not necessarily be the treatment of last resort, that the person need not be subjected to a long and arduous medical regimen before transplant is attempted. Giving a client the choice between transplant and dialysis while the choice is still realistic should be a treatment option.

Another issue in justifying transplants involves the cost/benefit ratio. This is particularly relevant when hearts are involved, but the principles apply also to kidney transplants. The costs in both time and money are enormous. Transplants are among the most expensive medical procedures done in the United States today (see Chapter 2). Can spending hundreds of thousands of dollars on transplanting a handful of organs be justified when entire generations of children could be immunized for approximately the same cost, when the money could be used for thousands of people dying of starvation, and when the same money might even lead to a cure for a type of cancer? A single life saved as a result of a transplant is dramatic and is of course gratifying to the organ recipient and his family. But is it worth it when compared to what *could* have been done with the same money?

Most heart and kidney transplants take place in large metropolitan medical centers that support vast research complexes. Therefore people in need of transplants must live close to these facilities or be attended by a physician who has a connection with the hospital. This eliminates many people, including those who have no physician, those who receive health care in clinics (except in rare instances when a condition is very unusual and can be used for teaching purposes), and those who live in rural areas—usually the poor. Once again, we see that sophisticated health care is available primarily to certain upper- and middle-class segments of society. Heart transplants have all but disappeared for the time being, but kidney transplants are fairly common. However, lower-class people are less likely to seek continued treatment for kidney disease, and if they are treated on an on-going basis, they are less likely to be viewed by physicians as appropriate recipients for transplant.[10] If other than medical criteria are used in the selection process for transplants, people from the lower class will score lower on criteria that are generally grouped into what is known as social worth, that is, education, occupation, past achievements, future potential, and so on. Therefore they receive fewer kidneys than people from the middle and upper classes. It would be an unfair oversimplification to state that recipients of kidney transplants are chosen solely on the basis of race or social class, but most transplants are performed after the person has been on dialysis for a period of time, often years. The reasonable criteria for choosing potential dialysis recipients are the ability to understand the treatment and cooperate with it, an atmosphere in the home of support and help, and the maintenance of prescribed nutritional requirements. It is more likely that an upper-class, educated person will meet these criteria.

SOCIAL AND PSYCHOLOGIC ASPECTS

Roger Coene, a management employee of the New York Telephone Company, wrote of his experience with a kidney transplant and his feelings about it. Coene, who is not an ethicist, philosopher, attorney, or physician, wrote with intelligence and insight.[11]

Coene had suffered from chronic glomerulonephritis for 10 years and knew he would have to choose between dialysis and a transplant; he realized that kidney disease dominated his life and placed all other life events in a different perspective. In 1975 Coene's father became seriously ill with a heart condition. Facing last-resort surgery, he insisted that his kidneys be given to his son if the surgery failed. Father and son were under treatment in distant states, and arrangements for kidney retrieval, perfusion, and transportation had to be made. The father's hospital seemed more interested in receiving payment and was inflexible and insensitive in making plans. Coene's father died immediately after the operation, but the team responsible for retrieving the kidney acted too slowly even though Coene made repeated frantic telephone calls. The kidney that was eventually removed had deteriorated so much that transplant would have been useless. Coene felt grief over the father's death, bitterness over the insensitivity of the transplant unit, and anger at the weaknesses in the system. He was also billed for services he did not receive, and he refused to pay. Coene thought the transplant unit acted as it had for several reasons: (1) they disliked the idea of transplanting the kidneys of a 71-year-old donor because his age decreased the success rate, (2) they were uncomfortable dealing with the actual recipient rather than his physician, and (3) they resented not receiving one of the kidneys for their own research.

Coene's kidneys deteriorated further, and he was placed on dialysis and his name added to a list of people waiting for a kidney transplant. About a month later he was again disappointed when a kidney that had been thought a good match turned out not to be. Two weeks later he was notified that another kidney was available, and he agreed to participate in a research study designed to minimize rejection by daily doses of placental gammaglobulin. The researcher requested consent during the 3 frantic hours in which Coene was being prepared for surgery. Coene thought he was well prepared for the physical aspects of postoperative care, but the psychologic factors were another matter. He said that each day after his kidney function tests he could tell by the expression on the faces of the physicians and nurses and by how much time they were willing to spend with him whether his new kidney was functioning well. All the transplant recipients in the unit lived a watch-and-wait kind of life, seeking support more from each other than from health professionals. On the 17th day after the transplant rejection seemed confirmed, and doses of immunosuppressive drugs were increased, also increasing the unpleasant side effects. Biopsy revealed irreversible rejection, and plans were made to remove the kidney. Coene was placed back on dialysis, but he experienced severe withdrawal symptoms when he was weaned from the immunosuppressive drugs. He described the symptoms as "depersonalization"; they sounded frightening but were controlled by tranquilizers. About 3 months later Coene was back to his pretransplant level of general health and began thinking about making another attempt at a transplant. "The fundamental choice, of course, is between continued dialysis or renewed transplant attempts in an effort to achieve the quality of life that I feel is essential."[11]

The crux of the decision for Coene and anyone else facing the issue indeed involves the quality of life. Dialysis can be difficult and unpleasant, and it surely restricts one's life to a large degree, but it is secure and predictable. Having a transplant is risky and emotionally exhausting. No guarantees exist that a transplant will not be rejected. Dialysis requires strength of character and a determination to follow through with the regimen. It also requires the support of family members, particularly if it is to be done at home. A transplant, if it is successful, will permit the person to lead a much less restricted life, and he will feel generally better than when on dialysis. Neither choice, however, provides a lifetime cure for kidney disease, and there is an increased risk of complications and death with either decision. There is one important advantage to dialysis: the technology is advancing more rapidly than that of transplantation. More efficient machines and filters are available, making dialysis faster and safer. Transplants have a low statistical probability of success and are accompanied by great anxiety and unpleasant physical symptoms.

Coene chose dialysis because he thought he could not justify the risk of another transplant attempt. The psychologic effect of choosing a treatment can take almost as great a toll as the disease itself. "The patient who chooses a transplant faces a greater risk of dying in order to gain a better chance for a normal, unrestricted life. The patient on dialysis is less likely to die but more likely to suffer further medical and psychological damage from the long-term effects of therapy."[12] The mortality rate for transplant recipients is 10% in the first year, and about 50% of all transplant cadaver kidneys fail within 2 years, forcing the person back on dialysis to await another transplant.[12] The poorer the person's general health, the higher the rate of failure; therefore, since twice as many people with kidney disease have other complicating factors, transplants do not hold a particularly bright promise of success. Knowing this (informed consent requires that the potential recipient know the facts) creates a psychologic strain that is difficult to bear, particularly in view of other frightening facts. Immunosuppressive drugs, which must be taken forever, cause serious side effects; malignancies occur within 10 years in 25% of transplant recipients; brain tumors are 35 times more common than in the general population; and psychiatric symptoms occur with predictable regularity.

Donors too experience a profound psychologic impact. Simmons and Klein[13] studied 130 donors and their families. One year after transplant, donors whose gift was still functioning in the recipient were interviewed. The authors acknowledge that the bias of interviewing only these donors downplays the negative reaction to kidney donation, but their purpose was to study the psychologic cost of a successful transplant. They concluded that people were more willing to donate than might have been assumed by the lay public and health professionals. Of the eligible family members of potential recipients, 57% volunteered to donate without having been asked; they appeared to volunteer as a spontaneous offer rather than as a result of careful deliberation. Even a year after the transplant, donors generally retained the positive feelings of increased self-esteem, happiness, and strengthened emotional ties with the recipient. Donors perceived their gift as not only a general saving of life but also the prevention of the death of a loved one. Of all the families, 25% had negative experiences. Most of the conflicts involved potential donors who did not volunteer and who became angry at family pressure to donate. Many of those who did not wish to donate were provided with a false medical excuse by the surgeon; the authors do not discuss the ethical implications of this practice. Many local physicians who were not involved with the transplant advised against donation by a potential donor who seemed ambivalent. Of all donors, 34% said they did not feel completely well even a year after surgery, and more than 75% could not go back to work for at least 2 months. All donors incurred large medical expenses.

Most people probably perceive the gift of a kidney as a gift of love and do not seriously consider the risk, expense, and other factors involved. Because of this it would be easy for the transplant surgeon to skip over some of the facts that are essential to informed consent. A person eager to donate is less likely to pay attention to the negative ramifications than a person who feels some degree of ambivalence. "For those who are ambivalent about the donation, who are subjected to family or professional pressures, or who are unable, because of age or other condition, to give a truly informed consent, the gift ought to be carefully examined before it is allowed."[12]

Fox[14] sees several sociologic issues involved in organ transplantation, such as problems of medical uncertainty, ambiguities about the developmental state of a relatively new treatment (concerning how experimental or therapeutic it should be considered), difficulties with informed voluntary consent, decisions regarding the allocation of scarce resources, conflicts among physicians about prolonging life, sociopsychologic relationships between transplant clients and the health professionals who care for them, and public interest in the experimental aspects of new procedures. Many of these issues have been discussed elsewhere in this book.

One of the most perplexing problems is the uncertainty resulting from the fact that the technology is new and mostly still experimental, especially the techniques to minimize the risk of rejection. Uncertainty takes a psychologic toll on both physicians and clients. Clients are also subjected to physical uncertainties. Physicians are necessarily forced to play the dual role of healer and researcher because they must use clients as sources of data for future clients while at the same time doing everything possible to assure a successful transplant in each client. The clients are thus patients and experimental subjects, even if they are not participating in formal research. They are aware that if a transplant is rejected by their body, the information gained from that failure will be used to attempt an improvement of the procedure for the next person. The major uncertainties in kidney transplant treatment result from a lack of knowledge about immunologic reactions. Immunosuppressive drugs work only sometimes, and the wait-and-see situation described by Coene can be nerve-wracking. Even after the immediate postoperative period has safely passed, the kidney can be rejected at any time. Living with that possibility requires social and emotional adaptation. Statistical projections of the likelihood of rejection are now too crude to be of much use, and a donor or cadaver kidney that appears to be histocompatible may be rejected. Until exact prognoses can be made, physicians and clients must adjust to this uncertainty.

Informed consent with kidney donation involves complex social relationships as well as ethical considerations. A living kidney donor not only is giving part of his own body to a relative, usually a close one, but is to some degree taking the fate of the recipient into his own hands. If a prospective donor refuses, the recipient can always fall back on dialysis for a while, but this is not the same. Refusing to donate a kidney is easily perceived as passing a death sentence. "One of the questions . . . is whether under the life-and-death circumstances that are preconditions for a live transplant, the gift of an organ can ever be said to be sufficiently voluntary, disinterested, and spontaneous to justify its acceptance."[14,p.414]

There is much controversy about the issue of undue influence by family pressure, guilt, and even coercion. There is no such thing as a disinterested kidney donor; even if the recipient were a total stranger, the idea of giving away a part of one's physical self is a decision not to be made lightly One can assume that a kidney donor is under some pressure even if it comes only from within. Having the power to save the life of someone loved will cause sleepless nights. Even the most voluntary act of donation must be tinged by the avoidance of guilt, an experience that in itself can produce guilt. Fox makes an effort to delineate those internal and external pressures that are "normal," "healthy," and "rational." She describes the modern family as small, intimate, and relatively socially isolated. Each relationship within the family operates at a high level of emotional intensity and is critically important to the family's stability. Even with no outside manipulation, each family member will feel intense pressure to donate; the kidney becomes a symbol of family loyalty. "The basic social and psychological significance of making such an exceptional gift is no different from gift-giving in more usual and less tragic conditions. A gift is a form of particularistic exchange that ideally expresses and reinforces a relationship between the person who gives and the one who receives."[14,p.414] Thus, Fox believes, if a family member refuses to donate an organ to another, the implication is that the ill person is being abandoned to his fate and the bonds that linked him to the family are broken. Fox reports that many prospective donors feel they have no choice and must give up a kidney or be unable to face themselves or their family. Donors who are turned down for immunologic, medical, or psychologic reasons often experience intense depression and feelings of failure. Many transplantation teams employ the services of a psychiatrist, probably as much to help physicians cope with family trauma as to help the family members themselves.

Fox also reports an interesting phenomenon that she describes as a "generalized norm." If a prospective donor is found to be "psychologically unsuited or incorrectly motivated," he and the family will be given a medical reason for his unsuitability. The truth will be withheld from even the prospective donor, who is told that he is not histocompatible. Physicians frequently withhold the whole truth from clients and families, but this deliberate deception on a routine basis is a relatively new medical practice. It is rationalized on the grounds that the truth would cause excessive psychologic harm to a family that is already in turmoil.

The ethical implications of this practice are far-reaching. On the surface it might seem a kindness, an act of justifiable paternalism, but by not knowing the truth the potential donor is discouraged from sharing his feelings with the ill person and with other family members. This may or may not be appropriate, depending on the family's coping mechanisms and their history of dealing with crises. One can understand why a physician might wish not to become embroiled in a family trauma, but it does not seem that he is justified in telling a lie for that reason. Is he justified in lying to protect the family, and is he in a position to know whether he *should* make a decision to lie, no matter how involved he is with the family? The fact that this kind of lying has become routine makes one wonder what other lies will become permissible in the future. It would seem psychologically healthier and ethically more correct to permit the potential donor to lie to his family if he chooses. He, however, should be told the truth about why he is being rejected as a donor, and he should be offered the services of the transplantation team psychiatrist. If he has strong feelings of ambivalence about donating or if his motivation is somehow questionable, he is already aware of these feelings, and helping him to ignore or deny them does him a disservice even though it may be easier for the physician to tell this lie than to deal with the traumatic scene that may follow the revelation of truth.

Recipients of a kidney transplant have also been known to experience profound psychologic shocks. They are not only gravely physically ill but will spend the rest of their lives hanging on the edge of kidney rejection. Their image of their body might be affected, although this is more likely with a heart transplant because the heart is imbued with more personalization and emotionality than a kidney. The recipient needs to cope with feelings of gratitude and indebtedness toward the living donor; he is likely to feel bound to the donor even if he had not previously felt particularly close to him. Family members do not always love or even like each other, although negative feelings may remain on a nonverbal level. Having to express gratitude to a sibling or parent with whom one was not particularly close before the transplant could engender feelings of resentment that will forever affect the relationship. Even if love existed previously, the relationship between the donor and recipient is bound to change. The recipient may come to believe that he can never again express an angry or negative feeling toward the donor because he owes his life to him. Because the situation is unprecedented in their previous personal experience, few people would anticipate future problems and seek guidance. If the recipient is lucky enough to come under the care of a sensitive transplantation team psychiatrist, some problems may be averted or dealt with as they arise. Most people are not this fortunate and are left with feelings of guilt, resentment, and fear.

Being a recipient of a cadaver kidney can bring its own psychologic trauma, including a "creepy" sensation of having a dead person's organ living inside one's body or a sense of revulsion. Most recipients of cadaver kidneys never know from whom the organ came, because matching is done by computer and is almost as impersonal as a blood transfusion. Consequently the problem of gratitude does not exist or exists in a different form: the recipient may need to express gratitude for the gift of life and is unable to direct those feelings toward a specific donor. The physician is then the usual object of gratitude.

Recipients of a heart transplant are subject to an even greater variety of psychologic stress. Because the heart is a metaphor for the seat of romantic feeling and a good deal of emotionalism, it may seem to some that the persona of the dead donor has been assimilated into the being of the recipient. The family of the dead heart donor may experience the strain of not being able to think of the person as dead as long as his heart is still alive. They may become unduly anxious about the health and fate of the recipient, may consider him a new member of their family, and may grieve afresh when he dies.

All people who require a heart or kidney transplant come close to death, and this in itself is a psychologically traumatizing experience; receiving a donor organ is an added jolt. It is likely that the recipient may view life from a different perspective, may assign new priorities to various life experiences, and may develop different attitudes towards death. The experience always creates psychologic changes, and many people grow and develop new sensitivities and awareness.

SUPPLY OF DONOR ORGANS

Organs for transplant come only from living donors and cadavers. The latter is the more common source, although the technologic difficulties in the transplantation of these are greater. It is almost universally required that living donors be genetically related to the recipient, and this greatly decreases the pool from which to draw. If no living donor volunteers or if no volunteer is histocompatible, the potential recipient is then placed on a waiting list for a cadaver organ (see Chapter 2 for a discussion of the ethics involved in the allocation of scarce health resources). Many more people require kidney transplants than there are kidneys available.

Although most people think of kidney donation as a purely voluntary act, especially in view of the psychologic overtones discussed previously, a recent event in Pittsburgh may force us to alter our thinking.[15] The case involved a bone marrow transplant, but the principles could apply equally to a kidney, blood, or any other tissue or organ that can be removed from a living person. Robert McFall, a 39-year-old unmarried man suffering from aplastic anemia, which is usually fatal, filed suit to compel his cousin David Shimp to donate bone marrow that physicians said was necessary to save McFall's life. This was the first suit in the United States and possibly in the world seeking to forcibly extract tissue from the body of someone unwilling to give it up.

Before an individual becomes a candidate to donate bone marrow, he must pass two tests for compatibility. Shimp voluntarily underwent the first, which showed that there was an excellent chance that he would be a suitable donor. Shimp changed his mind about wanting to donate and refused to undergo the second test. McFall then filed suit to compel Shimp to submit to the second test and to donate if the test showed that he was a compatible donor. McFall's attorney claimed that Shimp led McFall to believe that he would be a willing donor but then reneged, thus causing "a delay of critical proportions." Shimp was therefore responsible for McFall's precarious health, and the implication was strong that he would also be responsible for McFall's death.

Anglo-American common law has never imposed an obligation on a person to come to the aid of another unless he is responsible for the peril. For example, a passer-by is not legally required to jump into a lake to save a drowning person unless he pushed the person into the lake in the first place or in some other way caused him to be in danger of drowning. If a person has a heart attack or chokes on a piece of meat while you are in his presence, you are not *legally* obligated to go to his aid. If you calmly sit by and watch him choke to death, you cannot be prosecuted for complicity in his death, though the action may be morally reprehensible. McFall's attorney argued that Shimp was at first not legally obligated to come to his cousin's aid but once having set the wheels of aid in motion was then obligated to continue. As an analogy, if you assure a crowd of onlookers that you will jump into the lake to save the drowning person and remove your coat and shoes before changing your mind, the delay could make a critical difference to the drowning person. Once having taken action to save him, you would be legally responsible to follow through with your stated intention.

The court denied that Shimp was legally obligated to donate, saying, "Our society, contrary to many others, has as its first principle, the respect for the individual, and that society and government exist to protect the individual from being invaded and hurt by another."[16] McFall died 2 weeks after the judgment.

As a precedent this judgment could be short-lived. Someone else might attempt to compel a donation, and sooner or later a judgment may be made in favor of forced donation of body parts. It is not likely to happen in the United States in the immediate future, but it is another potential invasion of personal privacy and bodily integrity to concern us in the future.

There is considerable debate over the ethics of removing a healthy organ from the body of a living person to save the life of another. The principle of nonmaleficence applies most clearly to the situation. No matter how statistically insignificant the risk of donation, the donor is being harmed. He must submit to major surgery with its attendant anesthesia danger, and he must live the rest of his life knowing that if his one remaining kidney fails, the tables will be turned and *he* will be seeking a donation. No matter how eagerly a person volunteers a kidney, is it ethical for a physician to deliberately harm him by removing it? The physician often is the one who must request a kidney for the client. One wonders if it would be more ethical for the physician in this situation to remove himself from the negotiations involved in requesting a kidney and act only as technician and perhaps interpreter of medical facts, determining only who is or is not histocompatible.

As long as informed consent is obtained, there seem to be no major ethical roadblocks to removing a kidney from a living donor, but it is an issue that should not be ignored and the practice should not be undertaken lightly. If society were to assume the attitude that a person with kidney disease has a right to claim an organ from a living donor, the machinery would be set in motion for mandatory donation. Related to this is the issue of the donor's competence. Allowing children to donate has already been discussed, as has a case in which a family called for a kidney donation from a profoundly retarded man (see Chapter 2). In that situation a majority of physicians, nurses, and social workers surveyed said they would favor removing the retarded man's kidney even though he was unable to comprehend the surgery itself or its implications. That position disturbs people who seek to protect those who cannot protect themselves and raises the question, again, of mandatory donation, perhaps using prisoners on death row or the "hopelessly" mentally ill as donors. The issues involved in the donation of kidneys by living persons reach far beyond the immediate family of potential recipients.

Cadaver organs

The cadaver donor is involved in an entirely different set of issues. Most cadaver donors are young and die as a result of an accident or brain disease. With many other causes of death, including old age, kidneys are deteriorated or diseased and thus useless for transplantation. Persons in the process of dying are also considered potential donors, particularly if prior to the terminal illness they had expressed a desire to donate. In this situation, ethical principles have been established to ensure that different physicians care for the donor and recipient. Simmons and Fulton[10] raise an interesting question. If a dying person's fluid balance is neglected, as it frequently is, his kidneys are not usable for transplantation. Can the team of physicians caring for the potential recipient intervene in the care of the dying donor to ensure that his kidneys remain healthy? What if that intervention causes the donor to live longer than expected and the recipient dies or becomes more ill as a result? Where do the loyalties of each physician or health team lie?

Another major issue with potential donors who are dying concerns how long the life-support system of an irreversibly comatose person should be kept operating *solely* to preserve organs for a future transplant. The law is fairly clear about turning off the respirator too soon (see Chapter 12), but there is little precedent about preserving organs in an otherwise dead body. It is medically easier and safer to keep the organ inside a functioning body than to remove it from a cadaver and chill, perfuse, and store it. One can envision comatose individuals being kept indefinitely attached to respirators awaiting recipients while the family of the "cadaver" remains in limbo trying to deal with a death that is not yet official.

Most cadaver organs, however, come from people are who irrevocably dead. Ethical issues still exist, however. People exhibit great resistance to donating their organs. A 1968 Gallup poll revealed that 70% of American adults said they would be willing to donate an organ after death,[17] but very few actually make arrangements to do so and relatives are loathe to make the decision after death. Part of the family's reluctance stems from the fear of bodily mutilation discussed previously, and part is genuine puzzlement about what the dead person would have wanted.

One solution to the problem of organ scarcity and family indecision would be legislation that makes every cadaver a potential donor unless the person himself specifically objects in writing before his death. Family members would not be able to override the general law. Superstitions, taboos, and the privacy of religious practice, however, will most likely prevent legislation of this type in the near future in the United States.

A compromise position is now in effect in all 50 states. The Uniform Anatomical Gift Act permits any adult over 18 who is mentally competent to donate his organs for transplantation after death. Family members may not override the donor's decision. Many people feel that the Uniform Anatomical Gift Act is morally preferable to a general law that would consider every cadaver a potential donor, because the deliberate giving of an organ is an act of charity and has a higher moral value than that same organ being taken by legislative action. But if a general law were enacted, people would not be considered donors, as taxpayers are not now considered donors to government coffers. The routine taking of organs from every medically eligible cadaver, as is done in some European countries, would ensure a supply of organs that would more closely meet the needs of transplant recipients than would the Uniform Anatomical Gift Act, through which only a small percentage of the population donate organs. One purpose of the act was to extend the field of cadavers from which organs could be taken, because the supply of unclaimed bodies was dwindling and the competition with medical schools that needed intact cadavers for teaching purposes was increasing. The act is based on the principle of autonomy and can be seen as closely allied, at least in a legal context, with those precedents that allow an individual to refuse medical treatment even if his own death is likely to result.

There are, however, strong proponents (more in the medical profession than in the lay public) of the view that all organs should be salvaged after death unless the person has expressly prohibited that action in writing before death. Because young healthy people do not generally think about what will become of their organs after death, and because young people who die in accidents are the preferred organ donors, the supply of organs would be greatly increased by universal cadaver salvage. Dukeminier and Sanders[18] think that the routine salvaging of cadaver organs will best serve the interests of the community. They believe that leaving the decision to the individual is philosophically preferable only if the needs of the community can be met. But since the demand for organs far outstrips the supply, community need may override personal preference. The prevailing question concerns whether the personal preference of an individual should take precedence over the life needs of another who may die as a result. Dukeminier and Sanders do not conclude that all people must be compelled to donate after death, but their concession appears to result from an acknowledgment of religious freedom and constitutional rights. They believe that if the procedure of salvaging organs is made routine and legal, few people will object and the supply of organs will increase. The law should be based on four principles:

1. Leaving useful cadaver organs to putrefy should be seen as unusual.

2. Removal of organs should be performed under conditions that do not burden the bereaved family with the problem, and they should not be required to make a decision.

3. The donor's family should have no power of veto over the donor's express decision to donate or to refuse to do so.

4. If the donor has not stated an opinion and if the family seriously objects to removal of organs, the objections should be controlling. This concession is inserted to prevent legal problems, but it does somewhat negate the purpose of the law.

The major difference between the Uniform Anatomical Gift Act and a law routinely salvaging all usable organs is the way in which the burden of decision falls. With the former a person agrees to take a positive action to give a gift to society; with the latter one could only act to deny the gift. In both situations, however, a person is actively forced to think about the fate of his organs and must engage in a decision-making process. Dukeminier and Sanders think that asking the family of a dying person for his heart or kidneys is a "ghoulish request" and that it would be "macabre" for people to carry little cards saying that their organs should be donated at death. Many people already carry eye donor cards and attach no greater emotional significance to them than to their credit cards, and in some states a person can indicate on his driver's license that he wishes to donate his organs. What might be considered more ghoulish or macabre is taking cadaver organs without first knowing the wishes of the dead individual or discussing organ donation with the family. That secret practice could surely be labeled a form of desecration of the dead. Discussing what should be done with one's body is no more macabre than discussing the details of a funeral or choosing and buying a cemetary plot, both of which are common practices.

Before the tradition of separation of church and state became part of common law and secular courts arose, all burial practices came under the jurisdiction of ecclesiastical courts and neither the family after a death nor persons themselves before death had a voice in what was to be done with their bodies. When secular courts took responsibility for the disposition of the dead, a doctrine of a "quasiproperty right" to a body came into effect. This means that the person or his family can claim no commercial right to the body but that the family does have a right regarding disposition within certain legal bounds.[6] It was seen that the family has a duty to protect the body from violation, but the family members also are restricted in what they can do to or with the body. They are required to bury or cremate it in a legally sanctioned way (they may not keep it as their own property and bury it in the back yard), but they are given the right to have the body buried intact unless a criminal investigation intervenes. The state does not have property rights over a body, unless a crime is involved, and cannot hold a body as security against debt or compel an autopsy or any other kind of mutilation to be performed. There are, however, certain instances in which the state can claim property rights to a body because the wishes of the family are overridden by the needs of society. A medical examiner may detain a body for as long as required for investigation of a crime, and the state may exhume a body in a criminal investigation. In certain instances of highly virulent epidemics of communicable disease, the health department may require that a body be buried within a specified period of time or that the coffin be sealed.

Should the need for organs for transplantation be considered a situation in which the state may claim property rights over the dead? The question must be debated in terms of whether a body is property and if so to whom it belongs. It cannot belong to the individual himself because his personhood no longer exists and he cannot make a decision about disposal of the property. If property is whatever courts choose to protect, then an assertion has been made about

a legal positivism and the omnicompetence of legislatures and courts in making and unmaking legal rights. Factually, of course, this cannot be denied. Remembering, however, that the rights legally recognized in the past were founded upon familial duties and sacred trusts arising out of our common humanity and from respect for the dead, we may question whether legislatures or courts are omnicompetent to make and unmake legal rights without violating real human interests, concerns, and values. This is what was meant by saying that "a dead body belongs to no one and is therefore under the protection of the public"—under the protection of our legal tradition.*

This does not settle the question of to whom a body belongs. By invoking both tradition and legal precedent one can defend equally well the position that a body belongs to a family or to the state. Neither the Uniform Anatomical Gift Act nor a legalized routine of taking organs need disrupt the traditional ways of caring for the dead. The removal of organs is no more mutilating than an autopsy and in many instances is less so. Burial rights would not be affected, and the body would not look any different except for the incision.

The issue of respect for the dead has always been cloudy. Respect in this instance is directed toward a collection of organs and tissues rather than toward a person. The fact that we shy away from handling a cadaver roughly and cover it in a shroud stems more for, an atavistic fear of spirits than a realistic fear of hurting the cadaver. Respect for the body of the dead has an emotional rather than ethical basis.

If a body belongs to no one and will be buried or burned, what ethical issue could stand in the way of removing any or all usable organs for transplantation provided that the individual has not specifically objected before his death? Only one objection could be raised: those people who are not aware of the law or the medical routine may not have been given a chance to object. One can make an analogy, however, to dying without a will. Almost everyone has some property, even if it may have no great intrinsic value. If a person dies intestate and is not married, his property and other assets go to the state. There are people who do not know this and others who do but still refuse to leave a will. It can be said that by abdicating responsibility for the disposal of one's property, one permits the state to do with the property as it chooses and is permitted by law. If a law to salvage all usable organs is enacted, it will become common knowledge like the law about dying intestate. The responsibility to object in writing then becomes the individual's, not the state's. However, if the individual does not object, can the state be certain that he wanted to donate his organs or that he simply did not know he could object? The answer could not be legally determined, analogous to the situation of a person dying intestate. In the one instance the state benefits from a person's property, and in the other a human being could benefit from the donor's organ.

The gift may be greater in terms of philosophic or charitable value if it is freely and actively given as under the Uniform Anatomical Gift Act. Whether a legislative act is required to permit removal of the organ, however, is irrelevant to the saving of a life. Legislating the salvaging of organs depends to a great extent on the values of society and the balance it chooses to strike between the need to save lives and the respect it wishes to accord to the bodies of the dead. Dukeminier and Sanders

---

*Ramsey, Paul: The patient as person, New Haven, Conn., 1970, Yale University Press, p. 206.

favor routine salvaging of organs. Ramsey favors the Uniform Anatomical Gift Act for several reasons, the most compelling of which is expressed in the following:

A society will be a better human community in which giving and receiving is the rule, not taking for the sake of good to come. The civilizing task of mankind is the fostering, the achievement, or the shoring up of consensual community in general, and not only in regard to the advancement of medical science and the availability of cadaver organs in efforts to save the lives of others. Civilization means living our consensual communities, not living in communities in which consent and refusal go on, just as surely as we live our bodies, not in them. . . . The routine taking of organs would deprive individuals of the exercise of the virtue of generosity.*

Children and incompetents as donors

There is precedent for permitting the removal of a kidney from a child, but all cases involve identical twins who had not only given consent but were eager to donate and fully understood the implications. Most were adolescents and were children only in a legal sense. In addition most of the cases involved a benefit to the donor as well as the recipient; that is, if the donor were denied the opportunity to give a kidney, he would be permanently psychologically harmed.[19]

In 1969 a Connecticut judge allowed a transplant to take place between 7-year-old twins, and in the same year a Kentucky court granted permission for a transplant from a 27-year-old retarded donor to his 28-year-old brother. In both cases the court relied on the testimony of people other than the family and physicians that the potential donor would be psychologically harmed if the transplant were denied.[19] Other precedents also exist: in 1973 in Louisiana a court refused to allow a retarded child to be used as a donor for his sister, and 2 years later the Supreme Court of Wisconsin denied a request to remove the kidney of a catatonic schizophrenic man for his sister. Both opinions cited a lack of benefit to the donor.[19]

It seems that the underlying factor in all these cases involves whether the donor benefits. Some might justify taking an organ (almost always a kidney) from a child or incompetent when there is no probable benefit to the donor in the same way as some would justify nontherapeutic research in children. The principles are similar, and the justification is difficult to make in both. Fost[19] says that nonbeneficial research in children can be justified only when (1) the child is used only as a "last resort" (when no competent adults are available), (2) there is no more than a "trivial" risk, (3) there is a firm medical basis for expecting a benefit for others, and (4) consent is provided by a legally authorized representative of the child. All four conditions must be met.

If we use these criteria to justify a child or incompetent being an organ donor, we find ourselves back on a slippery slope. A child or incompetent is rarely a last resort; usually a living or cadaver donor can be found somewhere. Even if the most thorough computer search reveals not a single compatible cadaver organ, would it be better to take the organ of a child or place the recipient on a waiting list for a cadaver organ?

---

*Ramsey, Paul: The patient as person, New Haven, Conn., 1970, Yale University Press, p. 210.

Defining an acceptable risk as "trivial" is too subjective to be of much legal or ethical help in determining whether using a child as an organ donor is justified. Risk can be seen in psychologic as well as medical terms, casting it in an entirely different light. Imagine the terror of a young child or mentally retarded person who is wheeled off to the operating room after having been told that a part of him was going to be removed to help someone else. Is saving someone's life worth the possibility of creating terror in a child? What feelings of guilt and fear would remain with that person?

The third condition, the expectation of a medical benefit for the recipient, has not been sufficiently proved except in the case of identical twins. Receiving a kidney from a living related donor is only marginally more advantageous than receiving a cadaver organ. At the end of a 3-year period, 80% of the recipients of a sibling's kidney were alive, compared to 62% of recipients of cadaver kidneys.[19]

If moral justification cannot be based on the first three conditions, then the fourth, the consent of a representative of the child, is useless, because it is predicated on the first three. Let us assume for the sake of argument, however, that the conditions described above can be met, that a donation from a child can be justified on the basis of the first three conditions. The decision then rests with the parent or guardian who must give consent. If there will be no benefit for the donor child or incompetent, on what basis can a parent give away the organ of a nonconsenting child? One argument is that the child should consent to giving the organ because it is his moral obligation to do so. This is similar to McCormick's argument (see Chapter 9 for a discussion of children as research subjects) that a child ought to participate in nontherapeutic research because there are certain values to which he ought to subscribe to achieve full status in the moral community.

Another argument is that if the child or incompetent states that he wants to be a donor, his statement should be taken at face value even though it is highly unlikely that he understands the implications of his desire.

A third argument is that the judgment of the parent or guardian is substituted for that of the child and that the child's best interest is perceived by the adult. This assumes that the child or incompetent, if he had the same faculties as the consenting adult, would make the same decision as that adult. This argument denies the existence of the child's individualism and uses him as a means to an end.

Another argument uses studies to show that adults decide to donate kidneys more on an emotional basis than as a result of carefully weighing medical and statistical factors; therefore informed consent in the matter of organ donation is an elaborate ritual that has little or no real meaning in the decision-making process. Consequently a child's kidney could be removed without the consideration of informed consent. This is a specious argument. Informed consent does exist, and if individuals choose to disregard it, it is they who may make that decision. In a way, they are consenting to ignore consent. To take a right from a child because an adult chooses to abdicate the right would be to deliberately remove a great deal of a child's legal and moral protection. If an adult wishes to cut off his finger as a religious sacrifice, he may be morally permitted to do so, but he may not cut off the finger of his child.

If the absence of informed consent is a reason to exclude persons as renal donors, many adults would have to be excluded. A consistent position would be to say that only informed and consenting donors could be used, and then to administer a test to determine whether or not the prospective donor is actually capable of achieving a state of being informed. If the person passed the test, age should not be a barrier to donation.*

Even if one acknowledges that a child would definitely benefit from donating a kidney, there are reasons to keep children from being donors. If a twin has kidney disease, it is likely that the identical sibling will have a propensity for developing the same disease and will therefore need both kidneys. There might be family disturbances that are not known to the transplantation team and that could adversely affect the donor. If the recipient dies, the donor, especially if he is a young child, might feel guilt and blame. And one might question the donor's motives and understanding of the procedure simply because he *is* a child.

The greatest ethical problem involved in using children or incompetents as donors is that others decide what will or will not benefit them now and in the future. An 8-year-old twin has the emotional maturity of an 8-year-old; the decision he is being asked to make or that is being made for him might be viewed in an entirely different light if he were 5 years older, or 10 or 20. There is no way to ask a child to give up a kidney for a sibling without impressing on him the fact that the sibling will likely die without it. This alone makes the situation coercive even though there may be no deliberate maleficence. How much of a child's willingness to donate arises out of pressure or guilt rather than a sense of altruism? How much altruism can a child be expected to have? It does no good to agree that most adults donate to prevent feeling guilty, because we are not speaking here of adults with adult emotions. It is impossible to predict that a decision made by an 8- or 10-year-old will not be regretted when he matures. A parent may claim that he knows his child well enough to be certain of the child's feelings, but this is not so. No one can feel another person's feeling. There is reason to believe that a child donates his kidney in part to please his parents or to prevent his parents from blaming him for the sibling's death if he refuses to donate. Since a parent cannot make this decision with absolute certainty, it is unlikely that a psychiatrist could and even less likely that a court could know the child's mind.

One must look with great skepticism at those court decisions that permitted a child to donate a kidney because it was assumed that the donor would also benefit from the act. It may indeed be true that the child would be irreparably harmed if he were denied the opportunity to give the gift of life to a sibling, but to assume that a child wants to donate simply because he says he does would be to do him a great disservice. Instances in which a child, particularly a nonconsenting one, should be used as an organ donor are extremely rare. There are almost no situations in which it is morally acceptable to remove an organ from a mentally incompetent adult who cannot comprehend the implications of the procedure.

---

*Fost, Norman: Children as renal donors. Reprinted by permission from The New England Journal of Medicine **296**(7): 366, 1977.

Fetus as organ donor

Veatch[20] presents a case in which the conception of a fetus was planned for the purpose of creating a kidney to be transplanted to its father. The situation is important in and of itself, but it also has enormous future implications.

The case involved a 28-year-old engineer who had been on dialysis for 3 years and was becoming desperate because of the restrictions it placed on his life-style. He had been adopted as an infant and thus could find no genetically compatible donor. He had a rare tissue type that made the possibility of receiving a cadaver kidney unlikely. His mental and physical state continued to deteriorate, and he threatened to kill himself if he had to remain on dialysis indefinitely. His wife presented a novel solution to the transplantation surgeon: she could become pregnant, have an abortion after 5 or 6 months, and have the fetus's kidneys transplanted into her husband. The surgeon knew that this was technically feasible and that the graft probably would not be rejected. He did not, however, know if it was ethically correct to transplant kidneys of a deliberately conceived and aborted fetus.

The case is accompanied by the reactions of Mary Anne Warren, a philosopher at San Francisco State University, Daniel Maguire, a theologian at Marquette University, and Carol Levine, Managing Editor of the *Hastings Center Report* where the case first appeared.

Warren viewed the dilemma in terms of the moral status of a 5- or 6-month old fetus, that is, whether it should be considered a full human being with a right to life. In this situation the issue of abortion has nothing to do with the rights of the woman carrying an unwanted pregnancy but is a question of the moral correctness of killing a fetus at this age. If the fetus is considered a full human being, then the proposal is tantamount to murder and is not permissible. If the fetus has no significant right to life, there is no reason why the wife cannot put into effect the plan to save her husband (refer to Chapter 7 for a discussion of the status of the fetus). Warren does not view a fetus as a full person and therefore sees no serious moral objection to killing it.

Maguire proposes an alternative to abortion. Because the fetus also inherits genetic characteristics of the mother, it may not be an appropriate donor; thus the baby should be allowed to be born and then it can be determined whether its tissue is genetically suitable. If the match is suitable and if the baby has two healthy kidneys, one could be transplanted to the father. Maguire believes that the transplant would occur more successfully if the kidney were more mature, and the fact that no abortion took place would make the transplant more ethically permissible. Terminating the life of a fetus is not the same as using a baby as a donor, but either way the fetus or the live baby would be used as a means to an end. Maguire confesses he is uneasy with either solution. He says the proposed abortion is not moral, but he also states that we cannot assume that the baby would give permission to donate if it had the mental capacity to do so. He points out that the autonomy of the baby should be protected until it can make its own decision, though this would not help the father, who would probably be dead by then. Maguire makes the following, seemingly contradictory, statement about the baby as organ donor.

Relationship to the other and the capacity for sharing are present before we are aware of them, since they relate to our elementary humanity and not just to our subsequent maturity and volition. Part of the awesome grandeur of parental care is the right and duty to interpret sensitively what a baby's humanity entails. And it may entail the surrender of a paired organ when that surrender is "a gift of life." The inability to permit this has its roots in an isolationist individualist anthropology that ostracizes the baby from genuine humanness under guise of protecting its nonadult status.*

Maguire would not permit abortion in this situation, but neither is he able to take a definite position on the morality of taking the baby's kidney.

Levine objects to the planned action as an unwarranted manipulation of the procreative act as well as an abortion. Deliberately conceiving and aborting a child for an organ would not only be an affront to the dignity of the fetus as a potential human being but would also permit the wife to use herself as a means to an end. Levine does not see this situation as an issue of an altruistic sacrifice of one life to save another. The husband is not dying in a medical sense but is threatening to kill himself, although he may see being on dialysis indefinitely as a kind of death. Levine makes the point that even if a fetal kidney transplant could be successfully accomplished, it would probably not last for more than a few years. What then? Would the husband return to dialysis, or would his wife need to become pregnant again? Even in the unlikely event that the procedure could be accomplished successfully twice in a row, a permanent solution would not have been achieved. Levine also considers the wife. Is her offer to use herself as an organ incubator entirely voluntary, or is she being coerced by her husband's threats of suicide? Levine believes that the abortion should not be considered and that the husband should receive psychiatric help in dealing with his feelings about continued dialysis. Marriage counseling is also indicated.

CRITERIA FOR DEATH

The reader is referred to Chapter 12 for a discussion of the criteria for death and the ethical issues involved. What is important here are the issues involved with organ transplantation. Dedek expresses the problem succinctly: "Transplantation . . . is technically possible as long as the organ has not deteriorated. It is morally imperative that a heart donor be dead. But it is medically imperative that he not be so dead that his heart cannot be used for a transplant."[17,p.35] This statement is even more applicable to donors of kidneys because of the speed at which they deteriorate.

The vast majority of cadaver organs are removed from people who have died accidentally and about whose deaths there is no question. Requesting organs for transplant from the family of a trauma victim has become almost as routine as requesting permission to perform an autopsy on a person who has died in a hospital. The ethical dilemmas occur in the less common instances when the fact of death is in question.

---

*Warren, Mary Anne, Maguire, Daniel, and Levine, Carol: Can the fetus be an organ farm? Hastings Center Report 8(5): 24, October 1978. Reprinted with permission of The Hastings Center, © Institute of Society, Ethics and the Life Sciences, 360 Broadway, Hastings-on-Hudson, N.Y. 10706.

The crux of the problem concerns whether to discontinue artificial life-support systems when the criteria for irreversible coma have been reached. The most commonly used criteria are those of the Harvard Ad Hoc Committee, which define irreversible coma but do not equate it medically or legally with death. The decision to terminate life supports probably depends on one's values, the emotions evoked by the situation, and the prevailing legal climate. If an organ recipient is waiting in the wings while a comatose individual who is in essence dead is artificially maintained, whose needs should take priority? The answer lies in a personal balance of ethical values because either decision can be seen to be morally permissible or impermissible. In the end, the average person usually lays aside the ethical and medical criteria that influence his thinking and decides what he *feels* a person to be and whether the comatose individual has a greater claim to keep breathing or the potential transplant recipient to receive another chance to live.

Beecher makes the point that death occurs at various levels at various time intervals in all organisms. "Individuals die legally, spiritually, or physiologically, but many of their cells continue to metabolize . . . Which of these states are we to call death?"[21, p. 153] His point is that the answer is arbitrary—that there is no definite answer.

SUMMARY

Organ transplantation has had a long history of unsuccessful attempts, and only in the past 2 or 3 decades have researchers begun to solve the rejection problem. Many problems with transplantation still exist, however, and although kidneys are transplanted relatively often, the procedure cannot be viewed as completely routine. Although hearts and kidneys receive most of the publicity, other tissues are more frequently and successfully transplanted, such as corneas, bone, and blood. Liver and lung transplants are still in the early stages of research.

The central religious issue with organ transplantation concerns whether a person has a right to deliberately mutilate his own body to save the life of another. Traditional conservative religious views do not permit mutilation, but this position is far from absolute, especially when another human life is at stake. Organ transplantation is neither specifically permitted nor prohibited by conservative Catholics or Orthodox Jews. The Protestant position views the gift of an organ as an act of charity, and transplantation is therefore neither encouraged or discouraged by Protestant theologians.

Some ethical issues are similar to the religious ones, especially the concept of sacrificial obligation. Is preservation of self or preservation of others a higher moral duty, and is volunteering an organ purely a gift or an attempt to avoid guilt?

Another ethical dilemma involves the cost/benefit ratio. Transplants are among the most expensive medical procedures in terms of both the cost of surgery and the time the recipient gains. Dialysis is considerably less expensive, but it bears its own psychologic and medical problems. The cost of developing a totally implantable artificial heart would far exceed the current cost of heart transplants, but research is still in early stages. Society must begin to think about the priorities for its financial resources.

Many people are forced to choose between waiting for a donor kidney and spending the rest of their lives on dialysis. It is a difficult choice. A person with a transplant can lead a far less restricted life than one who undergoes dialysis, but transplants have a lower statistical probability of success and one may face repeated surgery or an eventual return to dialysis.

Donors too are faced with a crisis of conscience, even though studies have shown that they make the decision to donate more for emotional reasons than as a result of carefully weighing the facts and risks. Informed consent does not play a large part in the decision to donate, but most donors are pleased with their decision even though medical problems are common.

Organs for transplant come from living (usually related) donors and cadavers, and the supply of both is smaller than the demand. Legal precedents have established that no one may be compelled to donate an organ, and it is not permissible to remove an organ from a cadaver if the person has specifically objected before death. Since transplanting an organ from a living donor depends on the histocompatibility of one's immediate family and on their willingness to donate, the vast majority must wait for a cadaver organ. There are essentially three ways to obtain cadaver organs: (1) by requesting them on an individual basis at the time of death, (2) from a bequest that an individual makes before death through the Uniform Anatomical Gift Act that he wishes to have organs removed for transplantation, and (3) by proposed legislation to consider every person a potential donor unless he specifically refuses in writing before death. Arguments about advantages and disadvantages of each method generally center on matters of practicality and the degree and value of charity involved.

There is legal precedent to permit children and incompetents to act as organ donors, but most of these decisions involved close blood relatives and situations in which there was also a demonstrated benefit to the donor. It is difficult if not impossible to justify using a nonconsenting child as an organ donor or a fetus that was specifically conceived to be used as a donor.

REFERENCES

1. Nelson, James B.: Human medicine, Minneapolis, 1973, Augsburg Publishing House.
2. Hardy, James P., et al.: Heart transplantation in man: developmental studies and report of a case, Journal of the American Medical Association 188:1132-1140, 1964.
3. Jonsen, Albert R.: The totally implantable artificial heart, Hastings Center Report 3(1):8-11, November 1973.
4. Leach, Gerald: The biocrats, New York, 1970, McGraw-Hill Book Co.
5. Pope Pius XI, quoted in Dedek, John F.: Contemporary medical ethics, New York, 1975, Sheed & Ward, Inc., p. 31.
6. Ramsey, Paul: The patient as person, New Haven, Conn., 1970, Yale University Press.
7. Fletcher, Joseph: Our shameful waste of human tissue: an ethical problem for the living and the dead. In Cutler, Donald R., editor: Updating life and death, Boston, 1969, Beacon Press.
8. *Masden v. Harrison,* No. 68651 Eq., Mass. Sup. Jud. Ct., June 12, 1957.
9. DeWolf, L. Harold: Organ transplants as related to fully human living and dying. In Williams, Preston N., editor: Ethical issues in biology and medicine: proceedings of a symposium on the identity and dignity of man, Cambridge, Mass., 1973, Schenkman Publishing Co.
10. Simmons, Roberta G., and Fulton, Julie: Ethical issues in kidney transplantation. In Frazier, Claude A., editor: Is it moral to modify man? Springfield, Ill., 1973, Charles C Thomas, Publisher.
11. Coene, Roger E.: Dialysis or transplant: one patient's choice, Hastings Center Report 8(2):7, April 1978.

12. Levine, Carol: Dialysis or transplant: values and choices, Hastings Center Report 8(2):8-10, April 1978.
13. Simmons, Roberta G., and Klein, Susan D.: Gift of life: the social and psychological impact of organ transplantation, New York, 1977, John Wiley and Sons.
14. Fox, Renee C.: A sociological perspective on organ transplantation and hemodialysis, Annals of the New York Academy of Science 169:406-428, 1970.
15. Meisel, Alan, and Roth, Loren H.: Must a man be his cousin's keeper? Hastings Center Report 8(5):5-6, October 1978.
16. Quoted in Meisel, Alan, and Roth, Loren H.: Must a man be his cousin's keeper? Hastings Center Report 8(5):5, 1978.
17. Dedek, John F.: Contemporary medical ethics, New York, 1975, Sheed & Ward, Inc.
18. Dukeminier, Jesse, Jr., and Sanders, David: Organ transplantation: a proposal for routine salvaging of cadaver organs, New England Journal of Medicine 279:413-419, August 22, 1968.
19. Fost, Norman: Children as renal donors, New England Journal of Medicine 296(7):363-367, February 17, 1977.
20. Warren, Mary Anne, Maguire, Daniel, and Levine, Carol: Can the fetus be an organ farm? Hastings Center Report 8(5):23-25, October 1978.
21. Beecher, Henry K.: Research and the individual, Boston, 1970, Little, Brown and Co.

BIBLIOGRAPHY

Barnard, Christiaan: Human heart transplantation. In Frazier, Claude A., editor: Is it moral to modify man? Springfield, Ill., 1973, Charles C Thomas, Publisher.

Beecher, Henry K.: Research and the individual, Boston, 1979, Little, Brown and Co.

Coene, Roger E.: Dialysis or transplant: one patient's choice, Hastings Center Report 8(2):5-7, April 1978.

Dedek, John F.: Contemporary medical ethics, New York, 1975, Sheed & Ward, Inc.

DeWolf, L. Harold.: Organ transplants as related to fully human living and dying. In Williams, Preston N., editor: Ethical issues in biology and medicine: proceedings of a symposium on the identity and dignity of man, Cambridge, Mass., Schenkman Publishing Co.

Dukeminier, Jesse, Jr., and Sanders, David: Organ transplantation: a proposal for routine salvaging of cadaver organs, New England Journal of Medicine 279:413-419, August 22, 1968.

Fletcher, Joseph: Our shameful waste of human tissue: an ethical problem for the living and the dead. In Cutler, Donald R., editor: Updating life and death, Boston, 1969, Beacon Press.

Fost, Norman: Children as renal donors, New England Journal of Medicine 296(7):363-367, February 17, 1977.

Fox, Renee C.: A sociological perspective on organ transplantation and hemodialysis, Annals of the New York Academy of Science 169:406-428, 1970.

Frazier, Claude, A., editor: Is it moral to modify man? Springfield, Ill., 1973, Charles C Thomas, Publisher.

Leach, Gerald: The biocrats, New York, 1976, McGraw-Hill Book Co.

Levine, Carol: Dialysis or transplant: values and choices, Hastings Center Report 8(2):8-10, April 1978.

Meisel, Alan, and Roth, Loren H.: Must a man be his cousin's keeper? Hastings Center Report 8(5):5-6, October 1978.

Moore, Francis D.: Social investment and patient welfare in organ transplantation. In Williams, Preston N., editor: Ethical issues in biology and medicine: proceedings of a symposium on the identity and dignity of man, Cambridge, Mass., 1973, Schenkman Publishing Co.

Nelson, James B.: Human medicine, Minneapolis, 1973, Augsburg Publishing House.

Ramsey, Paul: The patient as person, New Haven, Conn., 1970, Yale University Press.

Simmons, Roberta G., and Fulton, Julie: Ethical issues in kidney transplantation. In Frazier, Claude A., editor: Is it moral to modify man? Springfield, Ill., 1973, Charles C Thomas, Publisher.

Simmons, Roberta G., and Klein, Susan D.: Gift of life: the social and psychological impact of organ transplantation, New York, 1977, John Wiley and Sons.

Smith, Harmon L.: Ethics and the new medicine, Nashville, 1970, Abingdon Press.

Veatch, Robert M.: Case studies in medical ethics, Cambridge, Mass., 1977, Harvard University Press.

Warren, Mary Anne, Maguire, Daniel, and Levine, Carol: Can the fetus be an organ farm? Hastings Center Report 8(5):23-25, October 1978.

12

Dying and death

DEFINITIONS OF DEATH

In the past the only cardinal indicators of death were the absence of blood flow, the cessation of respiration, and the presence of fixed and dilated pupils. Although a physician was and still is legally required to pronounce death, anyone using only these criteria could determine the difference between a live person and a corpse. But as technology has become more complex, so has the definition of death. Two major technologic developments of the past generation have complicated the definition of death. The first is the creation of machines that can artificially sustain heartbeats and respiration indefinitely, even when there is no discernible brain activity; the second is the various forms of transplant surgery that require fresh, well-preserved donor organs. The second creates a dilemma for the physician declaring death because he must not deprive the transplant recipient of the freshest possible organ but cannot declare death too soon for fear of removing an organ from a living person.

Defining death involves several different perspectives. Philosophically when we speak of death, we must decide if we mean the death of a body or of a person. If we use all or even some of Fletcher's criteria for personhood (see Chapter 1), the death of a person will be seen as vastly different from the death of a person's body. When we speak of body death, do we mean just the brain or the entire body? If one could satisfactorily solve the philosophic issues, there is still the medical dilemma of determining exactly when death has occurred and defining precise criteria that differentiate between a live person and a dead one. As we shall see, this is not an easy task. The lack of clear-cut criteria for death has led to legal problems, including accusations that physicians committed murder. Most states do not have a law that defines death, and when cases come to trial, the judge and jury must rely on possibly conflicting testimony of equally capable physicians as they describe the state of death.

Ethical problems abound. At what point can organs be removed for transplant if there is a question of when or if death has occurred? What weight or bearing should the client's or family's consent have on the decision about death? How long and for what reasons should one be supported on machines that artificially sustain life or that rather than sustaining merely defer the finality of death? Can an organ ever be removed prior to the declaration of death; that is, can one "life" ever be sacrificed for another?

Brain death

The term *brain death* has become popular though few people know precisely what it means. The brain stem is involved in many reflex activities, including respiration, which can be artificially continued even when the brain stem is temporarily or permanently not functioning, as in anesthesia, paralysis, or a drug overdose. As long as respiration continues, the heart will beat; a functioning brain is not necessary for heart action. The brain stem is only one part of the brain and is not usually associated with personhood. That function belongs to the neocortex, where higher human functions occur. The neocortex must also be determined to be dead before the *person* is considered dead. The person must not have use of any of his senses or faculties, he must not be able to take any protective reflex action (gagging, blinking, drawing away from pain), and there must be no reasonable hope of his ever being able to do any of these things again. Further diagnostic tests (measuring the enzymes released by cerebrospinal fluid or the amount of oxygen entering and leaving brain cells) may be able to pinpoint more precisely the time when death occurs and may provide a more accurate determination that death has indeed taken place, but for the present the absence of activity in both the brain stem and the neocortex is generally considered the major guideline.

Harvard Ad Hoc Committee. In 1967 an Ad Hoc Committee of the Harvard Medical School published a report as the result of an examination of the definition of brain death and irreversible coma.[1] It stated two reasons why a definition was needed: technologic improvements in procedures for saving the lives of those severely injured or gravely ill sometimes had only partial success, and the victims were left in a limbo of being neither completely alive or totally dead. The burden this placed on families, hospitals, and the legal structure was enormous; there had to be an attempt to resolve the dilemma. The other major reason was the need to have established criteria for the removal of organs for transplantation. The Ad Hoc Committee was not concerned with the cause of a coma, and they restricted themselves to only those individuals who exhibited no discernible central nervous system activity. The following characteristics define a *permanently* nonfunctioning brain:

1. *Unreceptivity and unresponsivity.* There is total unawareness to externally applied stimuli, even painful ones, and inner needs. Even the most intensely painful stimuli evoke no sound or movement.
2. *No movements or breathing.* Continuous observation for at least 1 hour in which there are no spontaneous attempts to breathe, move, or react to stimuli such as light, sound, touch, or pain satisfies this criterion. If the person is connected to a respirator, it should be turned off for 3 minutes. If during this interval the person makes no spontaneous attempt to breathe, the criterion is satisfied.
3. *No reflexes.* The pupils are fixed and dilated with no response to light, and there is no ocular response to the ears being irrigated with ice water. All the usual reflexes are absent, including deep tendon reflexes.
4. *Flat electroencephalogram.* This is the basis on which all the other criteria rest and is the indicator that no electrical activity exists in the brain. It is

suggested that at least 10 to 20 minutes of recording be done and that the same procedure be repeated 24 hours later.

The Harvard Ad Hoc Committee stated that brain death can be determined *only* by a physician and usually in consultation with one or two other physicians. They recommended that after this determination is made, colleagues should be informed and *then* the respirator turned off. The committee specifically stated that the physician is responsible for making the decision and that it is "unsound and undesirable" to have the family made the decision. Because 10 of the 13 men on the committee were physicians, it is understandable that they would give total power in the decision to the physician, but many people disagree with that stance, and in the decade and a half since the committee made its report, others as well have entered the decision.

Other aspects of defining brain death. A dramatic and well-publicized case points out not only that there is a need to define precisely when and if death has occurred but also that health professionals cannot blithely and complacently decree a person dead without looking at the human, philosophic, and ethical ramifications of death and dying.[2]

On May 24, 1968, a black man named Bruce Tucker fell and suffered a massive head injury. He was rushed to the Medical College of Virginia Hospital where he was found to have a skull fracture and other serious complications. Various surgical and medical procedures were performed, and by the next morning Tucker was attached to a respirator and was "mechanically alive" with no hope whatsoever for recovery. Also at the same hospital was a client, Joseph Klett, who was awaiting a heart transplant. David M. Hume, head of the heart transplant team at the hospital, saw Tucker as an ideal donor for Klett. Tucker had a flat EEG, but his other vital signs were normal. At 2:45 P.M. the day after his fall, Tucker was taken back to the operating room and prepared for the removal of his heart and kidneys. The respirator was turned off at 3:30 P.M. Five minutes later Tucker was pronounced dead, and the mechanical supports were immediately reconnected to preserve his organs. His heart and kidneys were removed even though his vital signs continued to be normal.

Tucker's organs were removed without informing his family, although his wallet contained the business card of his brother who had been in his office all day, only 15 blocks away. William Tucker, the brother, brought suit against the surgical team for wrongfully ending Bruce Tucker's life. The jury found in favor of the surgeons; subsequent coverage by legal and medical press commented only on the definition of brain death and did not seem to find the ethical issues important. The general public, except for the black community, seemed mostly undisturbed by the case and did not appear aware of any other issues involved in the decision.

Some philosophic issues in defining death. This case can be used as a basis for examining the ethical, philosophic, and practical issues involved in defining death.

The first issue concerns when one slips from irreversible coma into death. The Harvard Ad Hoc Committee defined coma as a criterion for death but did not say that irreversible coma was necessarily synonymous with death, although many have interpreted the report to equate the two. The difference may be slim, and one philosophic concept of death may rest on the cessation of neocortical functioning, but death and coma are not the same. The Harvard committee recommends that in the face of irreversible coma a physician take responsibility for disconnecting the respirator. The committee was very careful to assign responsibility *only* to the physician; thus it could be interpreted that the committee advocates causing death by disconnecting the respirator in view of the hopelessly irreversible coma, though surely the committee members did not see themselves as advocates of killing.

If one does not disconnect the respirator, how can it be determined whether the person is indeed dead or still in coma? Theoretically one can exist almost indefinitely in this mechanical limbo. With our technologic skill we may have created a phenomenon of living dead—a nightmare world of machines and vital function monitors but no humanity.

Another issue involves the philosophic concept of death. Veatch has proposed that death be defined as "a complete change in the status of a living entity characterized by the irreversible loss of those characteristics that are essentially significant to it."[2,p.22] He points out that the definition applies equally well to a human being, an animal, a single cell, and even a social system. To define the death of a human being, then, one must know what a human being is, that is, what characteristics are particularly human. People generally know what death is; they recognize it and understand the concept. It is only in isolated cases that the issue needs to be debated at all. But because the number of these cases is growing and because we do not know where technology will lead us next, the concept of death needs to be examined. Veatch[2] sees four approaches to define or determine death:

1. *Irreversible loss of flow of vital fluids.* It is not as much the functioning of the heart and lungs themselves as the *flow* of blood and breath that causes life to exist, although admittedly the function and flow are so intertwined it is impossible to separate them. This criterion of flow is shaky, however, because technology has guaranteed the ability to keep our blood circulating and breath entering and leaving our bodies.

2. *Irreversible loss of the soul from the body.* All religions speak of a soul though some do not use that word, and even people who are totally agnostic or atheistic acknowledge some vital force that is different and independent from the chemical and electrical forces that hold our body together. Judeo-Christian belief holds that the soul is the essence of a human being. It is what drives and motivates one to acts of good and evil, to accomplishment or slothfulness, and when the soul has left the body, the person is dead. This may seem an amorphous concept, and some may scoff at the idea of a soul as a separate entitiy that takes leave of the body at the time of death, but it has been an important element in the philosophic concept of death.

3. *Irreversible loss of the capacity for bodily integration.* Technology can keep alive parts of a body that would otherwise have died. A comatose person who is alive by means of artificial respiration and various drugs that keep his blood pressure at an acceptable level and regulate the rhythm of his heart may be alive in the biologic sense of the word, but he is not an integrated

human being. The various systems of his body may be functioning, but the body as a whole cannot integrate those functions.

We are not interested in the death of particular cells, organs, or organ systems, but in the death of the person as a whole—the point at which the person as a whole undergoes a quantum change through the loss of characteristics held to be essentially significant, the point at which "death behavior" becomes appropriate. Terms such as *brain death* or *heart death* should be avoided, because they tend to obscure the fact that we are searching for the meaning of death of the person as a whole.*

Bodily integration is both internal (such as the regulation of blood pressure, the flow of hormones in a menstrual cycle, and the rush of adrenalin during anger or fear) and external (adaptation to a social and physical environment). It is evident that people in irreversible coma are unable to achieve either kind of integration.

4. *Irreversible loss of the capacity for social interaction.* Probably the single most significant characteristic of a human being, outside of purely physical ones such as an opposable thumb, the capacity for language, and the ability to walk erect, is his consciousness, the capacity for social interaction. The capacity is particularly human and is the important element, not the choice or circumstance to act on that capacity. What is meant by the capacity for social interaction? Rationality? Sanity? Emotionality? Communication? Any of them? All of them together? It probably makes little difference how one precisely defines the term; what is important is the recognition that the capacity for social interaction exists in a person or is only temporarily lost. The locus of social interaction is most certainly the neocortex, and if it is nonfunctioning, the individual has lost the capacity for social interaction.

Other loci of death

It is inappropriate to speak of "the locus of death" as though a pathologist could find the precise place where death first occurred. The locus of death is primarily a philosophic issue and depends on one's concept of death. If one believes that death is caused by a cessation of the flow of vital fluids, one could pinpoint the heart or lungs or perhaps even a specific organ as the locus of death. If one believes that death occurs when the soul leaves the body, then the locus of death is more elusive; most people believe that the soul resides in the brain, but that is far from a certainty. If death is thought to occur when the body loses its capacity for physical integration, then perhaps the locus of death is the central or autonomic nervous system, both of which are connected inextricably to the brain by the spinal cord.

All these views are worthy of consideration, but it is likely that for the present and some time to come, the locus of death will be seen as the brain. Most philosophers, theologians, and physicians believe that the essential characteristics of humanness are those that are rooted in the neocortex of the brain and that regardless of what occurs elsewhere in the body, if the brain is dead, the person is dead.

---

*Veatch, Robert M.: Death, dying and the biological revolution, New Haven, Conn., 1976, Yale University Press.

Statutory definitions

Before considering what legally constitutes being dead, it is necessary to look at the issue of *who* should define death. By tradition and legal precedent it has been the physician, but in many instances death is not merely a technical matter of the absence of all the signs of life. The idea of death involves more than the physical, and physicians may not be qualified to deal with the philosophic aspects. They can describe the condition of deep coma and they can report an isoelectric EEG (no apparent electrical activity in the brain), but to call the coma irreversible and as a result pronounce a person dead is to engage in prophecy rather than diagnosis. The chance of a person recovering from such a coma may be enormously remote, but while the chance exists, the *legal* status of the comatose person is in doubt.

By enabling death to be postponed or prolonged the medical and scientific community has caused the dilemma. Should they be the only ones to resolve it, or should the public have a voice in defining death? Much public discussion has occurred in recent years, particularly in the wake of cases brought to the public's attention and dramatized by the press, notably the case of Karen Ann Quinlan. Though the public may discuss such cases at length, it is still physicians who define death, and the lay public has no official effect on the decision. Nurses in particular are impotent in deciding when death occurs and even how to treat the client while he is dying.

Allowing the judicial system to make the decision has the advantage of putting popular attitudes into practice, and each judicial opinion would help create a body of precedents that could influence decision makers. But each case of death now is decided on an individual başis, and the courts play a basically passive role; that is, they must await litigation by someone who seeks to define death in a particular instance. Litigation is costly, time-consuming, and emotionally draining. A judge or jury could be asked to define the death of an individual, but expert medical testimony would be required as part of the evidence and the court might not feel competent to make a decision and simply rubber-stamp the opinion of the testifying physician. Thus the de facto decision would be the physician's.

As a third alternative, defining death could be a legislative decision. A simple description of the transition between the state of being alive and that of being dead would not suffice. Capron and Kass[3] define four levels of definitions important in the creation of such legislation: (1) the basic concept, (2) general physiologic standards, (3) operational criteria, and (4) specific tests or procedures. The basic concept of death is a philosophic matter and offers no practical help in devising criteria but is important in how it influences the attitudes of those writing the standards. General physiologic standards are technical matters and are only descriptive of a person's condition, not *decisive* in defining that condition. Operational criteria further define what is meant by physical standards. Specific tests and procedures determine whether established criteria are met; if the tests are to be specific, the implication is that they will be physiologic, and if the definition of death rests on these tests, then the standard is purely physiologic and physicians make the decisions without popular or legislative input.

Those attempting a definition should be concerned with the death of a total human being rather than of his individual cells, brain, or other organs. It is with human beings that society and legislation are concerned, not the separate parts that make up a total person. Aside from defining the actual physiologic state of death, legislation could venture into other areas such as determining who should be charged with making the decision, how many people should collaborate, how the time of death should be fixed, and perhaps what it is permissible to do with a body after death.

The Kansas statute. In 1968 Kansas became the first state to enact legislation defining death. Alaska, California, Georgia, Illinois, Maryland, Michigan, New Mexico, Oregon, and Virginia have done so since. Because a legislative definition is important to society's relationship with death, and because many think that the Kansas law contradicts itself in places, it is stated here in its entirety:

A person will be considered medically and legally dead if, in the opinion of a physician, based on ordinary standards of medical practice, there is the absence of spontaneous respiratory and cardiac functions and, because of the disease or condition which caused, directly or indirectly, these functions to cease, or because of the passage of time since these functions ceased, attempts to resuscitate are considered hopeless; and, in this event, death will have occurred at the time these functions ceased; or

A person will be considered medically and legally dead if, in the opinion of a physician, based on ordinary standards of medical practice, there is the absence of spontaneous brain function; and if, based on ordinary standards of medical practice, during reasonable attempts to either maintain or restore spontaneous circulatory or respiratory function in the absence of aforesaid brain function, it appears that further attempts at resuscitation or supportive maintenance will not succeed, death will have occurred at the time when these conditions coincide. Death is to be pronounced before artificial means of supporting respiratory and circulatory function are terminated and before any vital organ is removed for purpose of transplantation.*

Although commendable for its attempt, this statute has several serious short-comings and inconsistencies. It requires only that a physician determine death, placing too much power in the hands of a single person. "Ordinary standards" of medical practice are not defined, and courtroom arguments about what could and should have been done for the client as part of ordinary practice could be long and bitter. The statute defines a dead person in two distinct ways—by cardiac and respiratory function and by brain function. The latter is not specifically defined though an acceptable standard was available in the Harvard Ad Hoc Committee report of 1967. The law seems to have been drawn up for the specific purpose of preventing litigation concerning organs removed for transplantation, and thus it does not consider any but the physical aspects of death. No effort is made to confront or even acknowledge the philosophic aspects. The wishes of neither the dying person nor the family are taken into consideration if the physician alone makes the decision.

Suggestions for a statutory definition. Drawing up a workable and humane stat-

---

*Quoted in Benton, Richard G.: Death and dying: principles and practices in patient care, New York, 1978, Van Nostrand Reinhold Co., p. 23.

ute to define death is such an awesome task that many wonder if it could be done. If the law is too general and not sufficiently definitive, it might as well not exist. If it is too specific, the criteria might soon be outmoded and the responsibility would be too concentrated. If it is too flexible, it defeats its own purpose; if it is too rigid, the definitions become unusable.

Capron and Kass[3] have enumerated five principles on which a statute should be formulated:

1. The statute should be confined to death of the individual as a whole being.
2. The statute should be confined to the question "Is he dead?" rather than "Should he be allowed to die?" It defines a condition, and although it may relate to an ethical issue, the issue itself is not the law.
3. The statute should allow for changes in methods to determine death but not for new concepts of life and death. The importance of separating the concepts is to prevent a "sliding scale of leniency" in the determination of death, depending, for instance, on the supply and demand of organs for transplantation.
4. The definition of death should be universally applicable to all people without regard to wealth, social usefulness, stature, or other variables.
5. The statute should be flexible enough to accommodate scientific advances without changing the law each time a new technology is found to be applicable.

One might wonder why a statutory definition of death is needed. Some think its sole purpose concerns organ removal, but there are other reasons as well. The major reason is to preserve the dignity and humanity of the dying or dead person and his family by avoiding the situation in which there is confusion about whether he is alive or dead and in which his family is forced to suffer agonies of false hope. As well, it must be absolutely certain that a person is not pronounced dead prematurely. There is an economic reason also, because keeping a body alive places a tremendous financial burden on the family or, more likely, the hopsital or state. A statute could also be used to prohibit physicians from capriciously declaring a person dead.

Any law must assign responsibility. In the Kansas statute the responsibility rests solely with the physician, a condition many find unacceptable. If death is to be legally defined almost entirely in physical terms, then the description of death should be within the province of those most qualified to describe it, physicians and scientists. But what about those people most affected by the application of the definition, the person and his family? What should their legal responsibility be?

PROLONGING LIFE ARTIFICIALLY
When is it appropriate to be permitted to die?

The question of when a person should be permitted to die is the crux of one of the most perplexing issues of this age. Volumes have been written about the subject, but there has been no satisfactory answer to the question of when and if people should be permitted to die if they choose. We can only scratch the surface of the issue of the quality of life, as it is often called.

There are two opposing positions regarding the artificial prolongation of life, the "death with dignity" and the "right to life" position. Advocates of the former believe that the decision to artificially prolong a life should rest with the dying person himself, in the form of a living will or by direct discussions, or his family if he is not conscious and has not left instructions. They believe that a person should not be forced to endure pain, suffering, humiliation, expense, and prolonged dying if he chooses not to, that in the absence of any reasonable hope for recovery he should be able to choose to die with dignity rather than linger and suffer with indignity. Opposing advocates believe that while there is still life there should be continued treatment, that hope should not be cast aside, and that no individual has a right to determine when life is over because only God can determine this.

The ethical issues here are related to the concepts of individual liberty and choice. If we as a nation believe in the right to privacy, as the Constitution specifies, and if that right includes controlling our own bodies, then how has the health care system over the years managed to transfer that right to physicians who generally decide whether we will be permitted to die? A physician is both a private citizen and a member of a specific group and is thus affected by the issue both as an individual who potentially may want to be permitted to die or let a family member die and as a physician in a position to make that decision for others. The issue involves not whether a particular physician is competent to make that decision but whether an individual has the liberty to control his own destiny as far as is humanly possible.

California Natural Death Act. In 1974 Representative Barry Keene introduced a bill into the California State Assembly that stated, "Every person has the right to die without prolongation of life by medical means." The wording of the bill is simple—too simple—but it sparked debates and hearings throughout the state. As a result of those hearings, the bill, known as the Natural Death Act, became law in California in 1976. The law gives adults the right to direct physicians to withhold or withdraw life-sustaining procedures on the grounds that they have a right to control decisions affecting their own medical care and lives. Among the specific provisions are the following:

1. The individual can ask that his life not be artificially prolonged in a terminal condition.
2. The physician must consult with at least one other physician to determine that the prognosis is terminal.
3. A terminally ill person must wait 2 weeks after learning the prognosis before signing a directive.
4. Only mechanical or other artificial means to sustain a vital function may be withheld or withdrawn and these only when death is imminent.
5. A written directive is a person's final statement of his wishes.
6. The directive must be signed by two witnesses who are not related or heir to the person or responsible for his physical care.
7. A woman may stipulate that the directive may be suspended if she is pregnant.

8. The directive is valid for 5 years and may be reexecuted as often as needed.

9. The directive may be revoked verbally or in writing at any time.[4]

The law settled a variety of legal controversies, most of them having arisen from questions of living wills and professional liability when it was thought that health professionals may have acted to hasten a person's death by discontinuing artificial life-support systems. According to the Natural Death Act death under this directive does not constitute suicide, a matter important in terms of insurance policies. Many people think that the law is too restrictive and circumscribed to benefit the vast majority and that the purpose of the law was mainly to protect physicians and other health professionals from malpractice suits.

The debate in California prior to the law being passed was a microcosm of the worldwide debate about the right to be permitted to die. The Catholic Church moved from a position of extreme opposition to a more neutral one when the bill's wording was changed. The phrase "life-sustaining procedure" was more acceptable than "extraordinary medical measures" in defining what a person could direct to be withheld or withdrawn. The Church also was appeased by the mention of mechanical measures to sustain vital functions, specifically excluding surgery, pharmaceuticals, radiation, and other forms of therapy. Ambivalence about the bill is still strong, and many see it as a first step toward legalization of euthanasia and oppose it for that reason. Some think the bill too narrowly limits the circumstances in which a directive is permitted and fear that a physician might not act on a client's behalf unless the situation fits exactly what is described by law. However, the purpose of the law is to provide a guideline for action.

Rights of the dying

When we speak of the rights of the dying, we are referring to option rights rather than welfare rights (see Chapter 1). The rights of the dying are intricately interwoven with the relationship of the dying person to professional caregivers, including nurses, family members, social workers, and other members of the health team.

Right to know the truth. Two questions are involved in the right to know the truth: does the client have the right to know the truth, and is the physician obligated to tell the truth? There are several dilemmas involved. If the client thinks he has the right to know and wants to know the truth and the physician does not think he is obligated to reveal it, where can the client go for information? Family members may or may not know more than the client, raising the issue of the right to privacy: if a physician tells a client's spouse of the impending death of the client but does not tell the client, the physician has breached his pledge of confidentiality. Nurses and other health professionals are unlikely to give the client information if the physician has chosen not to. The client is then in a position of being unable to obtain facts about his situation. If, on the other hand, the physician feels obligated to tell the client the truth and the client does not want to know it, should he force the client to listen and perhaps cause psychologic harm?

If one accepts the premise, as many people do, that a physician is as morally obligated to give a client full and honest information about his diagnosis and prognosis as he is to give complete and skillful care, then one must be certain what the truth is—and this is usually not a clear-cut matter. The truth about the nature and course of a disease can never be known with absolute certainty; we convey knowledge as we perceive it, not necessarily as it really is. The client perceives what another says is truth through the filter of his experiences, feelings, and expectations. If I am told that I have leukemia and will probably die in 6 months, my perceptions of what will happen to me are colored by my knowledge of the disease, my fantasies about dying of leukemia, what the physician has told me and how he told me, my experiences with the death of others, whether I choose to embark on a course of chemotherapy, and other variables in my life experience. The physician may tell me the truth as he knows and sees it; the way I interpret it is my responsibility.

Is it ever permissible for a physician to lie or withhold the truth from a dying client? Most ethicists say that lying to a terminally ill person is not morally correct even if the client says he does not want the truth. If a client wants to be deceived if his illness is serious or fatal but wants the truth in other health matters, how will he know when the physician is telling the truth or when an illness is serious? A "conscientious liar," one who lies only when he thinks it morally appropriate to do so, assumes that other people know when he considers it appropriate to lie. By implication he admits his lying, and it is likely that he will not be believed even when he is telling the truth.

There is inescapably a subversive result of occasional lying. It makes no real difference whether it is perpetrated by a direct commission of an untruth, or indirectly through omission of a truth. Lying troubles the waters of human relations and takes away the one element of mutual trust without which medical practice becomes a manipulation of bodies rather than the care of and for persons. The assumption made by the physician, when he has the *presumption* to withhold the truth, is that the patient is really no longer an adult, but rather either a child or an idiot, more an *it* than a *thou*.*

Those health professionals who have had even minimal experience caring for people with terminal illnesses know that in most instances the truth is withheld from clients to protect the emotionality of the caregiver rather than the clients. Physicians and nurses in particular often find it difficult to deal with the fact that the client will die and tend to see it as a personal affront to their professional skills and ability. A physician who says, "I lost a patient today," seems to be saying that he has somehow failed to save that person. The nurse who says, "I hope he doesn't die on *my* shift," appears to want to avoid any thought that she could have somehow prevented or delayed the death. Kübler-Ross and others have shown that the dying need to have an accurate idea of what they face so that they can deal with their impending death in a healthy adaptive way. People with cancer and other terminal illnesses seem to know without being told that they are facing death. How cruel it is to force them to pretend that they know nothing, when their emotional

---

*Fletcher, Joseph: Morals and medicine, Princeton, N. J., 1954, Princeton University Press.

energy could be better spent savoring remaining time with the knowledge that time is limited.

There is still a problem when a client who says he does not want the truth and the physician has every reason to believe that he means what he says. Should the physician force the truth on the client for his own good? Should the physician do nothing and hope the client changes his mind? Should the physician intimate or hint that there is something the client should know without actually telling him what it is? Or should the physician remove himself from the care of that client and urge him to seek care elsewhere? How would the client react? How could it be done in a professional manner, and what reason would the physician give for resigning? Either he would have to tell the truth that he is resigning because the patient refuses to let him explain his illness or he would be forced to lie about his reasons for withdrawing his care. Neither alternative is satisfactory. Fletcher[5] gives four reasons why a physician must disclose the truth:

1. If a person is denied knowledge that is available to him, a moral human quality is taken away.
2. Facts about a client belong to the client. The physician is entrusted with them, and if he chooses to keep the facts from the client, he is stealing from him.
3. The fullest possible treatment and cure depend on complete trust and confidence.
4. A client needs all the facts about his own life and death to carry out his life responsibilities, and a physician cannot assume those responsibilities by withholding certain facts.

Informed consent. Informed consent necessitates truth telling (see Chapters 9 and 10), and several characteristics of informed consent are important in relation to the dying person. Of greatest concern here are the person's rights to refuse treatment and to receive information about the consequences of that refusal. Refusing treatment differs from the act of removing someone from an artificial respirator or terminating his life by other means (active and passive euthanasia) because the client specifically and consciously refuses to be treated surgically, with drugs or radiation, by hemodialysis, or even by hospitalization. Clients choose to refuse treatment for a variety of reasons, including religious beliefs, the wish to put an end to their own or their family's suffering, an inability to continue to pay for treatment, a desire not to give up control of their body functions, and the wish to be done with it—to die. When a client refuses treatment, it is usually the physician who feels responsible to discuss the consequences of the refusal with him. Often, however, the nurse is the first to know the client's feelings and intentions. The way she handles this knowledge and the client's feelings can make a difference between calm and supported action on a conviction and disgruntled resentment of all health professionals.

The refusal of treatment when the alternative is death is considered by many an act of suicide or voluntary passive euthanasia. Regardless of the moral implications, however, the person still has a right to refuse treatment, and the physician and nurse are morally obligated to tell the client what will happen if he does so.

(See Chapter 10 for a discussion of the legal and moral implications of refusal of treatment.) A major problem with putting this belief into practice is that the consequences of the refusal are never certain. A client may "go home to die," have a sudden remission, and live for several more years; pain that was not thought likely to occur until much later in the course of the disease might flare up suddenly; or after it is predicted that the client should live for a year, he might die in a week. Anything can happen. Health care can do nothing to alter the course of a disease if treatment is refused, and a caregiver can only make certain that the client understands this fact and that he is free to change his mind and reinstitute treatment whenever he chooses.

Ordinary and extraordinary means to prolong life

To attempt to define the difference between ordinary and extraordinary means to prolong and preserve life is to engage in a semantic discussion in which there can never be a definitive decision. The usual definition of *extraordinary* involves the use of artificial means to prolong life without which the client would die. This generally involves mechanical means to keep the person breathing and his heart beating but also involves the use of certain drugs to maintain blood pressure and keep the chemistry of body fluids in balance. The problem of defining these measures as extraordinary is that they are routinely used in all hospitals; in fact, resuscitating a person who has "died" is so routine that most hospitals have a policy that a physician must write a specific order *not* to resuscitate. Many forms of treatment that seemed extraordinary a few years ago are quite ordinary today, such as the reconnection of a severed limb, hemodialysis, heart transplants, cardiopulmonary resuscitation, transfusion, artificial respiration, and even some pharmocologic treatments.

The concept of extraordinary treatment cannot be defined to everyone's satisfaction, and perhaps it is not the most important question. What *is* important to discuss concerns whether these forms of treatment should be given to a person who is already dying of a disease and who would die without their use. The real issue involves thwarting nature. Any intervention in any illness can be seen as thwarting nature (for example, "strep throat" might lead to a fatal condition if one refused to take antibiotics), but the essential problem concerns what to do and how far to go in saving and prolonging life—the issue concerning if it is ever, sometimes, or always morally right to withhold these forms of treatment.

Traditional medical practice requires that everything humanly possible be done to preserve and prolong life; failure to do so is the equivalent of negligence, malpractice, or euthanasia. When the actual process of dying has begun, it may then be permissible, or even obligatory if the client requests it, to cease trying to cure him and begin caring for the process of his dying. If one accepts this premise, what measures should be taken to care for the person? Which measures could be seen to prolong life and which only to make dying more comfortable and acceptable?

If food and drink are given orally or intravenously, will the nourishment they contain prolong dying? If the client is removed from the hospital to a nursing home or his own home, how will the dying process be affected? The concept of a reasonable hope for recovery can be compared with the legal concept of proving a person guilty "beyond a reasonable doubt," for there is no such thing as completely eliminating doubt. If the dying process is ignored and the client is treated as if there were a reasonable hope for recovery, is this not a form of lying to the client? What of the family? It is possible that the family out of a sense of love, guilt, grief, or confusion will request that everything be done to save the person's life. How is a physician to deal with this dilemma? If anyone has a right to choose what will or will not be done for a dying person, the family comes closer to having that right than the physician.

This may mean the prolongation of dying or the continuation of extraordinary life-sustaining measures beyond reasonable moral justification. At the same time, guilt-ridden people in their grief may be unable to bear the additional burden of a decision to discontinue useless treatment, and they are often relieved if this decision is not placed wholly on them. This means that the physician must exercise the authority he has acquired as a physician and as a man in relation to the relatives and take the lead in suggesting what should be done. In doing this, the doctor acts more as a man than a medical expert, acknowledging the preeminence of the human relations in which he with these and all other men stand. For this reason, the medical imperative and the moral imperative or permission are, while distinguishable, not separable in the person or in the vocation of the man who is a physician.*

Ramsey's view is consistent with that of many theologians, ethicists, and physicians. It seems humane and practical but contains unwarranted assumptions. The first is that the family is often relieved if the decision to discontinue treatment is taken from them. It is agreed that in most cases the family undergoes tremendous stress and in their anguish may think they wish to abdicate responsibility, but do they really? If a decision is made for them, will they then and in the future be relieved? One cannot know, but the physician has an obligation to do his best to find out what the family wants before he assumes they will be glad to hand the responsibility to him. In this age of highly specialized care it is likely that the attending specialist will not have known the client as a person before seeing him as a dying individual and will not know his family.

Second, Ramsey assumes that the physician can act more as a person than as a medical expert, that he can separate his human functions from his medical ones. This may not be a reasonable expectation. Third, Ramsey assumes the traditional viewpoint that the physician should take the lead in suggesting what should be done. He does not say the physician should make the final decision but strongly implies it by presenting a picture of a family being grateful to the physician for accepting responsibility that was certainly more theirs than his. This attitude perpetuates the paternalism of the health care system and ignores other health professionals, mainly nurses and social workers, who can and should play an important role in supporting the family during this crisis.

Most hospitals have a policy that requires the written directive of a physician if the client is not to be resuscitated. Hospital care has become so technologically

---

*Ramsey, Paul: The patient as person, New Haven, Conn., 1970, Yale University Press.

oriented that unless there is an order to the contrary all clients who die are immediately resuscitated, even 85-year-olds who die of terminal cancer and children with leukemia who have spent most of their lives on chemotherapy. Resuscitation is inappropriate in some instances in which it might be thought by some to be medically indicated and in all instances in which the client specifically requests that this technology not be used. If the client is reasonably healthy and competent to make a decision, as is often the case before surgery, the people caring for him might wonder how much he knows about the technology involved in resuscitation procedures. He should be told that sometimes resuscitation is a temporary life-saving measure (as with cardiac arrest during or after surgery) and to categorically refuse it might be to ensure death. In this case an order not to resuscitate (ONTR) would probably not be appropriate. If, on the other hand, the client faces imminent death from an illness that is terminal, ONTR would more likely be appropriate regardless of the age of the client.

The issue is pragmatic as well as philosophic. If a person is suffering from a terminal illness, especially if he has endured long bouts of physical pain, and he wishes not to suffer any longer than he would in the natural course of the disease, it would be inhumane and cruel to force him to stay alive to continue suffering. That would be akin to using technology as an instrument of torture. Many people disagree with this view, saying that health professionals are bound to preserve and protect life. Here there are two moral principles in conflict. The Socratic method of dealing with this dilemma would be to decide which moral rule has precedence over the other. Those who think that the preservation of life is the higher rule would resuscitate the client regardless of his wishes (except in California where health professionals are obligated by law to defer to the written directive of the client), and those who think that the client should not be made to suffer further would not resuscitate him.

The pragmatic view—that if a person has a terminal illness and will surely die in a matter of days or weeks, it is a waste of time, manpower, and materials to save him—may seem cold-blooded. But if a heart stops beating because the cancer is so invasive that vital organ systems are already beyond effective function, it does little practical good to start the heart artifically so that it can pump blood around a mostly dead body for a few more days.

So far ONTR has been discussed in terms of what the client himself would want. What if he is not competent to state his wishes, as may be the case with victims of an accident, sudden heart attack, or overdose of drugs? Most hospitals have a policy that the decision not to resuscitate or to turn off the apparatus if it was started is the responsibility of a professional committee in consultation with the family. The judgment of competence is a hazy area. Is the client able to understand anything, and if so, can he act on his understandings? Is he permanently incompetent, as in irreversible coma, or can his cerebral functioning be expected to improve? Is his judged incompetence the result of brain damage or drugs, or is his mind clouded by physical pain? Usually competence in a medical sense means that a person is able to understand the risks of and alternatives to a proposed treatment and that his decision reflects a deliberate choice. Tests of competence must be applied by more than one person and on more than one occasion or the judgment cannot be considered valid.

Can a competent person ever be legally forced to accept treatment against his will? Some believe so.

The rendition of emergency life-saving medical treatment on the person of the objecting adult patient is proper. It will be seen that neither the common law nor the "free exercise" of the First Amendment of the United States Constitution gives the individual a right to reject life-saving treatment. The law's traditional view of the sanctity of human life and the importance of the individual's life to the welfare of society deny the individual the right to, in effect, consent to his own death.*

The argument is that a person does have a right to refuse medical treatment but not life-saving treatment in an emergency. The line between the two situations is not clearly drawn, and the person refusing treatment in a nonemergency situation may be signing his own death warrant as surely as the one refusing emergency treatment. If a person refuses chemotherapy for leukemia, he will die. If a person refuses a transfusion when an artery has been severed in an accident, he will die. The two instances are similar if it is assumed that both people are equally competent to make the decision. If a client refuses treatment and the physician treats him nonetheless, the client can sue for battery; there are sufficient legal precedents to ensure that he is likely to win the suit on the grounds that he had not legally consented. If the victim of an accident is unconscious or otherwise unable to give consent for emergency treatment, the physician may treat him with impunity, the assumption being that if the client were conscious he would have given consent, as a majority of people would. There are so many legal precedents in this area that the physician does not need to obtain a court order in each individual situation.

The problem arises when a competent conscious adult refuses life-saving emergency treatment. The argument above maintains that in an emergency one cannot be certain that the client really means what he is saying when he refuses treatment; this is an understandable view. In an emergency no one is as rational as during calmer moments because the mind can be confused or clouded by pain, stress, the sudden rush of events, or a loss of blood. If the physician acts according to the client's wishes at the time of the emergency, how can he know what the client would have wanted if the same procedure were proposed during a nonemergency? If a client is in an accident that crushes his leg and it must be amputated to prevent his death from blood poisoning and hemorrhage, he might say, "I'd rather die than live with only one leg," and refuse to give consent for surgery. What is the physician to do? The physician knows that the client can be fitted with an artificial leg and after rehabilitation can live quite well. He can explain this to the client, who in a haze of anguish and confusion may still refuse. The same surgeon can explain the same procedure to a diabetic, who calmly and rationally contemplates the loss of his leg and his future adaptation to that loss and who may also refuse amputation.

---

*Comment: Unauthorized rendition of lifesaving medical treatment, California Law Review 53:860, 1965. Copyright © 1965, California Law Review, Inc. Reprinted by permission.

The preceding argument maintains that because the emergency or life-threatening situation makes a difference in what the physician should do, he should amputate the leg of the accident victim but not the diabetic's.

Who should make the decision?

The following examples illustrate the dilemmas involved in determining who should make what decisions about the prolongation of life. Matthew Donnelly was dying of skin cancer that had probably resulted from 30 years of doing research on x rays.[6] Several parts of his body, including his jaw, upper lip, nose, left hand, and part of the right hand, had been surgically removed, and he was blind and in unremitting physical pain. A cure was impossible, and the only further treatment was more mutilating surgery and analgesics. Physicians estimated that he had about a year to live. He wanted to die, and his request was repeated and unmistakable, especially to his youngest brother Harold. Donnelly was in the hospital in an agony of pain and wanted only to be released from that pain. He had made the decision to die, but since he was not in a position to act on that decision, should someone else act as the agent of Donnelly's decision?

The following discussion is concerned not with whether the decision to die is right or wrong but with *who* if anyone should act on the decision. Should the physician accede to Donnelly's request either by killing him directly or by letting him die by withholding nutrients and all medication except analgesics? The physician is faced with a conflict. He knows what the client wants and knows that the client will not be cured, that he faces a slow and painful death, but as a physician he has a moral duty to preserve life by adhering to the moral code of his profession. Does the code apply equally in all cases, or can the physician ignore it or set it temporarily aside when the situation in his opinion seems to warrant it? Is a professional code binding on all members of the profession including those who do not always accept it in whole or in part? Are there principles, such as nonmaleficence, that supersede codes of ethics?

Should Donnelly's brother Harold act as an agent either by killing his brother as requested or by making it possible for Donnelly to kill himself? If Harold did kill his brother, would it be an act of premeditated murder or would the court find him not guilty because of mitigating circumstances? Is it ever morally correct (except in cases of self-defense) to deliberately kill someone or aid in someone's suicide? The state by executing criminals condones the killing of people it considers a menace to society and in effect is saying that society will be better off if certain people are killed. Donnelly is saying the same thing; in his judgment he would be better off dead, and he is asking his brother to do for him what the state does for certain criminals. If Harold kills his brother, could he not use this reasoning as the basis of a legal defense?

A possible alternative is to convene a panel of experts to decide whether they should act on Donnelly's decision. Many hospitals engage in this sort of collegial decision making when vital issues are at stake. Collecting a group of concerned and thoughtful people is not difficult, but is it morally correct? Can a group be charged with deciding the fate of an individual? The foundation of our judicial system acts on the premise that a jury of twelve people can decide one's fate. The difference is that a jury determines the guilt of a person accused of a crime. Since Donnelly has done no wrong, is the determination of his fate properly left to a group of strangers?

Another important issue concerns whether Donnelly fully understands the impact of what he is requesting and whether death is the only solution for him. Has every possible combination of analgesics been tried, and are there any other palliative measures to be instituted? Does Donnelly really want to die now, or would he be willing to wait for death to come naturally if he could be relieved of all or most of his pain? Obtaining this information is the responsibility of everyone involved in Donnelly's care, the physicians, nurses, family, and a consulting panel of other health professionals. Carrying out Donnelly's decision without first looking at every possible alternative would be an immoral and irresponsible act.

The second example involves a man who was alone in the world, dying, and not conscious enough to decide for himself what his fate should be.[6] A 60-year-old man who could not at first be identified suffered burns on about 70% of his body. He survived the first week of hospitalization without dying of infection, but he faced months of agonizing treatment and the physicians were not certain he would survive. A neighbor who identified him reported that he had no family and complained of being alone in the world. He remained in a semicomatose state but moaned in agony each time the pain returned. He had brain function but was not conscious. The neurologist could not predict when if ever he would regain anything resembling normal consciousness. Two nurses in the burn unit approached the physician and asked if it were really necessary to continue treatment. The physician said that if he were in that condition, he would not want treatment to continue, but since the client had no family or anyone responsible for him, he was unsure of the best course of action. The physician as a matter of principle wanted to give the best possible care to the client, but he could see the futility of continuing treatment. Who should have authority to make a decision in a case like this?

In trying to resolve this issue one must first decide which moral principle is to guide the choice of action. Should one be concerned primarily with the greatest good for the greatest number of people (utilitarianism)? If this principle is chosen, treatment might have to be discontinued because the greatest good for the greatest number would come from allowing him to die. On the other hand, society could benefit by keeping him alive to learn more about the treatment of severe burns. Thus the greatest good for the greatest number would result from keeping him alive and giving him the best possible care.

The second principle that could be used to guide the choice is the traditional medical ethic as represented by the Hippocratic oath that binds the physician to do whatever he thinks will most benefit the client. This principle is concerned only with what is correct for the individual in question and not with society in general. In this instance the physician has no way of knowing what is best for the client and cannot help but consider other factors in his decision, such as the cost to the hospital, the demands on his own time, and his own beliefs about pain and death. If the decision is left solely to the physician, he can only guess what the client would want or apply some ethical standard such as the Golden Rule, but in either case the choice is made on the basis of what the physician wants rather than on the basis of what is best for the client, because the physician has no way of knowing this.

The third approach to the dilemma involves Kant's Categorical Imperative. Is there a moral rule that must be applied to this situation regardless of the consequences, and is the physician obligated to obey that rule even against the dictates of his own conscience? Is the physician-client relationship a moral contract requiring that certain rules of conduct be carried out? Does the right to life supersede all other claims, and does the physician give up other choices when he enters into a contract with a client? Does the physician also have a contract with society because the action he takes with an individual will affect society as a whole? And if he has a contract with both, which takes moral precedence?

In the situation of the burned man, it appears that the best course of action is for the physician not to make the decision alone. Who then is responsible for the client since no one has come forward to claim a relationship to him? One of two things would most likely happen: a committee of health professionals employed by the hospital would assume responsibility and perhaps even legal guardianship, or the court would appoint a person probably an attorney, to act as agent for the client.

The final case involves a 26-year-old jet pilot who was horribly burned when the gas tank of his automobile exploded in an accident.[7] His father was with him in the car and died en route to the hospital, but Donald never lost consciousness. He suffered mostly third-degree burns on 68% of his body and was blinded. During the 9 months after the accident he had repeated skin grafts, enucleation of the right eye, and amputation of the distal parts of all the fingers on both hands. His left eye was surgically closed to prevent infection. His hands were deformed and useless because of contractures, and every day he had to be immersed in tanks to control the massive infection. He was transferred to another hospital 9 months later, and 2 days after admission he refused to give permission for further corrective surgery on his hands and insisted that he be allowed to leave the hospital and go home to die. Every day since the accident he had firmly stated that he did not want to live, and now he wanted to take action on his stated intention. If he were to return home he would surely die of massive infection. His mother could not care for him at home, nor could she bear simply to watch him die. A psychiatrist was called in and found Donald stubborn and determined but also bright, articulate, logical, and coherent—by no means mentally incompetent. He simply did not want to continue living as a blind and crippled person and hired an attorney to obtain his release from the hospital by court order if necessary.

Should Donald be permitted to go home to die as he says he wishes to do, and who should make the decision to release him from the hospital to his certain death? Donald has not wavered from his decision in 9 months, and the fact that he has hired an attorney further emphasizes his determination. His mother (the only family member mentioned) is equally adamant that she will not stand by and watch her son die at home; her religious and personal convictions would not permit it. Physicians at the first hospital made the decision to treat Donald and ignored his request to die. Physicians at the second hospital are faced with a more complex situation because Donald has refused surgery and wants to be discharged. Can they hold him in the hospital against his will? It seems that the decision is now up to the court because Donald and the hospital are at an impasse. Donald too is in a difficult situation; he could sign a release form to leave the hospital but because he is totally physically dependent cannot leave the hospital unless someone agrees to help him.

Is this as it should be? Can a philosophic issue be decided in a court of law? Precedents show that it can. Most legal cases pertaining to life and health conflicts involve a philosophic component, such as the rights of the handicapped, rights involved in issues of abortion, contraception, and sexual acts, and others. The court not only can decide but would be required to if the case came to litigation. In making its judgment the court either would take away Donald's personal liberty by forcing him to remain in the hospital or could be seen as aiding in Donald's death. How can society treat an individual as a free agent while still seeing to his best interests? Which interest should take priority? How can the individual's autonomy best be served?

There are three options in this situation: (1) compel treatment and thus take away Donald's status as a free agent, (2) cease treatment and thereby allow him to die, or (3) try to convince Donald to change his mind, allowing him to remain a free agent and preserving the physician's commitment to treat him. If regardless of his seemingly unshakable determination Donald could be convinced to stay in the hospital, could it be said that he was coerced? According to one view the health care system has no right to interfere with the free choice of individuals, even if the individual freely chooses death over a life that to many others would be acceptable. This view holds that even if Donald could be made to understand what care and rehabilitation could do for him, he should still be free to choose death. Only a completely totalitarian and paternalistic society would take away that freedom.

The outcome of this case was in fact quite different from any of these speculations. The psychiatrist, attorney, and Donald entered into an agreement: if the court ruled that he had the right to refuse treatment, Donald could remain in the hospital and be kept as free of pain as possible until he died. Donald won his case without having to go to court by forcing the physicians to seriously consider his request. Having asserted his independence of will and counteracted the total helplessness he felt, he reversed his decision, had the surgery on his hands, continued the other treatment, and has been rehabilitated to the extent that he can walk and feed himself. Displaying remarkable determination and courage, Donald became an attorney because he wanted to provide legal help and advice to others in similar positions. The search for an understanding attorney was one of the most difficult tasks Donald had faced during his ordeal.

EUTHANASIA
Issues and definitions

The word *euthanasia* derives from the Greek for "good death," a term many see as contradictory. Until recently, the word meant the act of painlessly and mercifully putting to death someone who was incurably ill and had no hope of recovery. The phrase *mercy killing* was used by the lay public as a synonym for euthanasia, and many people regarded the physical act as similar to that of putting to death a beloved pet that has become old and sick. The concept of euthanasia is more complex, however, and involves the participation or knowledge of the person to be killed (voluntary euthanasia) and the deliberateness of the act, that is, the difference between intentionally causing a person to die (active euthanasia) and refraining from doing something that would permit a person to continue to live (passive euthanasia). There are four different types of euthanasia:

1. With voluntary passive euthanasia a person is permitted to die with his consent and knowledge. This is the kind of euthanasia generally referred to in a living will.
2. With involuntary passive euthanasia a person is permitted to die without his knowledge and consent. The parents of Karen Ann Quinlan requested this when they asked that she be disconnected from her respirator.
3. Voluntary active euthanasia, in which a person is killed with his knowledge and consent, is the form of euthanasia closest to suicide.
4. Involuntary active euthanasia, in which a person is killed without his knowledge and consent, is the form of euthanasia closest to first-degree murder.

Until about 20 years ago the issue of euthanasia mostly involved intractable pain. In almost all cases the reason given for performing or condoning euthanasia was to end the hopeless suffering of a dying person, usually a cancer victim. But advances in the prolongation of life have made the dilemma of euthanasia more complex. People are sustained by respirators and dialysis machines and their vital functions are more mechanical than natural; more organs are being transplanted, and intractable pain can be at least partially controlled by drugs, psychic methods, and surgery. There are now more reasons to live and more reasons to want to die.

The issue of euthanasia involves two questions and several major arguments. (1) Under what conditions if any is euthanasia morally justified, and (2) should it be legalized? There are several basic arguments for and against euthanasia. The first involves the individual's right of free choice and the liberty to end his life when and how he chooses; this has been called the "death with dignity" argument. The second argument involves the release from suffering that has become hopeless and uncontrolled; to some it seems uncivilized and cruel not to permit release from intractable pain. The third argument involves the sanctity of human life: does life belong to God, to society in general, to the state, or to the individual? Does an individual who occupies a body have a right to destroy that body, and do others have a right or moral obligation to do so? Another argument is that euthanasia in certain instances will lead to relaxed standards about whom society is permitted to kill; some see the legalization of euthanasia as a possible beginning for killing certain groups of people, for example, defective infants, the "useless" elderly, and certain criminals. Closely related to this argument is the possibility of an abuse of a legalized form of euthanasia by physicians who want to get rid of a bothersome client, by transplant surgeons eager for healthy organs, or by family members anxious for an inheritance. The last major argument involves the concept of hope, the possibility that a mistake has been made in the diagnosis, that a miraculous cure or remission will occur, or that a cure for the disease will suddenly be discovered. The argument is that a living person if he has nothing else at least has hope, but a dead person has none.

Discussion of the arguments

The difficulty in discussing euthanasia is separating the idea in theory from the contemplation of the death of a very real individual. One might agree with the concept in general but be unable or unwilling to put it into practice. One might also be against the concept for moral or religious reasons, but when faced with one's own suffering or that of a person dearly loved one might see the issue in an entirely different light. When dealing with death in general and euthanasia in particular, one often cannot apply the abstract concept to a particular or personal instance. Personal suffering can change one's beliefs.

Euthanasia can be examined first in terms of release from intractable pain. A few basic questions must be considered: how much pain is tolerable, is there a purpose for suffering, at what point should an individual be permitted to be released from suffering, and should anyone but the suffering person participate in the decision? Anyone who has been in severe pain even if only for a short period of time knows the effect of pain on one's functioning. It decreases perception and awareness, it impairs the ability to think rationally and make judgments, functioning changes from being cognitive and emotional to being almost instinctual, and one's entire being is devoted to escaping the pain.

One cannot be expected to make a life-or-death decision while experiencing intense pain. But when is the appropriate time to do so? It is not reasonable to expect a healthy, pain-free person to look into the future and define a point beyond which he no longer wants to suffer. He does not know and cannot imagine what the pain will *feel* like, how he will endure it, how much he can endure, or what other circumstances in his life will affect his reaction to pain. If a person's pain could be temporarily eased, could he then make the decision? The only way to relieve intractable pain sufficiently is to give large doses of narcotic drugs that so depress the central nervous system that the ability to think rationally is severely impaired, and a decision made in this situation cannot be said to have been made by a rational cognitive process.

A person who is suffering physical agony is likely to have moments, even hours or days, in which he is lucid and relatively free of pain. This might seem an opportune time to make a decision about euthanasia, but is it really? The pain has left the person physically and emotionally exhausted, and he is aware that at any time the pain may return with full or increased force. He may be relatively free from pain for the moment, but his mind still reels from the enormity of his suffering. He vacillates and wavers from hour to hour. A decision made at this time cannot be said to have been made by a rational mind.

When then can a person make his own decision that he wants to be released from his suffering by death? The question cannot be answered.

Kamisar[8] says there are other difficulties even if the person's choice could be seen as "clear and incontrovertible." Is this the kind of choice we want a gravely ill person to make? Are there not people who would choose death because they are tired of life or because they think others are tired of them? Some who might not really want to die would choose euthanasia because the alternative seems selfish or cowardly or because they do not want to become a financial or emotional burden on their families.

Some people think there is a purpose to suffering or something to be gained as a result of suffering. Some think that suffering is necessary to the attainment of a certain spiritual level or to psychoemotional growth, and some think there is a value to martyrdom even if no philosophic or moral principle is involved. These persons might point to the physical suffering of Christ or some of the Christian saints as an example of the value of suffering. One can also take refuge in God's will: if God has for some inexplicable reason decided that a person shall suffer, then the person should suffer as God intended. Perhaps God did indeed create suffering, but there is also the means to relieve suffering by chemicals or surgery or, if these fail, by the free will to choose euthanasia. Those who see a value in suffering oppose all forms of euthanasia. Those who see pain as a needless cruelty most likely favor euthanasia.

The concept of personal liberty and choice is central to the issue of voluntary euthanasia, as it is to the issue of suicide. Voluntary euthanasia and suicide, which are considered almost the same by many people, generally affect only the person involved and his family. Society in general is affected only peripherally if at all. This cannot be said of involuntary euthanasia or other forms of killing. How much should society control what we do with our bodies if our actions affect only ourselves and our families? If I wish to smoke, drink, or eat so much that my health and life are in serious jeopardy, and if by putting my life in danger in this way I jeopardize the happiness and livelihood of my family, should society intervene and prohibit me from doing so? The prevailing view is that it should not, no matter what effect my actions have on the people who depend on me. The health profession, my insurance company, and a few concerned others would prefer that I not destroy myself in these ways, but society as a whole does not care. However, when I have been stricken with a terminal disease I myself did not cause and did not want and am suffering such unbearable pain that I am no longer able to live a human life as I envision it, society suddenly takes a great interest in whether I live or die and takes steps to prevent my choosing death. Even those institutions that might have wanted me to remain away from alcohol, cigarettes, or too many calories might now look more positively at my death than at my continued life. My physician and others attending me in my pain see how I suffer; they too suffer in their helplessness at not being able to ease me. My insurance company might prefer to pay my beneficiaries rather than continue to pay for my health insurance, which is much more expensive in the long run.

One wonders what stake society has in denying a person the liberty of voluntary euthanasia. It could be argued that the life of each individual is the founding concept on which our society is based, but this concept or principle is capriciously applied. We might say that we cannot permit voluntary euthanasia or suicide because we can never be entirely certain whether the person really wants to die or whether he would change his mind the next day or even the next hour. Acting on the decision for voluntary euthanasia makes the decision irreversible. But there are instances in which we can be certain that death is indeed the first, last, and only choice of the suffering person. There are limits to human endurance, and it is often obvious to the person himself and to those who know him well when the limit has been exceeded.

The "wedge" argument that the legalization or common practice of euthanasia would pave the way for other forms of societally sanctioned mass death is a serious argument and, some think, the most important reason to prohibit euthanasia. It is the argument most frequently used by those opposed to euthanasia but is not particularly logical, because it assumes that the reasons for one kind of action (euthanasia for intractable pain in incurable disease) are the same as those for an entirely different action (for example, killing deformed babies). It is imperative to examine the different conditions or reasons for these two different actions.

A conservative moralist might say that death is death and that killing is killing and the reason is unimportant. But the reasons for killling are important, and the law looks closely at a defendant's motive and intent when considering whether he is guilty of murder. Putting someone to death because pain and disability make his life unendurable or because his life is no longer recognizably human because of irreversible coma is not at all the same as putting someone to death because he might have a life filled with hardship, physical disability, or even pain. The wedge argument is also used by some to predict the killing of elderly people who have been abandoned by society and who might be thought to have no further productive use and the killing of certain types of incorrigible criminals.

If euthanasia were legalized, it would not follow that entire segments of the population would immediately fear for their lives. It could be said that any proposed social act would lead to other, more restrictive social acts. One might say that establishment of traffic laws could lead to a restriction on one's right to travel freely, but being required to stop at a red light is not the same as being stopped and searched at interstate borders. One restriction does not necessarily lead to the other. It is important to understand the difference between degree and kinds of actions.

It is not unusual to hear opponents of euthanasia maintain that its legalization would start us down the road to the kind of behavior that characterized Nazi policy in Germany less than 50 years ago. This argument is highly emotionally charged; the mere mention of Nazis raises hackles. One must, however, look at the socioeconomic and emotional tone of Germany between the World Wars and compare it to that of the United States today. There are few if any similarities and one enormous difference: we have had the experience of watching the Nazi horror, and too many people are unwilling to forget it and are keeping that experience fresh in the American consciousness. The possibility of euthanasia leading to a repetition of Nazism is remote.

The distinction between active and passive euthanasia is important. Active euthanasia, the deliberate and conscious act of killing a person, is condoned less frequently and by fewer people than passive euthanasia, the act of letting someone die naturally by not engaging in "heroic" artificial means of sustaining life. The morality of the two cannot be finely differentiated, and condoning one while condemning the other can create a more complex ethical dilemma than being categorically for or against all kinds of euthanasia.

Again, we confront the issue of cruelty. If one is opposed to a lethal injection for the surcease of intolerable pain but is in favor of not resuscitating a person when he dies naturally, one could be said to be in favor of pain, a position that could be seen as unnecessarily cruel. The issue of active and passive euthanasia often hinges on a time factor. For example, a young woman who is not breathing and is in cardiac arrest is admitted to an emergency room. She is at once resuscitated, and while her injuries are being attended to, she suffers another arrest. Again she is resuscitated, and she seems to do well during and immediately after surgery. Her wounds are serious, but she will survive and recover fully. The day after surgery she suffers yet another arrest and this time slips into a coma that becomes irreversible as days pass. She is maintained on a respirator while her other wounds slowly heal. Now comes the decision, the hard part. No one questioned the wisdom of resuscitating her three times because she was a young healthy woman who could survive her trauma even though she was technically "dead" during all three arrests. A decision was made not to use passive euthanasia, but now she cannot be expected to function normally again. Because she has no brain function, she is a different person, perhaps not a person at all. The decision now is entirely different.

There may be no moral difference between killing a person and letting that person die, or there may be a difference depending on a variety of external circumstances. The following example illustrates this issue. Ken is swimming alone in a pond, begins to drown and shouts for help. Jonathan, an excellent swimmer, sees a drowning man and immediately jumps into the pond and begins swimming toward Ken. As he draws near, he recognizes Ken as the man who is having an affair with his wife. If Jonathan calmly and deliberately pushed Ken's head under the water, waited until he was dead, and then left, no one would deny that Jonathan killed Ken even though he was clearly in danger of dying on his own. But suppose Jonathan after recognizing Ken decides to swim back to shore leaving Ken to sink or swim on his own, though Jonathan knows he could have saved Ken. Ken then drowns. No one would deny that Jonathan let him die, but in the act of letting him die and in view of the fact that he had the power to save him, did Jonathan kill Ken? The motive and intent were the same, the end result was the same, but the means differed. Does the morality differ from that of the first situation? Did letting Ken die when he could have saved him make Jonathan less guilty than he would have been if he had pushed Ken's head under the water? Is there a difference in the moral behavior?

The American Medical Association (AMA) condemns the "intentional termination of the life of one human being by another" but condones the "cessation of the employment of extraordinary means to prolong the life of the body." In other words, the AMA approves passive but not active euthanasia, probably on the premise that killing a client is morally worse than letting him die and is therefore not to be permitted. Is killing always worse? Our feelings toward killing are almost always negative because we associate it with murder that involves an evil motive or a war that horrifies us with its brutality. Our associations with letting someone die are usually humanitarian. One learns to think of killing a person as worse than letting him die, but in the kind of situations we have been discussing letting him die may be the same or worse than killing him. In a moral context, when a physician lets a person die when he could keep him alive, he is killing that person as surely as if he had injected the fatal dose.

The decision to let a patient die is subject to moral appraisal in the same way that a decision to kill would be subject to moral appraisal: it may be assessed as wise or unwise, compassionate or sadistic, right or wrong. If a doctor deliberately let a patient die who was suffering from a routinely curable illness, the doctor would certainly be to blame for what he had done, just as he would be to blame if he had deliberately killed the patient. Charges against him would then be appropriate. If so, it would be no defense at all for him to insist that he didn't "do anything." He would have done something very serious indeed, for he let his patient die.*

Rachels makes the point that the decision to do nothing is a decision and therefore an action, making passive euthanasia a positive action—or active euthanasia. There is therefore no moral difference between passive and active euthanasia though the method differs.

Those who disagree with this view argue that the agent of death creates a moral difference in the responsibility for the death. If a person has cancer and is permitted to die, the cancer is the cause of death, not the lethal injection by a physician. If Jonathan does nothing and lets Ken drown, the death is the result of accidental drowning, but if Jonathan pushes Ken's head under water, the death is the result of murder.

Another argument against morally equating killing a person and letting him die concerns guilt. Society exacts a terrible price for the act of killing; the conscience of most people, unless they are amoral, exacts a worse price. One may feel less guilty having let someone die than after actually killing him. The physician's guilt is usually far less if he does nothing than if he acts to kill. This may reflect an internalization of society's standards.

The questions of whether euthanasia is moral and whether passive euthanasia is more or less moral than active euthanasia cannot be definitively answered. What is essential in understanding the moral argument, though, is that one's opinion be rational and based on full consideration of the arguments. Euthanasia may or may not be moral or correct, and its correctness may vary from one situation to another. But it is immoral for physicians, nurses, and

---

*Rachels, James: Active and passive euthanasia. Reprinted by permission from the New England Journal of Medicine **292:**78-80, 1975.

other health professionals to give no thought to the issue and simply accept the ethical positions of others.

SUICIDE
Definitions

Suicide is the voluntary and deliberate killing of oneself, but this short definition does not adequately characterize suicide. Societal and cultural factors play a tremendous role in differentiating between suicide and acts of sacrifice, martydom, and even courage. Engaging in behavior that may lead to death can be seen as brave (rushing into traffic to push a child away from an oncoming car), routine (a bomb squad policeman defusing a bomb), sacrificial (falling on a grenade with one's body to save a company of soldiers), or stupid (smoking three packs of cigarettes a day). On the other hand, these acts could be seen as suicidal since the person knew the likely outcome but did not desist.

Another factor in defining suicide is motivation. If a pilot crashes his malfunctioning aircraft in a field, knowing he will die, rather than landing on a highway where he could likely save himself but might kill others, is his motive suicidal or humanitarian? If a spy bites down on a cyanide pill, is his motive self-protective to avoid further torture, suicidal, or patriotic? If an adolescent plays "chicken" in his hot rod and dies in the process, is his motive a psychologic need for peer recognition or suicide? To be considered suicide must the death be completely intended, or can it be only partly intended? There are three kinds of conditions that may result in suicide:

1. When personal and social isolation becomes intolerable, one might intentionally terminate his life. When the usual ego defenses break down or loneliness closes in completely, the individual may see only hopelessness ahead and kill himself.
2. When the individual's position in society changes and the usual restraints against suicide are removed, one might kill himself without a definite intention. This can occur when a person is removed suddenly from his former status, as with the death of a spouse, loss of a job, loss of all one's money, old age, a serious illness, or another situational crisis.
3. When a person leads a life-style or engages in actions that he knows will or can lead to death, he can be said to be suicidal. This could involve a dangerous occupation, such as a bomb squad policeman or a high-wire acrobat, or forms of culturally sanctioned suicide such as hara-kiri or self-immolation as a form of religious or political protest.

Cultural and ethical considerations

The morality of suicide is often considered from a religious point of view: if life is given by God, then it is God's to dispose of when and how God chooses. This view holds that a person is simply a custodian of a life that belongs to God and that to kill oneself is to act in direct opposition to God's will. Suicide is considered a major sin by most Western religions. Until recently, Catholics and Orthodox Jews who killed themselves were not permitted to be buried in the consecrated ground of a cemetery belonging to the religious group. The sin of suicide was considered so serious that the person was abandoned by his religion for all eternity. Most religions have tempered this view and now do not prohibit suicides from being buried inside the cemetery. To say that life belongs to God, however, is too simplistic and ignores the variety of ways God is viewed and God's commandments obeyed. To give one's life in the service of God is sometimes seen as a great good, as with holy wars, choosing death rather than forced conversion, and the crucifixion of Christ.

Societal sanctions color the morality of suicide. In Eskimo culture the very old are expected to go off alone with a minimal supply of food to die shortly of exposure. In some Buddist societies a woman was expected to throw herself on the funeral pyre of her husband. (In India the practice was declared illegal by Indira Ghandi, but in some places it is still expected by members of the community.) Socrates was banished from the city by an Athenian court for political reasons and charges of corrupting youth, but he chose to drink hemlock because he saw exile as a worse form of death than actual physical death. The first examples show adherence to societal expectations. Many societies do not consider a death to be a suicide if it accomplished a purpose that is seen by the society as morally desirable, such as Japanese hara-kiri and the death of early Christian martyrs.

Sacrificial deaths are also sanctioned by society. A person who jumps overboard from an overcrowded lifeboat and a wounded soldier who remains behind to die rather than allowing his platoon to risk danger by attempting to save him are examples of a person not directly killing himself but putting himself in a position in which he will die by other causes. Is a death a suicide by reason of the death-causing agent (the elements rather than a self inflicted death) or the motive (an attempt to save others rather than the direct wish to die)?

Thomas Aquinas in *Summa Theologica* argues that for three reasons it is unlawful to kill oneself:

1. Everything naturally loves itself and naturally keeps itself alive; suicide is contrary to natural law and therefore is a mortal sin.
2. Every part belongs to a whole; a person belongs to a community and thus is part of that community. If he kills himself, he injures the community, which is unlawful.
3. Life is God's gift, and whoever takes his own life sins against God.

The third argument has been considered previously, but the first two arguments are more slippery and difficult to discuss. The premise that an action is or is not "natural" has been used to justify or condemn all manner of human behavior, including various sexual practices, contraception, violent human relationships, research into life processes, and even some medical interventions. One could say that anything found in nature—in life—is natural. Suicide may then be viewed as a natural result of pain, unhappiness, loneliness, or unbearable isolation. If the release from a life that is seen as no longer livable is preferable to the continuation of that life, then suicide can be seen as a natural conclusion. Because human beings are the only species that commits suicide, it may indeed be natural in humans.

The second argument depends on whether the individual is seen as responsible only to himself or to the community at large. Also important is the question of who is affected by suicide and in what way. If a woman who lives alone, whose parents are dead, and who has no husband, children, or particularly close friends or relatives kills herself, who will be affected? If a woman is married, has children, and has living parents, or is divorced but has children depending on her for emotional and financial support kills herself, the effect is far different. The morality of the suicide itself may be the same, but the effect on the community is different. Many people would not agree with Aquinas if they think that the morality of an action depends on its effect on other human beings.

An act considered morally wrong is not necessarily blameworthy—an important distinction when considering suicide. We may think a person had a poor reason for killing himself and that the act had tremendously negative consequences for his family, but at the same time we do not necessarily *blame* him or see the act as a sin. We might justify his act by saying that he was under great emotional strain, that his character was somehow faulty, or that he was temporarily deranged, but we may not condemn it as immoral. Even if one condemned suicide as an act of cowardice, others would not agree that suicide is always cowardly and everyone could not agree what is a cowardly act.

Suicide could be seen as wrong but excusable and therefore not morally wrong, as in the cases of someone terminally ill and in great pain or someone temporarily insane or not his usual self because of severe depression. The suicide in these cases can be seen as wrong, unnnecessary, and perhaps hurtful to others, but not sinful.

The morality of suicide is more circumstantial than absolute. Some think that suicide is never morally wrong (pointless and misguided perhaps, but not wrong), and even those who think suicide is always a sin acknowledge occasions when the sin may be mitigated by circumstances. There may be a moral obligation not to cause one's own death, but there are situations in which it may be morally permissible or even obligatory to act in a way that may lead to death, as in the examples of landing the plane in a field instead of on a highway and staying behind to die on the battlefield alone.

There is a prevailing ethic that suicide has nothing to do with morality because someone who kills himself is mentally ill and his sickness overrides his moral choice. Conventional psychiatric thinking sees the desire to kill oneself as essentially sick and maladaptive behavior and dictates that person should be prevented from doing so. But Szasz[9] says the suicidal person is not necessarily mentally disturbed and does not require hospitalization or even treatment. Szasz acknowledges that voluntary counseling or psychotherapy might help the suicidal person cope with life, but he does not agree that psychiatry must *always* prevent a person from killing himself. A psychiatrist who takes this position is saying that he values the client's life more than the client does and therefore feels obligated to save his life. Physicians do not do this in ordinary medical practice. If a client refuses to take insulin even though he knows he will die of diabetes, the physician will try to convince him to take it, but if the client still refuses, the physician will not hospitalize him and force the insulin upon him.

If a client states that he is suicidal, however, he may be hospitalized "for his own protection." Szasz says that psychiatrists view suicide as a direct refutation of what the medical profession believes in, life. For the suicide to choose death in preference to life is too much for the psychiatrist to bear, and he punishes the person by hospitalization. Szasz believes that such hospitalization is a direct affront to the individual's right to liberty and that if the individual has a right to life, his life belongs to himself and he has a right to commit suicide. A person has a responsibility to his family and society, and by commiting suicide he reneges on that responsibility, but he has a greater responsibility to himself and society has no right to curtail his liberty.

In language and logic we are the prisoners of our premises, just as in politics and law we are prisoners of our rules. Hence we had better pick them well. For if suicide is an illness because it terminates in death, and if the prevention of death by any means necessary is the physician's therapeutic mandate, then the proper remedy for suicide is liberticide.*

CARE OF THE DYING

For the most part people who die in hospitals go through the dying process alone, lonely, in pain, frightened, ignored by the professional staff, and unable to talk about their feelings. Care of the dying (not treatment of the illness of the dying) is generally ignored in medical schools because curing illness is emphasized and dying and death may be seen simply as failures to cure illness. Nursing schools often do little better, although when the subject of death is raised, the concern is more for the humanity of the client than for his illness alone. But nurses, like physicians, sometimes see death as a personal or professional failure, as the loss of a client. Nurses are as anxious to avoid death as physicians and are as uncomfortable in its presence as anyone else.

Responsibility for care

There are two basic issues concerning the responsibility for care of the dying. Who should be responsible, the client, his family, society, or the health care system? And how should the dying process be managed—where should death take place, and what are the elements of care that should precede death? Inherent in these questions are the matter of cost (the responsibility for paying costs if the client's insurance does not cover his expenses), the issue of how much care and what kind of care should be given the dying, and the question of how long the process should be permitted to continue.

In the United States it has become routine for death to occur in a hospital, for a variety of reasons. But often it is inappropriate or can have negative effects, as the following case illustrates. A woman who had cancer begged her husband not to send her to the hospital to die. He agreed but then changed his mind and reneged on his promise because he thought their adolescent daughter should not witness the dying process and its attendant pain and sadness. The woman was sent to a hospital to lie in a cool white bed for the last few days of her illness and the

---

*Szasz, Thomas: The ethics of suicide. In Beauchamp, Tom L., and Perlin, Seymour, editors: Ethical issues in death and dying, Englewood Cliffs, N.J., 1978, Prentice-Hall, Inc., p. 138.

daughter was sent to stay with friends and was not told her mother was dying (though she had known it for years). The husband slept alone each night. Mother and daughter never had a chance to say good-bye, and father and daughter could not share their grief and loneliness because they did not acknowledge the dying process. Whether the husband and wife were able to share their feelings was not known but seemed unlikely since almost 30 years later he still had not accepted and adapted to his wife's death. His and his daughter's life were forever negatively affected because the process of dying and the attendant needs and feelings of the family as individuals and as a unit were not acknowledged and met.

It is sometimes appropriate to enter a hospital when the dying process begins. If there is a chance for remission or palliation of the illness and the client wants that opportunity, the hospital is the best place for treatment. If the hospital staff have learned to deal with the dying client and his family with care, it can be a positive place to die. If the atmosphere in the home is not appropriate, as with a rejecting family, inappropriate physical facilities, or the presence of negative stimuli, then the client could be brought to the hospital. Single people with no close family often have no choice but to enter the hospital when their illness becomes so advanced that they cannot care for themselves, though their isolation becomes even more complete there. Frequently the family cannot afford to keep the dying person at home, since most types of health insurance will not pay for home care (or home care premiums are prohibitively expensive) but will cover the costs if the client enters a hospital or nursing home. Nurses can help apply political pressure and provide legislative testimony to change this situation.

When the management of care for the dying is planned, several areas need to be considered. First, how the person wants to manage his own death should be considered because it is only fair and humane to allow a person control over his death. Regardless of how passive a person has been during his lifetime and how much the course of his life has been directed by whim or circumstances or the will of others, his life itself has been his to live as he wanted and needed. It is inhumane to suddenly wrest control from a person in his last life process and tell him how to do this most important and intensely personal thing. Even if he wants to leave the mechanics of dying to his family or to health professionals, his personal preference should take priority.

It is easy to agree with this principle but difficult to act on it. To find out what a dying person wants one must ask, and to ask one must face the fact that a person dearly loved will die soon. Accepting this hurts so terribly that most people try to push away the pain by pretending it does not exist. Many people seem to unconsciously think that if they do not talk about the impending death with the dying person, the death might not occur. It is incredibly difficult to say, "When you die I will be devastated by loss. I love you and will miss you so much that I don't know if I can bear it. But I want our last times together to be peaceful for you and lovely for me to remember. Tell me what you want us to do." These feelings will bring forth emotion and tears. But it is much more comforting to cry with the loved one, enfolded by his arms, than to cry alone and in secret in the dark, pretending the tears are not there.

If control over one's death is the goal, the second decision concerns how to achieve that goal. In general, the less institutionalized the care is, the greater control the client and family have. Hospital staffs are geared to following procedures, performing life-saving measures, and keeping human emotions and reactions out of the way of physical care. If the person is to be cared for at home, family members need to know what is involved in the care. A scream of agony is searing to the soul, bowel incontinence smells bad, a dying person may be angry and hostile and may rage and rail at the unfairness of his situation and may make demands that are seen as unreasonable, and family members might fight with each other and show anger and hostility at the one who is dying in ways that would seem cruel if one did not understand the emotional dynamics involved. One cannot easily say, "I am angry at you for doing this to me, for going off and dying and leaving me alone with my grief." A family needs help in the process of interacting with the dying person and needs to understand that their reactions are normal. Physicians are not usually equipped to do this, and neither are the clergy or the vast majority of the family's friends. Professional help is needed.

The living will. The length of time one wants the dying process to continue is an issue with ethical and legal ramifications. One cannot predict the moment of one's death except in the case of voluntary active euthanasia, but one can ensure that the dying process is not prolonged beyond the limit of endurance. The living will is an instrument by which a dying person makes his wishes known to those who are caring for him. The will is addressed to all people who will care for the dying or have some responsibilty for him, including the family, physician, attorney, and hospital or other institution.

Death is as much a reality as birth, growth, maturity, and old age—it is the one certainty of life. If the time comes when I, _____ can no longer take part in decisions for my own future, let this statement stand as an expression of my wishes while I am still of sound mind.

If the situation should arise in which there is no reasonable expectation of my recovery from physical or mental disability, I request that I be allowed to die and not be kept alive by artificial means or "heroic measures." I do not fear death itself as much as the indignities of deterioration, dependence, and hopeless pain. I therefore ask that medication be mercifully administered to me to alleviate suffering even though this may hasten the moment of death.

This request is made after careful consideration. I hope you who care for me will feel morally bound to follow its mandate. I recognize that this appears to place a heavy responsibility upon you, but it is with the intention of relieving you of such responsibility and of placing it upon myself in accordance with my strong convictions that this statement is made. Signed _____*

Except in California, where the Natural Death Act became law in 1976, living wills have no legal validity; the physician and others providing care are not legally bound by the person's stated wishes. They may feel a moral obligation to honor the

---

*Concern for Dying: The living will, revised. Reprinted by permission, Concern for Dying, 250 West 57th Street, New York, N. Y. 10019.

will, but it is wise for the client to discuss his feelings before the terminal stage of the illness so that if necessary he can find someone who is more receptive and sympathetic to his needs. The only legal obligation of the physician is to practice medicine as he sees fit.

Many people think that the living will should be made legally binding because as the health care system presently operates, the control of care lies within the system and not with the client. McCormick and Hellegers believe in the concept of the living will but are opposed to it becoming law.

> Our opposition, then, to living will legislation does not stem from what such legislation seeks to achieve, namely the self-determination of the patient over his or her fate in the face of a potentially abusive use of technology. Rather, we question whether such legislation may not result in precisely the opposite effect. We have no objection to the living will as a signal sent in advance by knowledgeable persons to their potential physicians. Indeed, such informal documents can be immensely helpful and reassuring. Our profound misgivings stem from the notion of living wills as law. The very fact that a law is deemed necessary to assure patient's rights implies, and therefore tends to reinforce, an erroneous presupposition about the locus of decision making in the physician-patient relationship.*

This position has several weak spots. The presupposition about the locus of decision making is not erroneous. Although one would like to see all health care decisions in the hands of the client, for the most part this is not the case. Making the living will law would in many instances change that. Physicians would be compelled to comply with the wishes of their clients and as a result might tend to pay more attention to clients' needs in matters other than dying. The choice and the locus of control would move from the impersonal system to the client.

McCormick and Hellegers seem to fear a backlash effect. They admit that a law is deemed necessary to ensure patients' rights yet hesitate to favor passage of that law while agreeing in principle with its tenets. If a law is necessary and people cannot be convinced to behave in certain ways without it, why oppose it? It is naive to think that people will do right because other people think they should do so. It is an unfortunate fact that some people do not always voluntarily grant human rights to others.

The health care system in the United States is characterized by a high degree of paternalism, as is evidenced in part by the locus of control in the physician-patient relationship. To oppose the legalization of the living will is to approve of and reinforce this paternalism.

McCormick and Hellegers raise interesting legal and ethical considerations in the matter of living wills. The first concerns how the law would affect those who have not written such a will. It is possible that a person who did not write a will could be thought to request life-sustaining treatment because he did not say otherwise. Such an interpretation would force people to make a decision about their own death before they were ready to and even if they would have preferred not to. The presence of a living will also tends to exclude the family from the decision.

---

*McCormick, Richard A., and Hellegers, Andre E.: Legislation and the living will, America **136**(10), March 12, 1977.

Some think this is good, but others think that the family should take part in the decision. All legislation must involve a penalty for noncompliance, but having to set a penalty for overtreating or overresuscitating would be a dilemma that might be too complex to solve. In addition, the existence of a living will would be irrelevant in an emergency when the client is not likely to be in contact with his physician and when emergency room personnel must make quick decisions.

Though these points are well taken, it should be possible to write a law that would protect the physician from malpractice suits as much as possible and ensure that the dying person receives the kind of care he wants. If the system had devised a way to meet the needs of the dying without legislation, this discussion would not have been necessary.

The hospice concept

An alternative to traditional avenues of care for the dying is the hospice. In the Middle Ages a hospice was a way station where people could stop to rest, eat, and refresh themselves on long journeys. The term over the years came to mean a shelter for homeless people who were old or incurably ill. Hospices were usually established and run by religious organizations. How appropriate, then, is the use of the word *hospice* for a place for people who are dying to go, a place to rest and be refreshed on the journey from life to death.

St. Christopher's. St. Christopher's Hospice in London, established in 1967 and now the best-known hospice, has served as a model and teaching institution for those who wish to study the hospice concept. Money for its inception was provided by a young man dying of cancer who wished for better treatment of the terminally ill. The hospice is in the city of London but is located away from the noisy rush and has a garden in which neighborhood children play.

Dr. Cicely Saunders, a nurse, social worker, and physician, is the founder and medical director of St. Christopher's. Her vision and planning have made the hospice a haven for the dying, and she has assembled a team of professional and nonprofessional workers who are dedicated to caring for the dying and to the maintenance of the hospice's principles and programs. The primary purposes of the hospice are the support for the dying person and his family, the control of pain, the maintenance of clients' social involvement, and the absence of a feeling of institutionalization. All employees participate in care, including the newspaper deliverer, the hairdresser, orderlies, and kitchen workers. Family members are not merely tolerated as visitors but are welcomed as an integral part of the client's life, and their needs are as much ministered to as those of the dying person. Clients support each other, and those without families are often "adopted" by the families of other clients and no one feels alone. No one dies alone at St. Christopher's; caring people are there until the last breath.

A person who has been with seriously and terminally ill patients in other environments is likely to observe a different attitude among most patients at St. Christopher's. There is less anxiety and obvious suffering, more serenity and sense of security. Photographic documentation of St. Christopher's patients tends to support this impression, although to date there has been no definitive research to evaluate the apparent benefits of the hospice as compared with other modes of care. One also gets the impression that it is neither the general atmosphere, not the specific treatment procedures that provide the favorable effects. Rather, it seems to be the integration of the humane impulse and clinical expertise.*

The moment of death is not hidden or avoided in discussions. Curtains are not drawn around the dying person's bed unless he specifically requests it. It is thought that even at the moment of death a person is part of his community and can draw support from it. This also helps other clients and employess as well to understand death and fear it less because they become familiar with it.

A primary objective at St. Christopher's is to free a client from pain so that he can be free to enjoy the time remaining. The severe pain of most dying people can be controlled, and their goal is to anticipate the person's pain and give drugs before it occurs so that he never experiences serious pain. In most American hospitals, in contrast, pain medication is withheld until the person is truly suffering and is in the humiliating position of being a supplicant for relief. Withholding medication also results in a larger dose of the drug being required to control the pain than if it had been given before the pain became unbearable.

In their quest for happy and comfortable patients, the hospice staff has noted that there are different kinds of pain, and that fear and anticipation of pain can be as uncomfortable and as painful as the misery caused by the disease. Once the patient discovers that it is again possible to be relatively free from pain, he or she relaxes and the psychological causes of pain disappear.†

The medication at St. Christopher's is given orally in a liquid form so that the amount and proportion of drugs can be easily controlled. This solution, called Brompton's mixture, contains alcohol, a fruit syrup, cocaine, heroin, and chloroform water and is administered on a flexible schedule depending on the client's needs. This combination of drugs was devised to provide maximum relief from pain while allowing the person to remain alert. The problem of addiction to narcotics is not considered serious for two reasons: (1) it does not matter if a person becomes addicted to a drug if he is to die soon, and (2) in many cases the dose of narcotics required is below addiction levels because the drug is given before the pain becomes agony.

St. Christopher's aim is to provide excellent medical care enhanced by "tender loving care." The staff also sees the hospice as a teaching and training center for those who wish to know more about caring for the terminally ill. Preserving the client as a whole person is emphasized until the moment of death.

Branford Hospice. The Branford Hospice, now known as Hospice, Inc., in New Haven, Connecticut, was established to adapt the British hospice concept to the American health care system. A combination of factors made New Haven a logical place for this demonstration project. New Haven county has a large population (750,000), there are several teaching hospitals, and it is the location of Yale Uni-

---

*Kastenbaum, Robert J.: Death, society, and human experience, St. Louis, 1977, The C. V. Mosby Co., p. 227.
†Rossman, Parker: Hospice: creating new models of care for the terminally ill, New York, 1977, Association Press, p. 89.

versity with important medical, nursing, and divinity schools. Hospice, Inc., was started as a home care program but progressed to meet the needs of people who required full-time hospice care.

Dr. Elisabeth Kübler-Ross gave a symposium in 1966 on death and dying while Dr. Cicely Saunders was a visiting professor at Yale University School of Nursing. The catalyst was Rev. Edward Dobihal, a chaplain at Yale–New Haven Hospital, who on a sabbatical had studied the British system. He assembled a group of people in the health care system who were concerned with the American way of treating and caring for the dying. Florence Wald, Dean of the School of Nursing, studied the needs of the dying and published the results of her findings; she later became coordinator of inpatient planning for the Branford Hospice. In 1971 the hospice was incorporated, and in 1973 Dr. Sylvia Lack from England was hired as the medical director.

The philosophy of care at Branford is similar to that of St. Christopher's, and the routine by which medication is given before the pain becomes unbearable and the emphasis on decreasing anxiety about the recurrence of pain are the same as the British system. The prohibition of heroin in the United States makes the control of pain slightly different, however, but methadone and other narcotics are proving useful. Some people have been concerned that using too much "hospice mix" could be a form of passive euthanasia, but this belief is unfounded. The control of physical pain and the freedom from the expectation of pain are not the same as euthanasia.

The hospice concept in a general hospital. The Royal Victoria Hospital in Montreal has a palliative care unit, but the 1972 research that determined the need for that unit showed care for the terminally ill in North America was sadly lacking.[10] A questionnaire was given to professional and nonprofessional health workers asking their opinions about the care of the dying. Clients also were asked. A partial list of results follows:

1. Forty-three percent of physicians thought clients wanted to know it if they were terminally ill; 64% of clients said they wanted to know.
2. Of 700 nurses given the questionnaire, only 225 responded, and only 91 of 340 residents and interns responded. The staff seemed complacent about the care they offered, yet the following conditions were found:
   a. Staff relationships with the terminally ill were too impersonal.
   b. Families were frequently excluded from discussions.
   c. Physicians and nurses avoided the terminally ill and were embarassed when clients wanted to discuss their forthcoming death.
   d. The critically ill were overtreated.
   e. Staff lacked expertise in dealing with the emotional needs of the dying.
   f. Relatives were excluded at the time of death.

The report following this study had an explosive effect for a short time but has not done much to change the general way terminally ill people are cared for in North American hospitals.

There are isolated examples of effort, however, such as the hospice team at St. Luke's Hospital in New York City. The team takes responsibility for the care of dying people on certain floors of the hospital, and clients remain in their own units rather than going to a special "death ward." The hospice team is composed of three nurses who in addition to caring for the dying person try to establish a support system with the personnel on the floor, interpret the needs of the dying to the hospital staff, and help the staff deal with their own feelings about death. Many hospital staff members feel overworked and resent the demands of the dying on their time and emotional energy; thus good relationships have developed between the hospice team and the regular staff. The team also serves as an advocate for the dying, succeeds in having some hospital rules relaxed (visits by children and pets, walks in the garden, overnight visitors, and so on), and advocates the hospice concept to health professionals unfamiliar with the concept or opposed to it.

The Palliative Care Unit at the Royal Victoria Hospital is an example of a special section set aside for the dying. Clients may stay as long as they need, and meeting the needs of the clients, the control of pain, and support for the dying process are emphasized. The philosophy is the same as in a separate hospice, and clients are encouraged to return home for as long as they are able, although they are welcomed back whenever they feel the need.

A hospice home care program. Part of the hospice philosophy is the concept that the dying person should be where he is most comfortable and where he most wants to be. Many people who would prefer to stay home with their families go into hospitals only because the burden of caring for them at home becomes too much for their families to handle because of physical debilitation or uncontrollable pain. In 1975 a group of physicians, nurses, and social workers at Overlook Hospital in Summit, New Jersey, was formed to investigate the possibility of giving supportive care to the dying at home.[11] The group decided to expand the hospital's existing home care department to include the following:

1. Physician-directed services to prevent the client from feeling abandoned by his physician when he enters the terminal phase of illness. The medical director of the home care department serves as primary physician in planning medical treatment and acting as a resource person to other staff.
2. Control of symptoms, including pain relief (methadone is frequently used) and the meeting of psychologic, spiritual, and social needs.
3. Coordination and communication by the entire team, which is headed by a nurse.
4. Round-the-clock services to prevent the feeling of abandonment particularly at night and on weekends when pain, loneliness, and depression are likely to increase. The entire hospice staff is on call (on a rotating basis) 24 hours a day, 7 days a week, and clients are encouraged to call for help whenever they feel a need.
5. Collaboration with the inpatient facility because it is not always feasible or desirable to have the client stay at home. He may need to be admitted for short-term or terminal care, and the inpatient staff needs to know the goals and concepts of the hospice team if support is to be continued while the client is hospitalized.
6. Family participation in care for all the reasons cited previously.

7. Bereavement services because the needs of the family do not end when the client has died. Different needs, including grieving and learning to reorganize their lives without the family member who has died, may arise, and the hospice team can help meet them.

Candidates for the home care program are those for whom palliative rather than curative treatment seem most appropriate—those who have a person to provide care at home between professional visits, those whose primary physician is willing to participate in the program, and those whose families are willing and able to support them at home. Most referrals come from physicians, and the care is paid for by a variety of sources including private insurance, the American Cancer Society, Medicare, and a special hospice fund established by the Overlook Hospital Foundation.

The staff's emotional needs are met through weekly group meetings and consultations with a part-time psychologist. The program is still in its initial phase of development, but the hospice team has shown the need for it and has demonstrated the fact that it can work successfully.

The hospice concept is needed. Death can be a time of learning, sharing, growing, and acceptance if the dying are not shut away in dark places, abandoned to pain, loneliness, and misery, and rejected by society in general and health professionals in particular. The traditional way of treating the dying is inhumane and unethical. As caring health professionals, we are obligated to ease the emotional and physical pain of the dying.

SUMMARY

The increasing complexity of medical technology has led to a difficulty in defining death, most specifically because of the development of machines that can artificially sustain life and various forms of transplant surgery that make it even more necessary to define death precisely. One cannot always be certain that death has occurred.

A definition of death must involve more than just the body and should concern the entire person and his ability to function as a human being. In 1967 an ad hoc committee of the Harvard Medical School published a report defining brain death and irreversible coma. That report and others decided that the brain should be considered the locus of death. If a person's brain is considered permanently nonfunctional, he *may* be considered dead. The ethical dilemma then is whether to declare a person dead if he has an isoelectric EEG though his heart and lungs are still functioning with mechanical supports.

Veatch has proposed a definition of death based on the irreversible loss of four characteristics of a human being: the flow of body fluids, the soul in the body, the capacity for bodily integration, and the capacity for social interaction. Loss of these means loss of functioning as a human being and therefore death.

Guidelines must be established to legally define death. The physician has traditionally been responsible for defining death, but the decision could be put into the hands of the judicial system, the legislature, or even the general public. In 1968 Kansas became the first state to enact legislation defining death, and several others have introduced such proposals. The Kansas statute has some serious short-comings, the most important of which is that too much control is in the hands of the physician. It is difficult to write a workable statute that is definitive, flexible, and satisfying to the majority.

Probably the thorniest ethical dilemma involves the artificial prolongation of life and the question of when it is not appropriate. The "death with dignity" position advocates personal liberty and the desire for an acceptable quality of life as reasons for being permitted to die. The opposing "right to life" position is that life should be prolonged at all costs, that hope should never be cast aside, and that no one but God has the right to determine when life is over. The debate on this issue is emotional and often bitter.

A dying person has the right to know the truth about his diagnosis and prognosis, although this is interwoven with the physician's right to practice medicine as he believes he should, and the right to informed consent concerning his illness and treatment.

The difference between ordinary and extraordinary means to prolong life involves an issue of interpretation because what used to be considered extraordinary (using machines to sustain life) is now done routinely in all hospitals. The traditional medical ethic requires that everything be done to preserve life for as long as possible, but more people are now claiming the right to determine how they will be treated during the terminal phase of an illness. Another major ethical dilemma occurs when the client is not in a position to choose for himself and someone else then has to make the decision not to resuscitate him or to turn off the respirator.

Many people believe that a person can and should be legally compelled to accept medical treatment against his will. The usual rationale is that the life of an individual is so important to society that it supersedes the individual's right to consent to his own death. This argument appears most strongly when a person refuses a treatment on the grounds that his religion forbids it. The conflict between the individual's right to liberty and the state's right to protect the life of a citizen has led to legal battles.

Euthanasia is voluntary or involuntary, passive or active. There are two basic questions involved with euthanasia: (1) under what conditions is euthanasia morally justified, and (2) should it be legalized? The arguments for and against euthanasia concern the individual's right to liberty, the release from suffering that has become unendurable, the sanctity of human life, the question concerning to whom a person's life "belongs," the argument that legalizing euthanasia may lead to killing people who are thought a burden on society, the possible abuse of euthanasia by physicians, and finally, the question of hope, frequently the only positive thing a dying person has left.

Suicide is not simple to define. A person may kill himself because he no longer wishes to lead a life he sees as intolerable, but one may also commit suicide as a religious self-sacrifice, by working in an extremely dangerous occupation, or because of sociocultural pressure. Determining whether a death was suicide generally involves questioning the motive, although the intention of the person is not always possible to determine. The debate over the morality of suicide involves a variety of issues including religion, law, society and culture, psychologic factors, and individual liberty.

Care of the terminally ill is generally ignored in medical schools and to a lesser extent in nursing schools. For the most part the dying are left alone in hospitals, generally ignored by the staff, their pain inadequately controlled, and their emotional needs not met. Sometimes a hospital is an appropriate place for the dying, but more often it is not. The care of the dying should center on what the dying person himself wants and how much control he wishes to have over his dying. Helping the person achieve control and involving the family successfully in his care should be high priorities, but these are often ignored by the American health care system. A living will is one means to exercise some control, but it is not legally binding in any state but California and it involves complicated legal and ethical issues.

An alternative to the traditional care of the dying is the hospice concept, best demonstrated by St. Christopher's in London where helping the dying person achieve and maintain the quality of life he wants is emphasized. This is accomplished through controlling his pain, giving emotional support to him and his family, promoting social interaction, and preventing the feeling of institutionalization. The atmosphere at St. Christopher's is open, caring, and warm. Drugs for pain control are specially tailored for each person and are given *before* the pain appears, and thus the person is freed from the psychologic oppression of the fear of pain.

Several hospice units modeled on St. Christopher's are being developed in general hospitals in the United States, and hospice home care programs have been initiated.

REFERENCES

1. Report, Ad Hoc Committee of the Harvard Medical School, Journal of the American Medical Association **205**(6):337-340, August 6, 1968.
2. Veatch, Robert M.: Death, dying and the biological revolution, New Haven, Conn., 1976, Yale University Press.
3. Capron, Alexander M., and Kass, Leon R.: A statutory definition of the standards for determining human death: an appraisal and a proposal. In Beauchamp, Tom L., and Perlin, Seymour, editors: Ethical issues in death and dying, Englewood Cliffs, N.J., 1978, Prentice-Hall, Inc.
4. Garland, Michael: Politics, legislation, and natural death, Hastings Center Report **6**(5):5, October 1976.
5. Fletcher, Joseph: Morals and medicine, Princeton, N.J., 1954, Princeton University Press.
6. Veatch, Robert M.: Case studies in medical ethics, Cambridge, Mass., 1977, Harvard University Press.
7. White, Robert B., and Engelhardt, H. Tristam, Jr.,: Case studies in bioethics, Hastings Center Report **5**(3):9, June 1975.
8. Kamisar, Yale: Euthanasia legislation: some non-religious objections. In Beauchamp, Tom L., and Perlin, Seymour, editors: Ethical issues in death and dying, Englewood Cliffs, N.J., 1978, Prentice-Hall, Inc.
9. Szasz, Thomas: The ethics of suicide. In Beauchamp, Tom L., and Perlin, Seymour, editors: Ethical issues in death and dying, Englewood Cliffs, N.J., 1978, Prentice-Hall, Inc.
10. Rossman, Parker: Hospice: creating new models of care for the terminally ill, New York, 1977, Association Press.
11. Ward, Barbara J.: Hospice home care program, Nursing Outlook, pp. 646-9, October 1978.

BIBLIOGRAPHY

Alvarez, Walter C.: The right to die. In Visscher, Maurice B., editor: Humanistic perspectives in medical ethics, Buffalo, 1972, Prometheus Books.
Aquinas, Thomas: Whether it is lawful to kill oneself (From Summa Theologica, 1259). In Beauchamp, Tom L., and Perlin, Seymour, editors: Ethical issues in death and dying, Englewood Cliffs, N.J., 1978, Prentice-Hall, Inc.

Beauchamp, Tom L.: Suicide and the sanctity of life. In Regan, Tom, editor: The value of life, New York, 1978, Random House, Inc.

Beauchamp, Tom L., and Perlin, Seymour, editors: Ethical issues in death and dying, Englewood Cliffs, N.J., 1978, Prentice-Hall, Inc.

Beecher, Henry K.: Ethical problems created by the hopelessly unconscious patient, New England Journal of Medicine 278:1425-1430, June 27, 1968.

Behnke, John, and Bok, Sissela, editors: The dilemmas of euthanasia, New York, 1975, Anchor Press.

Benton, Richard G.: Death and dying: principles and practices in patient care, New York, 1978, Van Nostrand Reinhold Co.

Black, Peter M.: Definitions of brain death. In Beauchamp, Tom L., and Perlin, Seymour, editors: Ethical issues in death and dying, Englewood Cliffs, N.J., 1978, Prentice-Hall, Inc.

Bok, Sissela: Personal directions for care at the end of life, New England Journal of Medicine 295:367-369, August 12, 1976.

Brandt, R. B.: The morality and rationality of suicide. In Perlin, Seymour, editor: A handbook for the study of suicide, New York, 1975, Oxford University Press.

Cantor, Norman L.: A patient's decision to decline life-saving medical treatment: bodily integrity versus the preservation of life, Rutgers Law Review 26 (2):228-264, Winter 1973.

Capron, Alexander M., and Kass, Leon R.: A statutory definition of the standards for determining human death: an appraisal and a proposal. In Beauchamp, Tom L., and Perlin, Seymour, editors: Ethical issues in death and dying, Englewood Cliffs, N.J., 1978, Prentice-Hall, Inc.

Comment: Unauthorized rendition of lifesaving medical treatment, California Law Review 53:860, 1965.

Douglas, Jack D.: Social meanings of suicide, Princeton, N. J., 1967, Princeton University Press.

Durkheim, Emile: Suicide (J. A. Spaulding and G. Simpson, translators), New York, 1951, The Free Press.

Epstein, Charlotte: Nursing the dying patient, Reston, Va., 1975, Reston Publishing Co.

Ferguson, Faye: Children's cognitive discovery of death, Journal for the Association of Care of Children in Hospitals 7(1):8-14, Summer 1978.

Fletcher, Joseph: Morals and medicine, Princeton, N.J., 1954, Princeton University Press.

Garland, Michael: Politics, legislation, and natural death, Hastings Center Report 6(5):5-6, October 1976.

Hook, Sidney: Ethics of suicide, International Journal of Ethics 37:173-189, 1927.

Hume, David: On suicide. In Beauchamp, Tom L., and Perlin, Seymour, editors: Ethical issues in death and dying, Englewood Cliffs, N.J., 1978, Prentice-Hall, Inc.

Kamisar, Yale: Euthanasia legislation: some nonreligious objections. In Beauchamp, Tom L., and Perlin, Seymour, editors: Ethical issues in death and dying, Englewood Cliffs, N.J., 1978, Prentice-Hall, Inc.

Kastenbaum, Robert J.: Death, society, and human experience, St. Louis, 1977, The C. V. Mosby Co.

Kohl, Marvin: The sanctity-of-life principle: a philosophic background for the consideration of euthanasia. In Visscher, Maurice B., editor: Humanistic perspectives in medical ethics, Buffalo, 1972, Prometheus Books.

Kübler-Ross, Elisabeth: On death and dying, New York, 1969, Macmillan, Inc.

Kübler-Ross, Elisabeth: Death: the final stage of growth, Englewood Cliffs, N.J., 1975, Prentice-Hall, Inc.

Margolis, Joseph: Suicide. In Negativities: the limits of life, Columbus, 1975, Charles E. Merrill Publishing Co.

McCormick, Richard A., and Hellegers, Andre E.: Legislation and the living will, America 136(10), March 12, 1977.

Menninger, Karl A.: Man against himself, New York, 1938, Harcourt Brace Jovanovich, Inc.

Montagne, Charles H.: Informed consent and the dying patient, The Yale Law Journal 83(8):1632-1634, July 1974.

Perlin, Seymour, editor: A handbook for the study of suicide, New York, 1975, Oxford University Press.

Rabkin, Mitchell T., et al.: Orders not to resuscitate, New England Journal of Medicine 295:364-366, August 12, 1976.

Rachels, James: Active and passive euthanasia, New England Journal of Medicine 292:78-80, 1975.

Ramsey, Paul: The patient as person: explorations in medical ethics, New Haven, Conn., 1970, Yale University Press.

Rossman, Parker: Hospice: creating new models of care for the terminally ill, New York, 1977, Association Press.

Schwager, Robert L.: Life, death, the irreversibly comatose. In Beauchamp, Tom L., and Perlin, Seymour, editors: Ethical issues in death and dying, Englewood Cliffs, N.J., 1978, Prentice-Hall, Inc.

Smith, David H.: Fatal choices: recent discussions of dying, Hastings Center Report 7(2):8-10, April 1977.

Smith, Harmon L.: Ethics and the new medicine, Nashville, 1970, Abingdon Press.

Strauss, Anselm L., and Glaser, Barney G.: Chronic

illness and the quality of life, St. Louis., 1975, The C. V. Mosby Co.

Szasz, Thomas: The ethics of suicide. In Beauchamp, Tom L., and Perlin, Seymour, editors: Ethical issues in death and dying, Englewood Cliffs, N.J., 1978, Prentice-Hall, Inc.

Veatch, Robert M.: Death, dying and the biological revolution: our last quest for responsibility, New Haven, Conn., 1976, Yale University Press.

Veatch, Robert M.: Case studies in medical ethics, Cambridge, Mass., 1977, Harvard University Press.

Veatch, Robert M.: Death and dying: the legislative options, Hastings Center Report 7(5):5-8, October 1977.

Ward, Barbara J.: Hospice home care program, Nursing Outlook, pp. 646-649, October 1978.

White, Robert B., and Engelhardt, H. Tristam, Jr.: Case studies in bioethics, Hastings Center Report 5(3):9, June 1975.

Williams, Glanville: Euthanasia legislation: a rejoinder to the nonreligious objections, New England Journal of Medicine 292(2):1-12, January 1975.

Index